Removable Prosthodontic Techniques

Dental Laboratory Technology Manuals

Removable Prosthodontic Techniques

Dental Laboratory Technology Manuals

John B. Sowter, D.D.S., M.Sc.

Roger E. Barton, D.D.S., EDITOR

REVISED EDITION

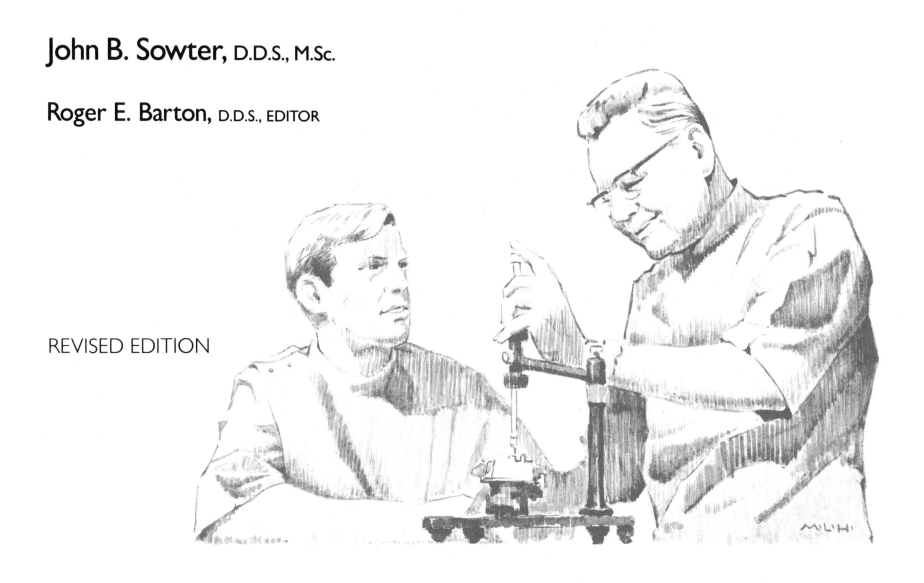

© 1968, 1986 The University of North Carolina Press
All rights reserved
Manufactured in the United States of America
This book, or parts thereof, may not be reproduced
in any form without permission of the publisher.

Library of Congress Cataloging-in-Publication Data

Sowter, John B.
  Removable prosthodontic techniques.

  (Dental laboratory technology)
  Editor: Roger E. Barton.
  Rev. ed. of: Prosthodontic techniques. c1968.
  Includes index.
  1. Complete dentures—Laboratory manuals. 2. Partial
dentures, Removable—Laboratory manuals. I. Sowter,
John B. Prosthodontic techniques. II. Barton, Roger E.,
1922–   . III. Title. IV. Series. [DNLM: 1. Prostho-
dontics—laboratory manuals. 2. Technology, Dental—
laboratory manuals. WU 500 S735p]
RK656.S58   1986   617.6′92   86-7065
  ISBN 978-0-8078-4166-2 (pbk.)

  11 10 09 08 07   11 10 9 8 7

Dental Laboratory Technology Manuals:

Dental Anatomy

Gerald M. Cathey, B.S., D.D.S., M.S.

Fixed Restorative Techniques

Henry V. Murray, B.S., D.D.S.
Troy B. Sluder, D.D.S., M.S.

Laboratory and Clinical Dental Materials

Karl F. Leinfelder, D.D.S., M.S.
Duane F. Taylor, B.S.E., M.S.E., Ph.D.

Removable Prosthodontic Techniques

John B. Sowter, D.D.S., M.Sc.

PREFACE

This revision retains the same "flavor" as the first edition, an attempt to present the basic laboratory techniques of removable prosthodontics. These basic techniques provide a foundation upon which more refined techniques and superior skills can be built.

The addition of a section on *Single Complete Dentures* fills a void left in the first edition. The use of materials which have made techniques either more refined or more simple without any sacrifice in quality have been included in this edition.

This manual is divided into two parts: **complete denture techniques** and **removable partial denture techniques**. In both parts sequential steps are outlined in detail. In addition, some clinical steps are shown to clarify the relationship of dental technology and clinical dentistry.

The technical procedures shown in this manual were done as "real" appliances were being constructed. The student is actually invited to "look over the shoulder" of the dentist and technician, following each technique from start to completion. Every step is shown; there are no hidden secrets.

Illustrations of clinical procedures are designated by letters A, B, C, etc.; technical procedures are numbered in order of performance.

It is impossible to give credit to all the people or publications which have contributed to this manual. There are many texts available which will help students of dental laboratory technology. The following will help expand theoretical knowledge in the area of removable prosthodontics.

Boucher's Prosthodontic Treatment for Edentulous Patients
by Hickey, Zarb, and Bolender.
The C. V. Mosby Company, St. Louis, 1985

Synopsis of Complete Dentures
by Ellinger, Rayson, Terry and Unger.
C & J Publishing Company, Lexington, KY, 1983

Treatment of Partially Edentulous Patients
by Boucher and Renner.
The C. V. Mosby Company, St. Louis, 1982

McCracken's Removable Partial Prosthodontics
by Henderson, McGivney and Castleberry.
The C. V. Mosby Company, St. Louis, 1985

Every effort has been made to use modern dental terms. Wherever possible, definitions have been quoted from *Boucher's Current Clinical Dental Terminology*, Third Edition, by Thomas J. Zwemer, published by the C. V. Mosby Company, St. Louis, 1982.

A few review questions are included at the end of each section. These questions cover the objectives of the particular section.

The technical procedure photographs from the first edition were done by Mr. William G. Blanton, C.D.T. Original artwork was rendered by Mr. James C. Handy, under the direction of Dr. M. Lamar Harrison. The new photographs were done with the assistance of Mr. Jerome D. Harrison, C.D.T.

The author, Dr. John B. Sowter, is in private practice; his practice is limited to prosthodontics. He received his dental degree from the University of Pennsylvania and his specialty training from Ohio State University. He is a diplomate of the American Board of Prosthodontics.

Roger E. Barton
Editor

CONTENTS

Removable Prosthodontic Techniques

Dental Laboratory Technology Manuals

SECTION I

Introduction to Removable Prosthodontic Techniques

The loss of permanent natural teeth is not a normal process but results from disease or accident. Tooth loss leads to changes in the face which must be understood by dentist and technician before successful replacements can be constructed.

Prosthodontics is "the branch of dental arts and science pertaining to the restoration and maintenance of oral function by the replacement of missing teeth and structures by artificial devices." (Current Clinical Dental Terminology) The term *prosthodontics* is a combination of the words "prosthesis" and "dentistry," and is used synonymously with prosthetic dentistry. A *prosthesis* is defined as "the replacement of an absent part of the human body by an artificial part." (CCDT) Thus, any dental restoration is a prosthesis. In common usage, however, the term prosthesis, when applied to dentistry, is used to designate an artificial replacement of a tooth or teeth and associated structures.

Prostheses are not restricted to dentistry. A prosthesis is a substitute for *any* natural part which has been lost. Artificial eyes and artificial limbs are both forms of prostheses, as are metallic joints or protective headplates which are implanted into the body. Prostheses have different functions. An artificial eye does not restore sight, but it does help a person's appearance. An artificial leg does not function as well as a natural leg, but its primary purpose is to restore function. A removable

Note: The designation (CCDT) throughout this manual indicates a definition quoted from *Boucher's Current Clinical Dental Terminology* by T. J. Zwemer; C. V. Mosby Co., St. Louis 1982.

dental appliance has the qualities of both an artificial leg and artificial eye in that it restores both function and appearance, but usually does not attain the efficiency or appearance of the natural part it replaces.

A denture is "an artificial substitute for missing natural teeth and adjacent structures." (CCDT) There are many types of dentures, but we are interested primarily in two; the complete denture and the removable partial denture.

A complete denture is "a dental prosthesis that replaces all of the natural dentition and associated structures of the maxillae or mandible." (CCDT) A partial denture is "a prosthesis that replaces one or more, but less than all, of the natural teeth and associated structures." (CCDT) A removable partial denture is "a partial denture that can be readily placed in the mouth and removed by the wearer." (CCDT)

It is interesting to note that in these definitions there is a reference to the teeth and associated structures. By definition, a removable prosthesis replaces more than just teeth; it also replaces bone and soft tissue which may have been destroyed by traumatic injury, by disease, or through natural processes.

The primary difference between a complete denture and a removable partial denture is the method by which the prosthesis gains support. A complete denture is supported by bone covered by soft tissue (mucosa). A removable partial denture gains support from the bone covered by mucosa, and from the remaining teeth. A removable partial denture is more stable and retentive than a complete denture due to the remaining teeth. Because of their better support, removable partial dentures are conceded by all authorities to be more efficient than complete dentures.

REVIEW OF ORAL ANATOMY

The teeth, tongue, lips, cheeks, and other oral structures with which we are concerned have several functions, among which are mastication, speech, and appearance. One cannot say that one function is more important than another. Mastication, or chewing is the first stage of digestion. Chewing is not confined to the teeth alone, but involves action of the tongue and cheeks, and all the swallowing muscles. Speech is also a function of the oral cavity. While speech is produced in the larynx, the structures in the oral cavity, along with the lips, help to make sounds intelligible.

The structures around a person's mouth also lead to a pleasing appearance. Throughout history the mouth has been important to a person's appearance.

A dental technician must be familiar with the structural form of the dental arches and the associated structures. Without understanding the natural structures it is difficult to recognize the changes which take place with the loss of teeth. The inclination and relationship of the anterior teeth to the lips are important factors in the restoration of normal lip contours and facial appearance. Knowledge of the natural condition is essential before the edentulous conditions can be understood. A review of the normal structures in the Dental Anatomy Manual, or a good dental anatomy text, will be worthwhile at this time.

ANATOMICAL CHANGES
ASSOCIATED WITH LOSS OF TEETH

The loss of a tooth produces many changes other than just leaving a gap in the dental arch. These changes may not be apparent to the casual observer or to the indifferent patient, but an observant person will notice these changes. When a tooth is lost, the supporting bone shrinks or, in dental terminology, resorbs. Resorption is most noticeable when several teeth have been lost, and is more apparent in the mandibular arch than in the maxillary.

The face changes greatly in appearance when all the teeth are lost. The changes are due to the loss of teeth, resorption of the alveolar bone, the ability of the patient to move the mandible closer to the nose (loss of vertical dimension), and lack of support for the facial muscles.

The description of the changes associated with the loss of teeth has been separated into two parts for ease of explanation.

CHANGES ASSOCIATED
WITH LOSS OF MAXILLARY TEETH

The form and structure of the alveolar process of both the maxilla and mandible change when the teeth are extracted. The casual observer may think there are fewer changes in the maxillae than in the mandible after the teeth are lost. This may be true; however, the changes often are of the same magnitude in both arches, but the presence of the hard palate makes changes in the maxillae less noticeable.

Most dentists agree that the function of the alveolar processes is to provide a foundation and attachment for the teeth. When the teeth are lost, the primary function of the alveolar process is destroyed and they resorb or atrophy as does any part of the body which no longer functions (for example, muscles which are inactive decrease in size). In addition, the intraseptal portions of the alveolar process which remain after the extraction of several teeth become rounded. The combination of the elimination of sharp edges (a natural process in all organisms) and atrophy causes changes in the gross contours of the alveolar bone. The internal architecture of the bone in the alveolar processes is reoriented, becoming finer and less dense after the teeth are lost.

Figures 1 and 2 illustrate the bony changes which take place in the maxillae following extraction of the teeth. In Figure 1, "a" is the arch before extraction and "b" is a cast of the edentulous arch three months after extraction. Figure 1, c and d are duplicate casts which have been sectioned. The two sectioned casts have been joined in Figure 2 using anatomical landmarks in the palate to align the two halves anteroposteriorly. This is dramatic proof that bony changes occur after the extraction of the teeth. The improper placement of artificial teeth without consideration of the bony changes will result in improper support for the lips and an unnatural esthetic result.

All of us have seen a horse shake his skin in one area when he is bothered by a fly. A horse can move his skin without moving another part of or any bones in his body because there are muscles in the horse's skin. If a man has a fly on his back, he has to make a skeletal movement (move an arm or twist his body) in order to dislodge the fly. However,

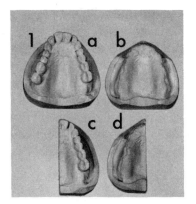

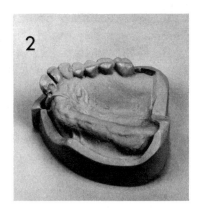

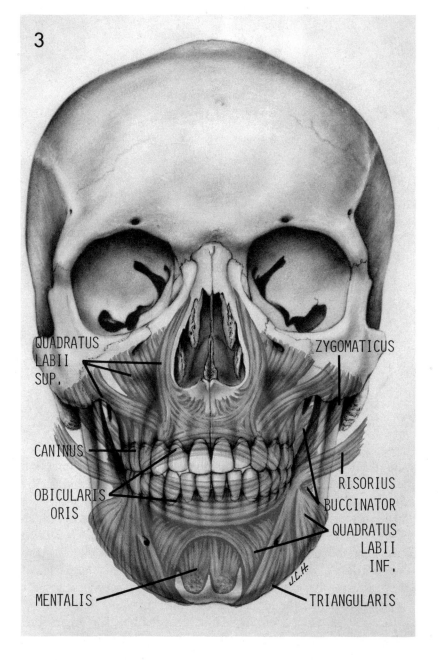

muscles are present in the facial region which allow a person to change his facial expression independent of any skeletal movement. We do this when we smile, frown, squint our eyes, or, in some people, wiggle our ears. The muscles of facial expression most important to the dentist and dental technician are those around the mouth (**Figure 3**). These muscles are supported by the teeth and the alveolar processes. The loss of teeth removes support from these muscles and without support the muscles do not function normally. If dentures do not restore lost structures and normal contours, the change around the mouth gives the individual the typical "denture look." Proper placement of the teeth, with proper contouring of the base, will aid in eliminating this unattractive appearance.

CHANGES ASSOCIATED WITH LOSS OF MANDIBULAR TEETH

The bony changes occurring after the extraction of mandibular teeth appear greater in the mandible than in the maxillae. The resorption of the alveolar process may result in having the tissues of the cheek (buccal mucosa) more or less continuous with the floor of the mouth. Reduced area for denture support accounts for patients having more problems becoming accustomed to mandibular dentures.

Figures 4 and 5 illustrate the changes which take place in the mandible after the teeth are extracted. It is not uncommon to find the genial tubercles at the crest of the residual ridge. When an individual has his

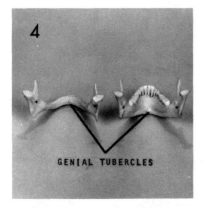

GENIAL TUBERCLES

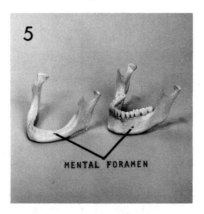

MENTAL FORAMEN

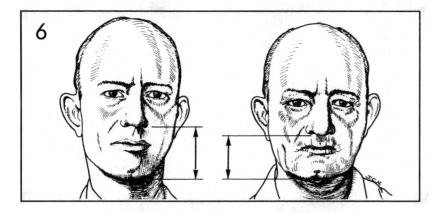

on the superior surface of the mandible. In instances of severe resorption, these muscles may originate on the crest of the residual ridge.

The clinical significance of these anatomical soft tissue changes is often overlooked. Normal contours can be restored with a maxillary denture, but it is almost impossible to restore *all* normal contours and expression with a mandibular denture because the attachment of the muscles to the crest of the mandibular ridge changes the action of these muscles. Proper placement of the mandibular teeth *helps* restore normal appearance and function, but it is impossible to duplicate the original contours of the lower lip.

ANATOMICAL CHANGES AND ESTHETICS

The loss of one or more teeth affects appearance in several ways:

(a) The unattractive appearance we see when a person has lost one or more anterior teeth, the "picket fence appearance."

(b) The change in shape of the lips or cheeks due to loss of support by the teeth.

(c) The change in a person's appearance due to conscious or subconscious efforts to avoid smiling or otherwise showing unattractive teeth.

(d) The changes in facial contour resulting from the loss of support for the muscles of facial expression.

(e) The illusion of a prominent chin which results from the mandible being closer to the maxillae (lost vertical dimension) as a result of the loss of all the teeth in one or both arches.

Many of the facial changes associated with the loss of the teeth are illustrated in **Figure 6**. The lips have lost their support with the result that the vermillion border (red portion) of the lips is thinner and creases have developed around the lips. Note the pronounced loss of support in the canine regions. The chin is closer to the nose due to a lack of vertical support which also causes the chin to be more prominent.

The degree of appearance which can be restored is dependent upon factors other than the loss of teeth and degree of resorption. The thickness of the lips and the development of the facial musculature are also factors in appearance. Men with beards and heavy lips are less likely to show the esthetic effects of severe resorption than are people who have thin musculature and tissue in the facial area. Elderly women

teeth, the genial tubercles are about one and one-half inches inferior to the incisal edge of the teeth. Thus, one can see how much vertical loss of tooth and bone may occur after the mandibular teeth are lost.

The soft tissue changes which occur following the loss of teeth are different in the mandible than in the maxillae. The maxillary muscles of facial expression attach above the alveolar process. Thus the attachment or origin of these muscles remains constant, even after the maxillary teeth have been lost and the maxillary alveolar process resorbs. Proper contours may be restored to the upper lip with a denture.

The same situation does not exist in the mandible. The origin of the triangularis, mentalis and quadratus labii inferioris muscles does *not* remain constant after the teeth have been lost. When teeth are present these muscles attach to the facial surface of the mandible. After the teeth are lost and the alveolar process resorbs, these muscles originate

with thin, fragile, parchment-like skin are difficult to treat with complete dentures in that it is hard to restore normal contours and good esthetics.

Proper facial contours, proper vertical dimension, and tooth selection are factors for which the dentist is responsible. It is important for a technician to understand them so that he can more intelligently follow the dentist's prescription (work authorization) and thus work in unison with the dentist to help achieve good results.

THE TEMPOROMANDIBULAR JOINT AND JAW MOVEMENTS

The mandible articulates with the skull at the temporomandibular joints (**Figure 7**). The condyle of the mandible fits into the *mandibular fossa* on the underside of the temporal bone, thus the name *temporomandibular articulation or joint.*

The *articular tubercle* or *eminence* is a rounded projection which forms the anterior boundary of the mandibular fossa. The *articular disc* is composed of tough fibrous tissue and lies between the mandibular fossa and articular eminence above and the condyle below. The disc is attached to the *capsular ligament* which surrounds the joint and is also attached to part of the external pterygoid muscle, one of the four major muscles of mastication. *Synovial cavities* filled with a lubricating fluid lie above and below the articular disc.

The structure of the temporomandibular joint permits the mandible to make many movements. There are two basic movements, a hinge or rotary movement and a sliding or translatory movement. The hinge movement takes place between the condyle and the articular disc while the translatory movement takes place between the articular disc and the mandibular fossa.

The mandible is shifted from side to side and opened and closed by coordinated movements of the muscles of mastication (masseter, temporalis, internal pterygoid and external pterygoid and other muscles). In lateral excursions of the mandible, one condyle is held in position while the other slides forward down the articular eminence. A slight side-shift (*Bennett movement*) accompanies these excursions. The lateral excursions of the mandible permit food to be grasped and crushed between the teeth.

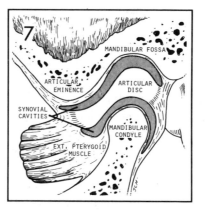

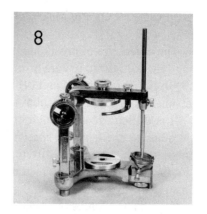

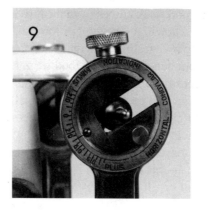

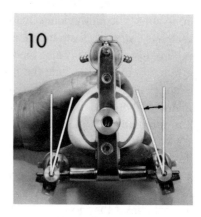

The teeth, muscles, and joints all work in harmony or decreased function and/or pain result. Likewise, denture teeth must be in harmony with the joints and muscles. For this reason, jaw movements are considered when planning the occlusion for artificial replacements.

Adjustable and semi-adjustable articulators simulate jaw movements. The Hanau H-2 articulator (**Figure 8**) is a widely used semi-adjustable articulator. This instrument has adjustable horizontal condylar guides (**Figure 9**) which, when adjusted by means of a protrusive jaw relationship record, represent the inclination of the mandibular fossa. The lateral condylar guidance, a mechanical equivalent of Bennett movement, is introduced by rotating the posts of the articulator (**Figure 10**).

OBJECTIVES OF PROSTHODONTIC TREATMENT

The objectives of prosthodontic treatment are (1) to restore masticating function, (2) to restore or improve the appearance of an individual, (3) to improve speech, and (4) to carry out these procedures in such a manner as to cause the patient no harm or discomfort.

It is difficult to say which of the three functions restored by dental prostheses, mastication, speech, or esthetics, is most important. Even though each patient has different ideas as to what a prosthesis should do, the dentist attempts to restore all three of these functions and to do it in such a way that the patient is comfortable.

Physicians, dentists and nutritionists agree that teeth are necessary for good digestion and optimal health. Chewing makes eating more enjoyable. The enjoyment of eating a good steak comes from the flavor which is extracted from the meat while chewing. Chewing of food and mixing it with saliva is also the first step in digestion, and must be done efficiently in order to gain the maximum benefit from the food we eat. Some people disagree that teeth are necessary for good digestion. They maintain that modern methods of refining and preparing foods have all but eliminated the mechanical need for chewing. The millions of people who have no teeth, natural or artificial, seem to support this view. To date, no one has studied how the presence or absence of teeth affects a person's health or his life expectancy. In this context, it is interesting to note that man is the only animal that can live without teeth. Other animals die if they lose their teeth.

The effect of teeth on appearance has been discussed earlier in this section. We may reiterate here that few people without teeth are considered attractive.

Effective speech requires teeth. Many sounds are formed by the tongue contacting or valving against the teeth. Proper placement of artificial anterior and posterior teeth is necessary to restore good speech. A constricted arch in a complete denture will squeeze the tongue, which produces whistling or hissing. Improper positioning of the anterior teeth inhibits the tongue and the lips from producing good sounds. The length and the labiolingual position of the anterior teeth should duplicate as nearly as possible the position of the natural teeth in order to obtain the best possible speech and appearance.

No dental prosthesis can function satisfactorily if it causes discomfort. An uncomfortable patient is unhappy. Furthermore, discomfort is usually a symptom of a harmful response to improper technique, to a change in the supporting structures of the prosthesis which has occurred since its delivery, or to psychological problems. It must be recognized that a patient has to accept the dental prosthesis psychologically in order to be comfortable. Some psychological problems may be triggered by the loss of teeth so that these problems become apparent concurrently with the delivery of a denture.

DIAGNOSIS AND TREATMENT PLANNING

The construction of removable dental appliances requires teamwork between the dentist and the dental laboratory technician. The dentist is responsible for all diagnosis and treatment, whereas the proficiency and skill of the technician make the treatment more efficient and effective.

The first step in prosthodontic treatment is to determine what conditions exist. The next step is to determine what to do. These steps are called diagnosis and treatment planning. A dentist uses various aids to arrive at a complete diagnosis. A *history* of the patient's physical, dental and, sometimes, emotional ills is necessary; a questionnaire or a properly directed conversation between patient and dentist are effective methods of obtaining a history.

Examination is essential to every diagnosis. The *clinical examination* usually precedes the *X-ray examination*, but this order may be reversed. Securing diagnostic casts is a part of the examination procedure. With the patient's history and the results of the examination at hand, the dentist can arrive at a diagnosis.

With the diagnosis completed, the *treatment plan* follows easily. The treatment plan acts as a blueprint for treatment. Naturally, in routine instances, diagnosis and treatment planning are done quickly, and often concurrently. A great deal of time may be consumed in these procedures for difficult, out-of-the-ordinary patients.

SEQUENCE OF PROSTHODONTIC TREATMENT

Some type of appliance is usually required for patients needing prosthodontic treatment. Clinical and laboratory procedures are necessary to produce the desired result. The clinical procedures are those done at chairside, while laboratory procedures are those which may be done in a dental laboratory. This manual is devoted to laboratory procedures. Certain clinical procedures are discussed briefly so that the technician will be able to see the importance of laboratory procedures for a beneficial overall result. It is essential for a dental laboratory technician to be knowledgeable about the clinical procedures, not so he will accomplish these procedures, but that he may be of more help to the dentist and work with him as a good team member.

A logical method of describing the laboratory procedures involved in dental prostheses is to describe the clinical procedures and then to describe the laboratory procedures which follow each appointment.

COMPLETE DENTURE TREATMENT PROCEDURES

The most common complete denture treatment sequence is one which involves five appointments for the patient. Each of the first four appointments requires laboratory support. In order to make this procedure readily understood, a brief description will be given of each clinical procedure, followed by the laboratory procedures needed to be done before the subsequent appointment.

The actual construction phase of complete denture treatment is usually preceded by several preparatory appointments. At these appointments the diagnosis and treatment plan are developed. The patient is prepared through surgical procedures and the oral tissues are returned to optimal health during these preparatory appointments.

APPOINTMENT ONE

Clinical Procedures: Preliminary impressions are made at this appointment. It is presumed that the clinical examination, X-ray examination, history, and any necessary preparatory treatment have been completed prior to this appointment.

Laboratory Procedures: The preliminary impressions are poured in plaster or dental stone to produce preliminary casts. Custom trays are then constructed on the preliminary casts.

APPOINTMENT TWO

Clinical Procedures: Secondary impressions, usually called final impressions, are made.

Laboratory Procedures: The final impressions are poured to form the master casts. These casts are an accurate negative reproduction of the final impression and serve as a foundation for the following phases of denture construction. Baseplates, also called trial bases, are constructed on the master cast and occlusion rims are placed on the baseplates. The occlusion rims and baseplates are used to record jaw relationships (vertical dimension, centric relation) and are used subsequently for arranging the artificial teeth.

APPOINTMENT THREE

Clinical Procedures: The vertical dimension is determined, the centric relation is recorded at the determined vertical dimension and a facebow transfer may be made. The size, shape and color of the teeth also are determined at this appointment.

Laboratory Procedures: The casts are mounted utilizing the facebow record and the interocclusal jaw relationship records made with the baseplates and occlusion rims. The teeth are then tentatively arranged and the wax bases contoured.

If an intra-oral or extra-oral central bearing device is used, an extra appointment is necessary. These devices are set up and adjusted using the preliminary mounting on the articulator. They are returned to the dentist where more accurate jaw relationship records are made. These records are then returned to the laboratory where the lower cast is remounted on the articulator and the articulator is adjusted through the use of eccentric jaw relationship records. The use of this procedure depends upon the personal preference of the dentist.

APPOINTMENT FOUR

Clinical Procedures: At this appointment the dentist will try-in the teeth which have been set up in the dental laboratory. He will check the teeth for proper placement and arrangement, proper appearance, and also will check the jaw relationship records made at the previous appointment. Final jaw relationship records may be made and are used by the dental laboratory technician to remount the mandibular cast on the articulator and to adjust the articulator.

Laboratory Procedures: The set-up of the teeth is completed and the denture bases are contoured to simulate the natural gingival tissues. The dentures are then flasked, packed with resin denture base material and processed. After processing the dentures are returned to an articulator and errors in occlusion which may have occurred during processing are removed. An occlusal index is made to preserve the articulator mounting, and the dentures are removed from the casts and finished.

APPOINTMENT FIVE

Clinical Procedures: At this appointment the dentures are delivered to the patient. The procedures which a dentist chooses to do at this appointment will be dictated in part by his method of constructing the dentures.

Some delivery appointments are very short, while others are lengthy requiring fine adjustment of the occlusal surface of the dentures. There are generally no procedures requiring the services of the dental laboratory technician at this time unless a dental laboratory technician is employed in a dental office, at which time he may aid the dentist in making occlusal adjustments after the dentures have been remounted on the articulator.

TREATMENT PROCEDURES
FOR REMOVABLE PARTIAL DENTURES

APPOINTMENT ONE

Clinical Procedures: At this appointment the examination (X-ray and clinical), and diagnosis and treatment plan are developed. The same procedures are followed as were discussed in the section on Diagnosis and Treatment Planning. The clinical procedure of most interest to the dental laboratory technician is the making of a preliminary or diagnostic cast. The production of this cast is an essential factor

in proper treatment planning. A simple jaw relationship record should be made at this time in order to mount the diagnostic casts.

Laboratory Procedures: The dentist is responsible for surveying and designing a preliminary cast for removable partial dentures. He should do this procedure himself, but it may be done jointly by the dentist and his laboratory technician. This preliminary survey and design will form a basis for restorative treatment of abutment teeth and may indicate to the dentist certain procedures which need to be done before a final impression is made. The proper use of the diagnostic cast will enable a dentist to make an intelligent treatment plan and to produce a more satisfactory result. Areas which require recontouring and preparation of occlusal rests should be indicated on the diagnostic casts along with required restorations. A custom tray may be made on the diagnostic cast if one is prescribed by the dentist.

APPOINTMENT TWO

Clinical Procedures: The mouth is prepared before a final impression is made. This may involve simple recontouring of the teeth, preparation of occlusal rests, or multiple appointments for extensive dental treatment. Upon completion of the preparatory phases a final impression is made. This may be made either in a stock tray which the dentist has available in his office, or may be done in a custom tray which is constructed in the laboratory on the preliminary cast.

Laboratory Procedures: The cast is poured in the final impression in the dental office or may be done in the laboratory if it is located close to the dental office. Pouring the master cast is done *immediately* after the impression is made. The partial denture framework or skeleton is made on this master cast in the laboratory. This is done through a process of surveying, designing, preparation for duplication, duplication, production of the refractory cast, production of the wax patterns, casting and finishing.

APPOINTMENT THREE

Clinical Procedures: At this appointment the casting is tried in the patient's mouth and any necessary adjustments are made. An impression of the ridge areas in a free-end extension partial denture is made and jaw relationship records are made. The proper mold and shade of teeth are selected by the dentist, and this information, along with the framework and jaw relationship records, is returned to the dental laboratory.

Laboratory Procedures: If a composite impression of the edentulous ridges has been made, the master cast is corrected. The casts are then mounted with the jaw relationship records on an articulator. The teeth are set, the gingival portion is waxed, festooned, and the partial denture is invested and the plastic base areas are processed. The partial denture is then returned to the articulator for removal of processing errors, and is then removed from the cast and completed.

APPOINTMENT FOUR

Clinical Procedures: The appliance is delivered to the patient and any necessary adjustments are made. These procedures may be extensive or simple, depending upon the dentist's techniques and the complexity of the partial denture.

This brief description of procedures for making complete and partial dentures is presented to give an idea of the importance of the dental technician in prosthodontic treatment. The clinical procedures are illustrated briefly in appropriate places in the text to give the technician an overall idea of where his work fits into routine prosthodontic treatment.

PROSTHODONTICS IN THE FUTURE

The past two decades have seen a decline in dental disease. The inclusion of fluoride compounds in water supplies and their use in dental practice have drastically reduced the incidence of dental decay. The inclusion of fluoride in water supplies appears to have far-reaching beneficial effects in that decay rates appear to be lowered even in "non-fluoride" areas, probably through inclusion of fluoride compounds in the food chain.

Newer treatment modalities have also reduced the incidence of decay. The use of pit and fissure sealants by dentists (along with the application of fluoride compounds to tooth surfaces) has further re-duced the incidence of dental decay. In some areas it appears that dental decay has almost been eliminated. These changes have affected the character of dental practice.

Now, there is an increasing effort to better control periodontal disease and progress is being made in this area. If the incidence of dental caries continues to decline and periodontal disease is controlled, what will happen to prosthodontics?

Prosthodontics is here to stay. Unfortunately, there will always be those people who are ignorant or foolish enough not to take advantage of preventive measures. If past experience is any indicator, many of these people will need prosthodontic treatment. Prosthodontic treatment also will be required to treat people who have lost teeth and adjacent structures through disease, neglect, or accident. People with congenitally missing teeth and other hereditary defects will require prosthodontic treatment. Defects caused by mutilative surgery to eradicate disease, primarily cancer, will need prosthodontic treatment to restore these people to productive membership in society. Even if dental disease is controlled in future years, the need for prosthodontic treatment will persist.

This manual introduces the basic techniques used in removable prosthodontics. Knowledge of and competence in these techniques will enable the ambitious and interested technician to develop proficiency in more advanced areas such as precision attachment partial dentures, speech devices for congenital deformities and appliances for surgically compromised patients.

REVIEW QUESTIONS

1. Define dental prosthesis.
2. What are the three main functions of the mouth and oral cavity?
3. List four ways the loss of several teeth affects appearance.
4. What are the four objectives of prosthodontic treatment?
5. What are the laboratory procedures associated with the first appointment for complete denture treatment?

SECTION 2

Preliminary Impressions and Casts

Preliminary impressions are the first clinical material a dental laboratory technician handles in complete denture construction. Preliminary impressions include all areas to be covered by the finished denture. The technician retains the accuracy of the impression by making well-formed preliminary casts.

Examination is the first step in denture construction. The dentist's training and experience enable him to assess the conditions in the patient's mouth and plan his course of treatment. Abnormalities must be recognized when present and either be removed or changes made in the treatment plan to accommodate them.

A thorough examination includes an X-ray examination. X-rays enable the dentist to determine the presence of embedded teeth, roots, cysts or tumors. Usually these objects or lesions are removed before the construction of the dentures is initiated, although in some instances, at the discretion of the dentist, they may be left in place. The quality of the bone which will support the dentures also may be evaluated through the use of well-made X-rays.

A complete denture is made of material which is stable dimensionally. However, the tissues which support the denture change with time. This decreases the accurate adaptation of the denture base to the tissue and may result in some of the supporting tissues being displaced. Before making impressions for new dentures, the dentist institutes treatment to be sure the supporting tissues recover from any displace-

ment and are in their normal resting condition. The treatment to allow the tissues to recover their natural contours will vary depending upon the condition of the mouth and needs of the individual patient.

Preliminary impressions are usually made of alginate or impression compound. Either material is satisfactory, although there are times when one is preferable to the other. The technique for pouring compound impressions is identical to that used for pouring alginate preliminary edentulous impressions.

Figures A through F illustrate steps accomplished by the dentist which lead to the development of preliminary impressions. **Figure A** shows the dentist, with a dental assistant, making the preliminary examination. **Figure B** shows the presentation of a treatment plan to the patient. After acceptance of the treatment plan by the patient, the dentist modifies the stock trays (**Figure C**) to make them more accurately fit the patient's mouth. Then the alginate is mixed (**Figure D**). **Figures E** and **F** show mandibular and maxillary impressions of alginate being made.

The objective in making preliminary impressions is to produce overextended impressions. This large impression distends the border tissues and covers all of the anatomical landmarks to be included in the denture base. The dentist or laboratory technician will place an outline for a custom tray on the preliminary cast through recognition of the anatomical landmarks (Section 3). The resulting custom tray will have an outline similar, but not identical, to the completed denture.

Preliminary casts may be made of either plaster or stone. The mate-

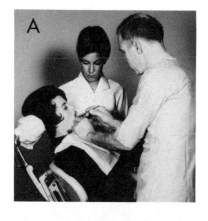
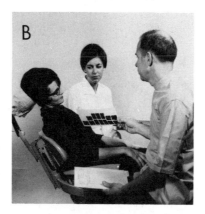
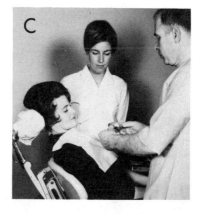
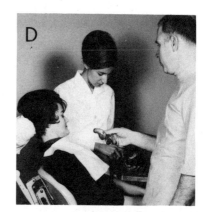

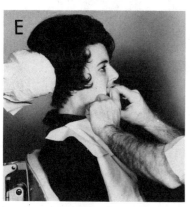
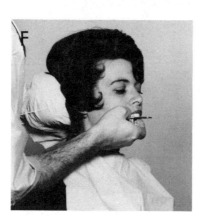
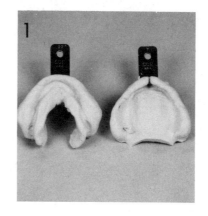
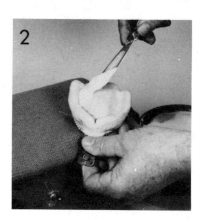

rial used is dictated by the preference of the dentist and/or technician and the cost of the various materials. The casts shown in the following sequence were made of plaster.

Figure 1   The preliminary impressions as they arrive in the laboratory.

Figure 2   Plaster is mixed to a thick consistency, such that it will not flow unless vibrated. The impression is held in the left hand by the tray handle with the base of the handle resting on the vibrator. The plaster is picked up on a spatula and placed into one corner of the impression. The plaster is allowed to flow around the impression to avoid trapping air bubbles. (Note: All impressions will be easier to pour if the surface is damp.)

Figure 3   The entire tissue surface of the maxillary impression is filled with plaster. Additional material is added to the impression so that all the impression is filled and the borders of the impression are covered.

Figure 4   A patty of plaster is placed on a glass slab. This mass of plaster should be about the size of the base of the cast. The filled impression is inverted onto the patty of plaster. Note that the plaster is thick enough to stand by itself and does not spread over the slab.

Figure 5   The plaster is pulled up around the borders of the impression with a plaster spatula or knife. The two spots on the surface of the impression tray are where the dentist held the impression in the patient's mouth. You can also see the utility wax which was placed along the posterior border of the tray to make the stock tray more accurate and help confine the impression material within the tray.

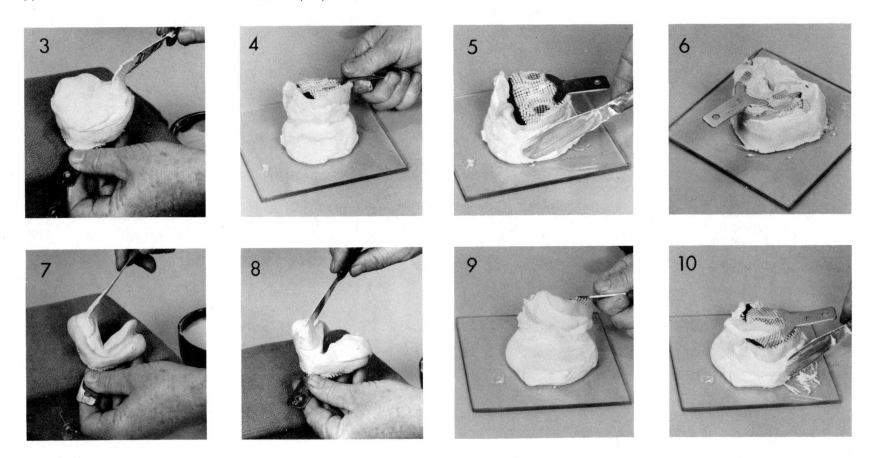

Figure 6 The poured maxillary impression is allowed to set until the heat is gone from the cast. To be safe, impressions should not be separated from their casts for at least 45 minutes to insure complete setting. A rough surface will result if an impression is separated from the cast before the gypsum has set. A cast with a rough surface is not accurate.

Figures 7 through 10 The same procedures are used for pouring a mandibular impression. Note in Figure 10 how the patty of plaster has been smoothed to make a smooth tongue space in the completed cast.

Figure 11 Care should be exercised that plaster does not build up on the lingual surface of a mandibular impression. This build-up will lock the tray to the cast and will make separation difficult. This illustration shows a plaster spatula being used to scrape out any excess plaster which may pile up on the lingual side of the impression tray.

Figure 12 The poured mandibular impression is allowed to set.

Figure 13 The maxillary impression is removed from the cast after the plaster has completely set. Maxillary impressions are best removed by lifting the posterior end and removing the impression in an anterior direction. This is particularly important when there is a deep labial undercut.

Figure 14 The mandibular impression is best removed by raising the anterior portion and then slipping the posterior portion of the impression from the cast.

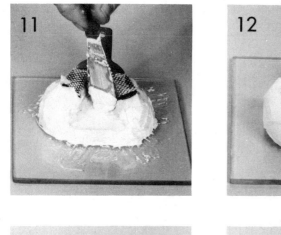
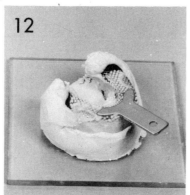
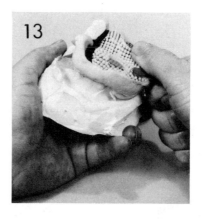
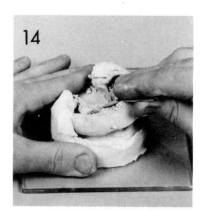

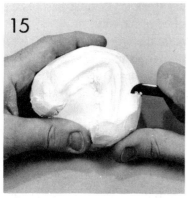
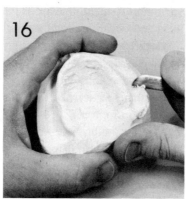
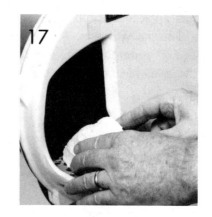
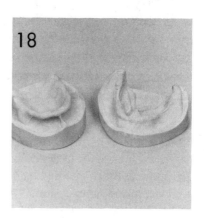

Figures 15 and 16   The excess plaster is trimmed down to the broadest point of the border roll on the cast. Trimming beyond this point reduces the accuracy of the cast. Additional trimming is acceptable after the outline of the custom tray is placed on the cast (Section 3).

Figure 17   The casts are then trimmed on a cast-trimmer so that a uniform ledge or land area three millimeters wide is produced around the cast.

Figure 18   The completed preliminary casts.

REVIEW QUESTIONS

1. What dental materials are commonly used in making a preliminary impression for complete dentures?
2. What is the recommended width of the land area around a trimmed preliminary cast?
3. What is the consistency of a plaster mix for pouring a preliminary cast?
4. What is the minimum time a plaster cast should set prior to separation from the impression?
5. What is the best way to remove a maxillary impression from a plaster cast?

SECTION 3

Custom Impression Trays

 A custom tray enables a dentist to make an accurate impression of the tissues upon which a complete denture will rest. A dental laboratory technician must recognize and understand the significance of anatomical landmarks on the preliminary cast to make satisfactory custom trays.

 An impression tray is "a receptacle or device that is used to carry the impression material to the mouth, confine the material in apposition to the surfaces to be recorded, and control the impression material while it sets to form the impression." (CCDT)

Impression trays are of two varieties:

(1) *Stock trays* are produced by dental manufacturers in a wide variety of shapes and sizes and are designed to fit most mouths. They are commonly made of metal, but some are made of resin materials. Stock trays are usually designed for a specific impression material, i.e., perforated or rimlock trays for alginate, water-cooled trays for agar-agar hydrocolloid, metal trays for plaster or compound, and resin trays for impression materials used in fixed prosthodontics (crown and bridge).

(2) *Custom trays* are made on preliminary casts, and are designed to enable a dentist to make a more accurate and detailed impression than is possible with stock trays. Custom trays are constructed for a specific impression procedure for one patient and are discarded after use.

Double thickness shellac baseplate material may be used to construct custom trays. The same technique shown in Section 5 for constructing shellac baseplates is used to make the shellac custom tray. The only variations in technique are (1) that double thickness shellac baseplate is used and (2) a handle is generally attached to the tray.

Modified methyl methacrylate resins are the most widely used materials for making custom impression trays. Trays may be made utilizing a "roll-out" technique, a "sprinkle-on" technique, or a wax pattern may be constructed, flasked, packed and cured. The "roll-out" technique is the most common.

Another method of making resin custom impression trays is through the use of a vacuum or pressure forming machine. This technique is covered in Section 15. They may also be made by using light-cured resins.

There are many acceptable variations in the construction of custom trays reflecting the personal preferences of the dentist. For example, some dentists prescribe a wax spacer to be left in the impression tray upon delivery, while others will want it removed. Some dentists may wish the wax spacer to be of a particular shape or to have the spacer varied in thicknesses in different parts of the tray. Some dentists will not use any spacer in the tray, but will relieve the tray at the time the impression is to be made. The type of handle placed on the tray also will vary from dentist to dentist. Variations in trays *may* be dictated by the type of impression material the dentist intends to use.

Some denture techniques do not utilize resin custom trays made on preliminary casts. These techniques require an impression compound preliminary impression. Dentists using this technique modify their preliminary impression and use it as a custom tray. The advantages of using an impression compound tray are that it involves one less visit by the patient to the dentist's office, and laboratory construction of custom trays is eliminated. The disadvantage is that the single appointment usually lasts longer than the combined time of the two appointments required for preliminary and final impressions utilizing resin custom trays. In addition, compound trays are usually bulkier than trays made out of resin material, and are more difficult to handle, particularly for those dentists who do not make many dentures. They may also warp if not handled properly.

The technique shown in this section, with the variations mentioned previously, is suitable for most situations you may encounter. Most impression tray materials currently on the market are adaptable to this technique. These materials are all "dead soft"; that is, they do not spring back or have elastic memory when being formed on the cast. Tray materials come in various colors; the tray generally is made of a material which will contrast in color with the impression material used by the dentist, permitting easier determination of pressure areas.

OUTLINE OF CUSTOM IMPRESSION TRAYS

The shape of a custom impression tray is most important. It should be as nearly the shape of the completed impression and denture as possible. The more accurate the tray, the more accurate the impression.

The outline of the custom tray should be placed on the preliminary cast by the dentist. When the outline is not indicated by the dentist, it must be done by the dental technician. The outline may show some variation, depending upon the preferences of the dentist and the materials which he uses. The outline described in this section is well accepted and adaptable to most impression techniques.

Figure 1 The preliminary casts are ready for custom tray construction.

Figure 2 The outline form is drawn on the preliminary cast with an indelible pencil. The descriptions of tray outline assume that the casts are viewed in anatomical positions, i.e., the maxillary cast with the ridge below (and the base superior) and the mandibular cast as it rests on the bench top.

Maxillary cast: The outline starts at the labial frenum, rises over the incisor and canine regions, down around the facial frenum (which may be indistinct as is the one on the cast in the illustration) up over the

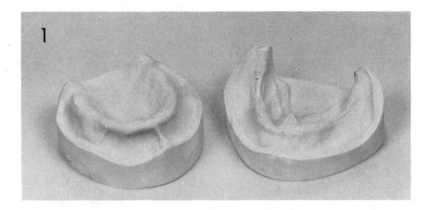

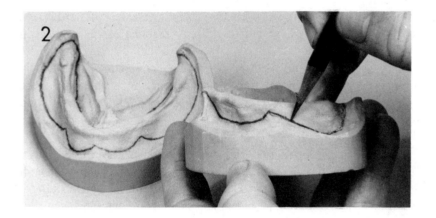

molar region around the posterior corner of the impression and through the hamular notch. It then crosses the posterior portion of the cast through the fovea palatina (usually two small depressions in the posterior portion of the cast). The hamular notch is the depression *behind* the maxillary tuberosity and the impression tray *must* cover this area. The outline is continued in a similar manner on the other half of the cast.

Mandibular cast: A line is drawn from the distal aspect of the retromolar pad to the external oblique ridge at a 45° angle to the crest of the ridge. The line then runs forward along the external oblique ridge to the superior aspect of the mandibular facial frenum. Anterior to the facial frenum the line drops over the canine and incisor region, then rises over the labial frenum. The same outline is drawn on the opposite side of the cast. The lingual portion of the outline follows the depth of the impression but rises over the lingual frenum (see Figure 19). The

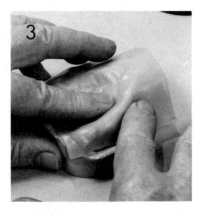
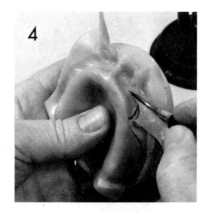
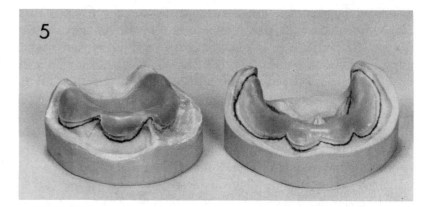

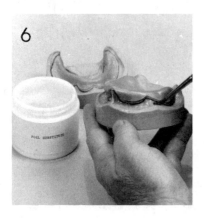
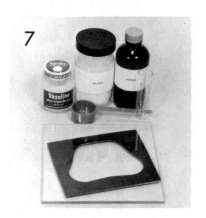
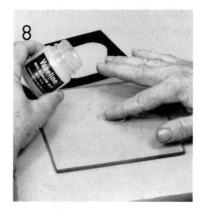
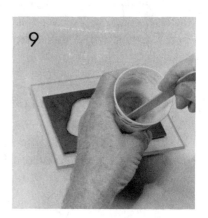

distolingual aspect of the outline should be carried far enough distally to insure proper coverage and will include coverage of the retromylohyoid depression and the retromolar pad. The accuracy of a completed final impression is determined to a large extent by proper outline form of the custom tray. When in doubt, the tray should be left long so that the dentist may reduce it.

Figures 3 and 4 A layer of baseplate wax is adapted over the cast as per the instructions of the dentist. The spacer shown is adapted just short of the indicated outline by approximately two millimeters. In the event a spacer is not prescribed, this step will be omitted.

Figure 5 The wax spacers are completed.

Figure 6 Tinfoil substitute is painted on all exposed portions of the cast. This is necessary to insure separation of the resin tray material from the gypsum cast.

Figure 7 The materials required for construction of a custom tray—powder and liquid components of the tray material, measuring devices, Vaseline, a glass slab and a form for the tray material.

Figure 8 The glass slab is lubricated by applying a moderate coat of Vaseline.

Figure 9 The manufacturer's instructions for mixing the tray material should be followed. A paper cup and wooden tongue blade are satisfactory for mixing the material and both may be discarded after use.

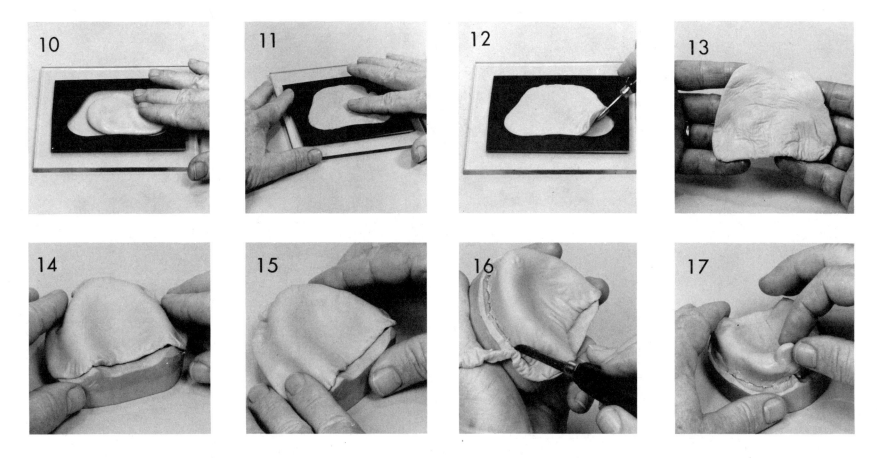

Figures 10 and 11   The mixed tray material is placed within the form on the glass slab. It is patted out to form a wafer of uniform thickness. A little Vaseline on the fingers will prevent the material from sticking to them.

Figures 12 and 13   The wafer of tray material is lifted from the slab. The wafer is handled so that a uniform thickness is maintained.

Figures 14 and 15   The soft tray material is adapted to the cast with light finger pressure. Excessive pressure will cause thin areas in the tray. Be sure that the material is adapted to the cast throughout the palate and around the borders. If a bubble appears, puncture it with a sharp instrument, expel the air and complete the adaptation to the cast.

Figure 16   A warm knife may be used to trim the soft material from around the borders of the cast. Do not attempt to cut the soft material to the tray outline, but remove only the gross excess. Be sure the material is adapted to the cast around the borders after trimming. Final trimming is done after the tray has cured.

Figure 17   The excess material is formed into a handle of the desired shape. The handle must be placed so that it will not interfere with any movements of the patient's lips during the impression procedures. The handle should be shaped so that it is easy to hold.

Figure 18   An L-shaped handle or a simple vertical handle is satisfactory; both avoid lip interference. The small vertical handle is usually preferred.

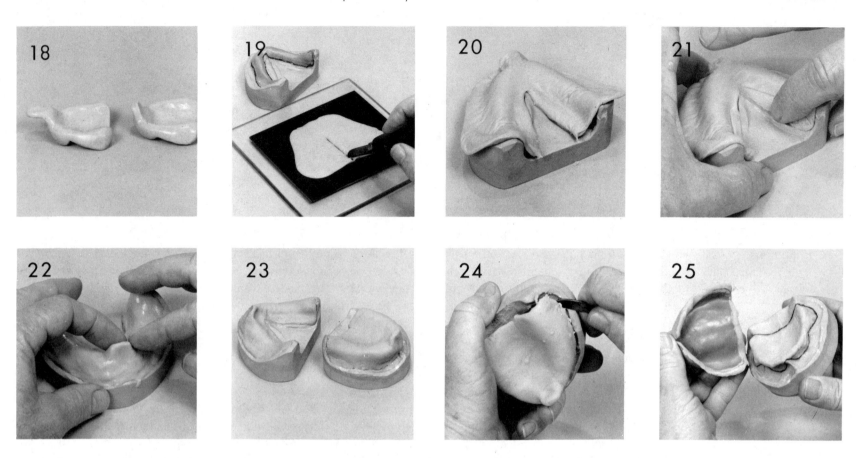

Figure 19   Mandibular custom trays are formed in a similar manner. The tray material is slit in the middle before the wafer is removed from the glass slab.

Figure 20   The material is centered on the cast leaving some excess on the lingual portion.

Figure 21   The material is adapted to the borders in the same manner as was done on the maxillary tray. The material on the lingual border is doubled back so that the lingual border will have additional thickness.

Figure 22   The excess material on the facial aspect of the tray has been trimmed with a warm knife. The handle has been placed and the surface of the tray is smoothed, using a little of the tray material liquid on a finger. Note the placement of the handle on the crest of the ridge.

Figure 23   The casts and impression trays are set aside until the material cures. The trays should not be separated from the casts until the heat of polymerization has dissipated.

Figures 24 and 25   The maxillary tray is removed from the cast by inserting a knife and gently lifting it from the cast. The tray is first lifted in the posterior region when anterior undercuts are present on the cast. The tray is then removed by lifting it from the cast in an anterior direction.

Figures 26 through 28   The mandibular tray is removed from the cast by inserting a knife blade in the anterior region and then slipping the posterior region from the cast. When undercuts are present in the retromylohyoid region, the mandibular cast must be fractured before the tray is removed. A sharp blow with a plaster spatula on the base of

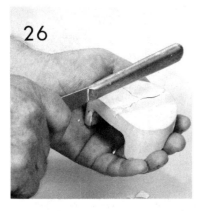
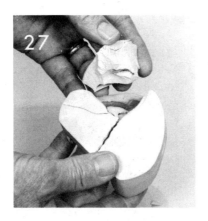
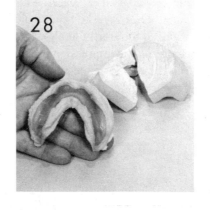
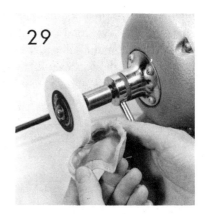

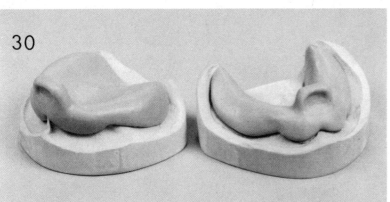

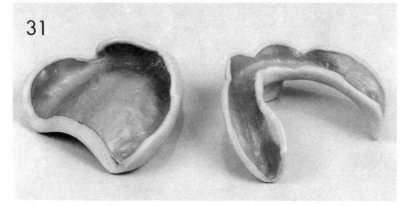

the mandibular cast will usually fracture it into two or three pieces which can then be removed from the tray. The pieces can be assembled for future reference during the trimming procedures. Note that in both the maxillary and mandibular trays the wax spacer adheres to the tray and not to the cast. The outline of the tray is transferred from the cast to the tray, but *this will occur only if an indelible pencil has been used to place the tray outline*. If the outline does not transfer to the tray, you must refer to the cast throughout the trimming procedures.

Figure 29 The tray is trimmed to the outline using a lathe and a large coarse cutting stone. The excess around the border is removed to the outline before any shaping of the external surface is attempted. Finer trimming may be done with smaller fine-grit wheels, arbor bands and acrylic burs.

The surface and borders of the tray must be smooth before it is delivered to the dentist. The tray may be smoothed using polishing wheels and pumice or some of the tray material liquid may be rubbed on the tray in order to produce a smooth surface.

Figure 30 The completed trays are now ready for delivery to the dentist. The outline on the cast is just barely visible under the border of the impression trays. The shape of the impression tray closely approximates the shape of the completed impression and denture. The handles on the trays are concave in form so that they will be easier to hold and not tend to slip from the fingers when the impression material is placed into the tray. Sometimes small handles are placed in the molar region of the mandibular tray to hold the tray in position while the impression material is setting.

Figure 31 The tissue surface of the impression trays utilizing this technique is almost completely covered by a wax shim or spacer. This spacer does not extend beyond the border of the tray. The mylohyoid region of the mandibular tray has been relieved arbitrarily to allow for movement of the tissues under the tongue during the impression procedure. This modification is usually done in the dental office and is the reason for leaving the lingual borders of the tray thicker than the facial borders.

REVIEW QUESTIONS

1. What is the purpose of a custom tray?
2. What type of impression material is used with a perforated or rim-lock tray?
3. What are the disadvantages of an impression compound custom tray?
4. Describe the construction steps of a custom tray made of "dead soft" material on a maxillary cast.
5. Name four techniques for constructing a custom tray and indicate the most common technique.

SECTION 4

Master Casts

This section begins to show the benefits of teamwork between dentist and technician. The dentist uses the custom tray made by the technician to make a final impression. In turn the technician uses the final impression to make a master cast which is the foundation for all techniques leading to the finished dentures.

Custom trays are used by the dentist to make final impressions which should be accurate in every detail and should reproduce the surface and border areas exactly as they will be in the completed denture. The pouring of casts into final impressions must be done accurately in order to maintain all of these areas, as the denture will be fabricated on these casts.

The dentist will check all areas of the custom tray before making the final impression. **Figure A** shows the dentist trying the mandibular custom tray in the patient's mouth to check for border extension and proper adaptation. The final impressions are made after the trays have been checked and corrected where necessary. **Figure B** shows a final mandibular impression being made, while **Figure C** shows a maxillary final impression being made.

The material which is used for final impressions will vary from dentist to dentist because of his personal preferences. The most commonly used materials for final impressions are plaster or other gypsum products, mercaptan rubber base impression material, silicone rubber base impression material, zinc oxide-eugenol impression paste, alginate, and, sometimes, waxes. The impression tray technique described in Section 3 produces trays satisfactory for use with all of these materials. Suitable adhesives are necessary for some of these materials.

The master cast produced from the final impression must include all

tissue and border areas which will be covered by the denture base. The border areas are particularly important in complete dentures because they form the seal which helps maintain the denture in place. Loss of the border, either in the impression, in the cast, or by overpolishing, will result in a denture having inadequate retention.

Careful handling of an impression is as essential as using a good technique for pouring the master cast. Do not handle the surface or border areas of the impression.

The impression must be beaded with a strip of wax or other suitable material, or the impression must be boxed. Boxing an impression produces a container into which stone can be poured, resulting in a denser cast. Boxing an impression also permits the use of a mounting plate which in turn permits the master cast to be repositioned accurately on the articulator after the dentures have been cured. Boxing also eliminates any risk of the stone pulling away from the impression which may happen when an impression is inverted. Alginate final impressions are poured without boxing or beading in the same manner as preliminary impressions. Alginate final impressions may be poured and not inverted as shown in **Figure 22**.

All master casts must be poured in stone. Regular stone is satisfactory for this purpose, but some dentists and laboratories prefer to use the harder die stones. Mechanical spatulation, preferably under vacuum, produces a better mix of stone and a denser cast. If mechanical spatulation equipment is not available, the stone should be mixed thoroughly to a thick consistency.

Three techniques may be used for pouring master casts: boxing, inverting the impression on a patty of stone without boxing, or pouring the impression without boxing but not inverting the impression. Each method produces satisfactory results.

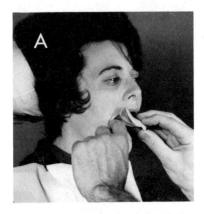

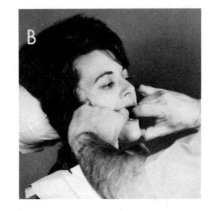

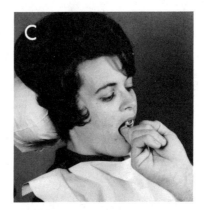

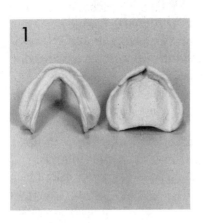

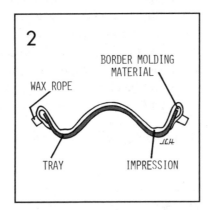

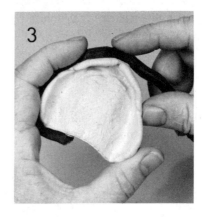

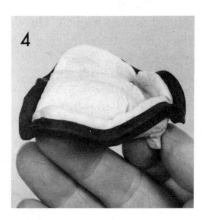

POURING FINAL IMPRESSIONS AND INVERTING

Figure 1 These final impressions have been made of zinc oxide-eugenol paste and are shown as they arrive from the dentist's office.

Figure 2 This drawing illustrates the proper placement of the wax bead on the final impression. It is placed at the greatest height of contour on the outside border of the denture. If there is any question as to the placement of this bead, it should be placed so that there will be a greater amount of the border showing. If it is placed too far away from the border, it is a simple matter to trim the cast. If it is placed too close to the border, the cast may be unsatisfactory.

Figure 3 The wax bead is adapted to the maxillary impression. The

wax used in this illustration is a square rope of utility wax which adheres to the zinc oxide-eugenol impression material.

Figure 4 The beading is completed for the maxillary impression. Note that the beading across the posterior border of the denture does not cover any tissue surface, but rather preserves the posterior border of the impression.

Figure 5 The beading is completed on the mandibular impression. Note the amount of the impression border which is visible below the beading wax. None of the tissue surface is covered by the beading wax.

Figure 6 The beading has been completed for the maxillary and mandibular impressions. Note the piece of baseplate wax which has been

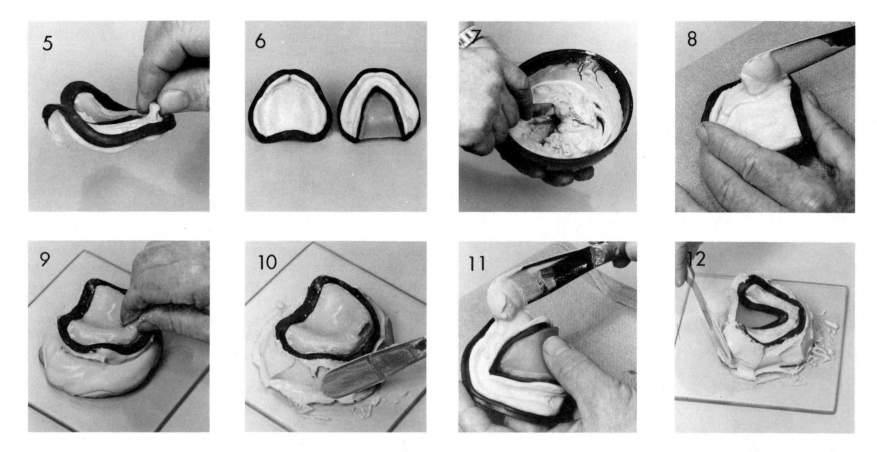

placed in the tongue space of the mandibular impression. The wax is on the inferior side of the wax bead but does not touch the impression surface. This piece of baseplate wax will produce a smooth tongue space on the completed cast and will eliminate the need for trimming in this area. Note that none of the tissue surface in either the mandibular or maxillary impression is covered by the beading wax.

Figure 7   The stone is mixed thoroughly to a thick consistency to insure a strong, dense cast.

Figure 8   The beaded impression is held on the vibrator as is illustrated, and the stone is placed into one corner of the impression allowing the stone to flow around the impression so that air is not trapped. The stone will flow more readily if the impression is damp, not dry. The impression is filled with stone in this manner.

Figure 9   A mound or patty of stone is placed on a glass slab. The filled impression is then inverted onto the patty of stone. It should be placed firmly but gently into the patty so that the poured part of the impression adheres firmly to the patty of stone. The impression is pressed until the deepest part of the impression is approximately one-half inch from the glass slab. This will produce a cast which is one-half inch thick in its thinnest area. The impression should be parallel to the glass slab.

Figure 10   After the impression is positioned, the spatula is used to pull some stone up around the wax bead. Very little manipulation is necessary. The cast is then allowed to set before any further work is done on it. Note that the stone was mixed to a consistency such that it did not flow over the glass slab.

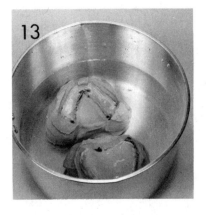
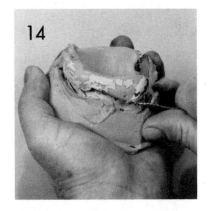
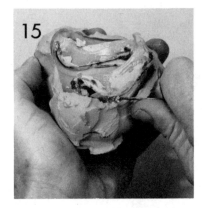
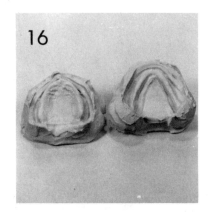

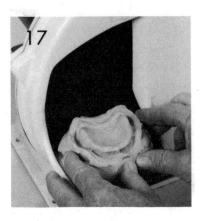
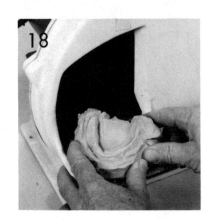

wax in the tongue space of the mandibular cast are removed. The casts are then placed in a pan of hot water, approximately 150°F., to soften the impression material. This shows the impressions in the hot water. A thermostatically controlled water bath is better used for this procedure. The casts are left in the hot water long enough to soften the impression material. Most zinc oxide-eugenol pastes soften in a period of four to seven minutes.

Figures 14 and 15   The impressions are removed from the cast by gently lifting the impression tray with a knife. Maxillary impressions are best removed by lifting from the back as is shown in **Figure 14** and then removing the impression tray in an anterior direction. Mandibular impression trays (**Figure 15**) are best removed by lifting one side of the impression tray gently and then removing it with a rotating movement. If the impression is so undercut that a tray cannot be removed safely by this method, a Hanau torch is used to soften the tray near the mid-line. This allows the tray to bend so that it comes off the cast easily.

Some impression material will adhere to the cast. This can be removed easily, and should be done with a blunt instrument to prevent scoring the master cast.

Figure 16   The impression trays have been removed from the casts and the casts cleaned of excess impression material. The casts are now ready for trimming.

Figure 11   A similar procedure is used to pour the mandibular impression using a vibrator. The stone is placed in one side of the impression, and is allowed to run to the opposite side. The impression is filled in a manner similar to that used for the maxillary impression.

Figure 12   A patty of stone is placed on the glass slab as was done with the maxillary impression. The mandibular impression is inverted onto the patty and the stone is pulled up around the wax beading. When using this method for pouring master casts, it is essential that enough stone be placed on the posterior part of the poured impression as is shown in this illustration. Note that a thick mix of stone is essential.

Figure 13   Both casts are allowed to set until the stone is hard. Allow the stone to set a minimum of forty-five minutes before any further manipulation is done. After the stone has set, the beading wax and the

Figures 17 and 18   The gross excess is removed from the casts on the cast-trimmer. Enough excess is left in order to provide a good border or land area on the cast which protects the anatomical surface of the cast.

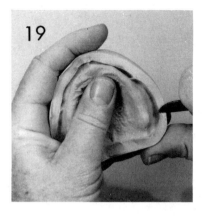

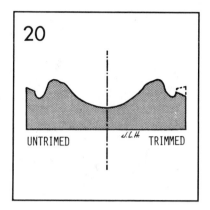

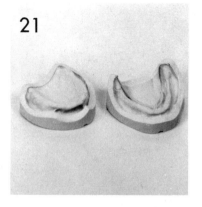

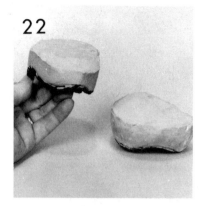

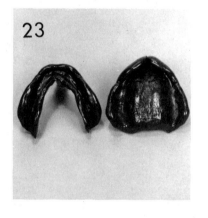

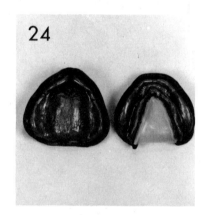

Figure 19　A knife is used to flatten the land area on the master cast. The land area should be reduced until the border of the denture area is exposed to its widest diameter. After the land area is completely trimmed, the cast may be returned to the cast-trimmer and additional trimming done to make the land area uniform around the circumference of the cast.

Figure 20　This drawing shows the level to which the land area should be trimmed. The anterior portion is beveled to permit better access for adaptation of base plates.

Figure 21　The completed mandibular and maxillary casts.

POURING FINAL IMPRESSIONS WITHOUT INVERTING

Many technicians and dentists believe that a more accurate cast is produced if the impression is not inverted on a patty of stone. An impression may be poured without inverting or boxing if a thick mix of stone is used. The same beading technique is used for maxillary and mandibular impressions as was used in the previous section. The stone is vibrated into the impression and is then built up over the impression. The impression and casts are set aside without inverting and the stone allowed to set.

Figure 22　Shows a maxillary and mandibular impression poured in this manner. Trimming procedures are identical to those shown in **Figures 17–20** in the previous section.

BOXING FINAL IMPRESSIONS

Boxing impressions is the most satisfactory method for making a master cast. The primary disadvantage of this method is that it is more time consuming. The advantages far outweigh the disadvantages. Boxing produces a dense, accurate master cast of predetermined thickness. It also allows the easy insertion of mounting plates into the base of the cast. These mounting plates permit a cast to be removed and repositioned accurately on an articulator during denture construction.

Figure 23　Maxillary and mandibular impressions are shown which have been made using mercaptan rubber base impression material.

Figure 24　A wax bead is placed around the impressions in exactly the same manner as was done for the zinc oxide-eugenol impressions in the

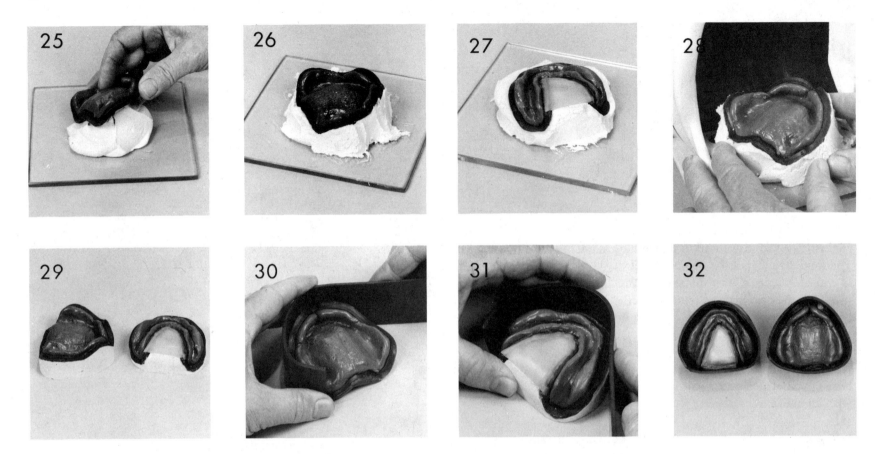

previous exercise. The tongue space is similarly filled in. One variation is necessary: Utility wax will not adhere to the rubber base impression material. Therefore, it is necessary to dab hot, sticky wax where the utility wax will be attached.

Figure 25   A patty of impression plaster is placed on a glass slab and the impression is seated into the plaster.

Figure 26   The impression should be made level with the glass slab and the plaster pulled up to the wax bead.

Figure 27   The mandibular impression is treated in a similar manner. The plaster extends behind the posterior border of the mandibular impression. Note the baseplate wax position in the tongue space.

Figure 28   The plaster bases are trimmed to the wax bead on a cast-trimmer.

Figure 29   The plaster bases on the mandibular and maxillary impressions have been trimmed.

Figures 30 and 31   A strip of boxing wax is wrapped around the prepared impression. The plaster base provides a firm attachment for the boxing wax and assures that the sides of the cast will be vertical. The boxing wax is wrapped around the entire impression and the junction between it and the utility wax bead is sealed.

Figure 32   The boxing of the maxillary and mandibular impressions is completed. The boxed impressions are always handled by their bases.

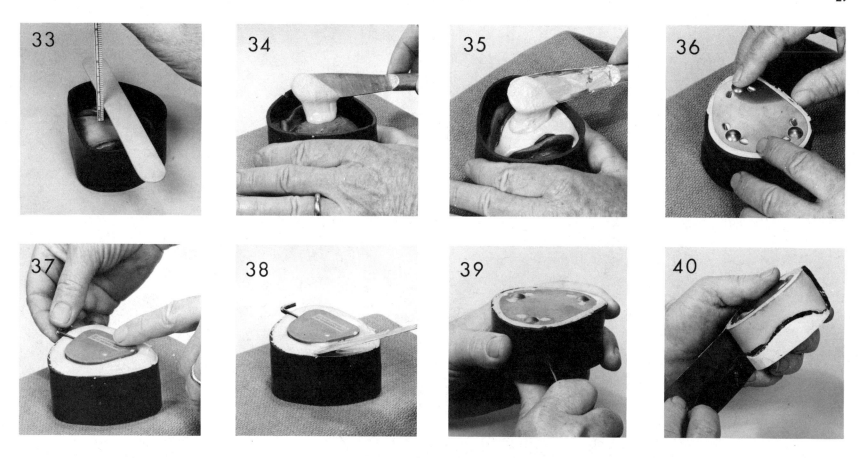

Figure 33 The base of the cast should be between three-eighths and one-half inch thick. This is easily determined when an impression is boxed.

Figures 34 and 35 The impressions are poured in stone.

Figure 36 This illustrates the use of a Stansbury mounting plate. This plate is placed on the surface of the stone and pressed to place until it engages the stone.

Figures 37 and 38 These figures illustrate the use of a Hanau split mounting plate. This plate is placed on the surface of the stone and the stone is teased around the edge until it engages the edge of one of the mounting plates. Usually the same type of mounting plate would be used on both maxillary and mandibular casts. Different mounting plates were used on these casts for illustrative purposes.

Figures 39 and 40 After the stone has set thoroughly, the boxing wax is removed from the casts.

Figures 41 and 42 The plaster base is removed from the impression tray by sectioning.

Figure 43 The wax bead is removed from the casts.

Figure 44 The casts are placed in hot water to soften the impression material. The rubber base impression material will not soften but the compound used to mold the border will soften and permit easier removal of the impression trays from the casts.

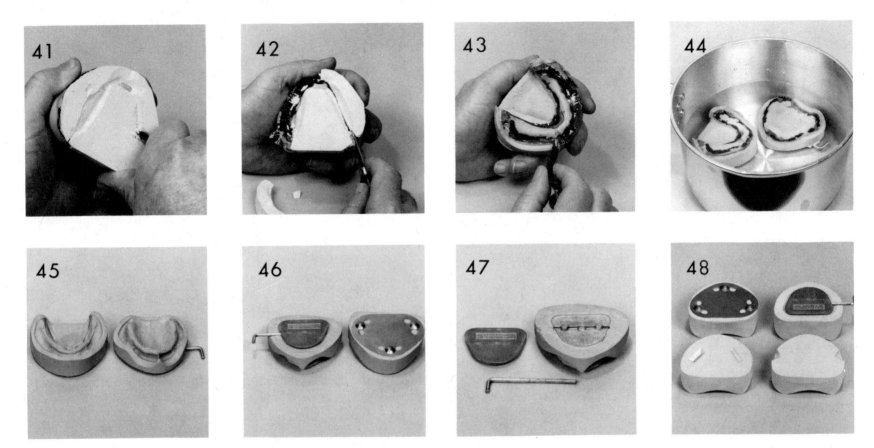

Figure 45   The completed casts.

Figure 46   The bases of the casts showing the Hanau and Stansbury mounting plates.

Figure 47   The Hanau mounting plate has been disassembled. When the cast is mounted on the articulator, the upper portion of the Hanau plate will be retained in the mounting plaster. The cast may be removed and replaced on the articulator by removing the pin which holds the plate together.

Figure 48   Several types of indexes or mounting plates may be used on the base of master casts to permit their removal and accurate replacement on an articulator during denture construction. The two casts in the foreground have had index grooves or notches carved in the base. These indexes also allow the casts to be replaced and removed. However, the removal will not be as easy as when mounting plates are used and the replacement will not be as accurate.

SUMMARY

Three methods of producing master casts from final impressions have been described. Each technique has its advantages and disadvantages. Each will produce an accurate master cast. Slovenly technique or improper handling of materials will produce casts which are inaccurate and inadequate.

REVIEW QUESTIONS

1. What is the proper thickness of the thinnest portion of a master cast?
2. What are the advantages of boxing an impression prior to pouring a master cast?
3. Name three techniques for pouring a master cast.
4. Draw a cross section of a maxillary master cast showing the proper placement of the land area.
5. What is the purpose of mounting plates?

SECTION 5

Baseplates

DLT 101 5/3/10 (Materials we discuss)

A baseplate is not a portion of the completed denture. It is a temporary base used to record the relationship of the mandible to the maxillae and upon which the teeth are arranged in wax for trial insertion in the patient's mouth. Baseplates must accurately fit the master casts and the mouth.

A baseplate is "a temporary form representing the base of a denture and used for making jaw relation records, arranging artificial teeth, or trial placement in the mouth." (CCDT) *(don't recomend) —flexible maybreak unged*

Baseplates are made from a variety of materials: wax, shellac baseplate material, auto-polymerizing resin, or a combination of these materials. Baseplates are temporary devices used during the construction of dentures and do not become a part of the completed denture. Even though baseplates are eventually discarded, they should be made to fit the master cast as accurately as possible. An inaccurate baseplate will result in inaccurate jaw relationship records and a false idea of the appearance of the teeth at the try-in stage.

Most baseplates are stabilized with a lining material to make them fit more accurately. By definition, a stabilized baseplate is "a baseplate lined with a plastic or other material to improve its adaptation and stability." (CCDT) Auto-polymerizing resin is the most commonly used material for stabilizing baseplates, although some impression materials may be used for this purpose.

A baseplate must fit the master cast accurately. An inaccurate baseplate will prevent the master cast from seating properly into the baseplate when the casts are mounted and will result in mounting errors and

eventual errors in jaw relationships. Inaccurate baseplates may appear to fit well in the patient's mouth because of the resiliency of the soft tissues, but such appearances are deceiving and result in inaccuracies unless the baseplates also fit the casts.

Since baseplates are temporary devices used in denture construction, care must be exercised that the master cast is not marred during their construction. When auto-polymerizing resin is used to construct or stabilize baseplates, all undercuts must be relieved. The relief used when a baseplate is stabilized should be conservative, but must eliminate all undercuts, even those in the rugae area, over the crest of the mandibular ridge, etc. Failure to provide relief in these small undercut areas will result in fracture of the cast. On mandibular casts, the retromylohyoid area must be blocked out to prevent the baseplate from flexing upon insertion and removal. Flexing in any kind of baseplate, be it resin, baseplate wax or shellac baseplate, will warp the baseplate.

Some denture techniques do not use baseplates but use the final denture base during the construction phases. In these techniques the denture base is constructed and then used in the same manner as a baseplate during construction. Instead of being discarded, it becomes an integral part of the denture. Bases used in this type of technique may be made of resin or cast metal.

During the construction of dentures, baseplates are not used alone, but are used as bases for occlusion rims, central bearing devices, or for a tentative arrangement of the teeth. An occlusion rim is a temporary occluding surface built on a baseplate to help determine the proper shape of a person's mouth, the placement of the dental arch, and aids in determination of proper jaw relationships. A central bearing device

Atlanta Technical College Bookstore
1560 Metropolitan Parkway SW.
Atlanta, GA 30310
t 404.225.4722
f 404.225.4725

Sale

Receipt: 0111078
n.jones   05/03/10 10:16

2 PENCIL RED/BLUE CHECKPOINT S1
   10014967

                          Y $1.98

                    Subtotal: $1.98
Tax:
  Sales Tax $0.16

                      Total: $2.14
Tender:

VISA $2.14
XXXXXXXXXXXXX9017
XXXX
150389

Change Due $0.00

NO RETURNS OF COS/BAR SUPPLIES,
HEALTH CARE SUPPLIES, AND USED
          TEXTBOOKS.
THE HOPE/PELL CHARGE PERIOD
ENDS SEVEN (7) BUSINESS DAYS
   FROM THE BEGINNING DATE
      OF THE QUARTER!

0111078

- Textbooks with plastic shrink-wrap must be unopened. If opened, the merchandise will be returned at the used price!

All sales of used texts, cosmetology/barbering supplies (includes mannequins, smocks, and jackets), and health care supplies are FINAL!

Atlanta Technical College Bookstore

Textbook/ Merchandise Return Policy

New textbooks, clothing, and office supplies may be returned within fourteen (14) calendar days of original purchase date, provided the following conditions are met:

- The original receipt must accompany the return.

- Merchandise must be in new, unused, resaleable condition!

- Textbooks with plastic shrink-wrap must be unopened. If opened, the merchandise will be returned at the used price!

All sales of used texts, cosmetology/barbering supplies (includes mannequins, smocks, and jackets), and health care supplies are
FINAL!

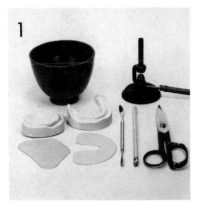 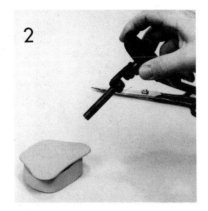 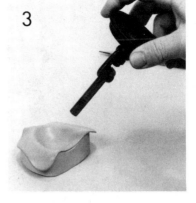 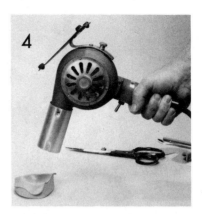

aids in the determination of jaw relationships. A baseplate is generally used for setting the teeth so that the teeth may be placed in the patient's mouth and the arrangement, mold and shade checked in the natural surroundings of the patient's mouth. These uses of baseplates are covered in following sections.

Three techniques for the construction of baseplates are illustrated in this section. Proficiency in and an understanding of these techniques will permit a technician to make satisfactory baseplates and to easily acquire skills in any other baseplate technique which may be required.

SHELLAC BASEPLATES

Shellac baseplates are made from preformed blanks which are composed of a resinous material which softens upon heating and hardens when cooled. Shellac baseplate material is brittle and comes in pink sheets. Shellac baseplate material comes in two thicknesses: the regular thickness and the double thick variety. The single thickness is used for baseplate construction, and the double thickness is used to construct custom trays. Shellac custom trays are constructed in the same manner as baseplates, except that a handle is added for ease of manipulation.

The same technique illustrated for shellac baseplates can also be used to construct wax baseplates. The techniques for adapting wax are the same as for shellac. A hard baseplate wax must be used for wax baseplates; softer waxes will not maintain their shape.

Shellac and wax baseplates do not reproduce all the detail on the master cast. They also tend to warp and cause mounting errors and,

later, errors in occlusion. For these reasons they must be made well by the technician and handled carefully by the dentist.

Figure 1 The materials required for construction of shellac baseplates are the master cast, shellac baseplate material, bowl of water, Bunsen burner, wax spatula, a wooden pencil with a good eraser, and a pair of scissors.

Figure 2 Before adapting the shellac baseplate, the cast must be treated so that the shellac baseplate will not adhere to the cast. This may be done in several ways: the surface of the cast may be dusted with talcum powder, the cast may be dampened, or a light coat of petrolatum jelly may be applied to the tissue surface of the cast. After the separating medium is applied to the cast, the shellac baseplate blank is centered on the cast. The Bunsen burner is inverted and the flame played on the surface of the shellac material, moving the flame back and forth so that the shellac blank is heated uniformly.

Figure 3 As the shellac material becomes softened, it will sag. If the blank has not been centered properly, the softened material can be moved on the cast until it is centered.

Figure 4 An alternate method for adapting the material is to use a heat gun. This is used in the same manner as a Bunsen burner, and produces good results. This piece of equipment is nice to have, but is not essential for the construction of shellac baseplates. (Some hair dryers may work but they must produce relatively high heat.)

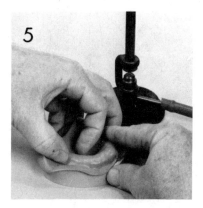
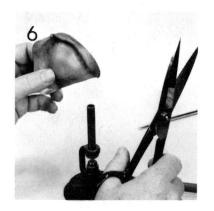
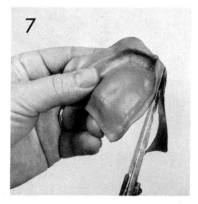
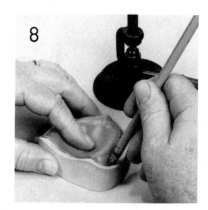

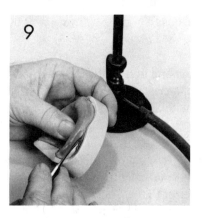
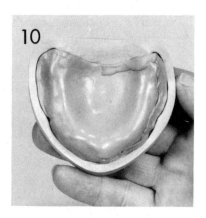

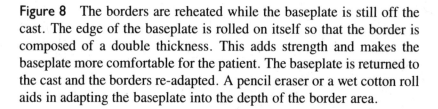

Figure 8   The borders are reheated while the baseplate is still off the cast. The edge of the baseplate is rolled on itself so that the border is composed of a double thickness. This adds strength and makes the baseplate more comfortable for the patient. The baseplate is returned to the cast and the borders re-adapted. A pencil eraser or a wet cotton roll aids in adapting the baseplate into the depth of the border area.

Figure 9   The double thick border is sealed by using a very hot spatula to seal the junction of the material around the border. The spatula should be cleaned periodically to avoid discoloring the baseplate with burned baseplate material which may adhere to the spatula.

Figure 10   This illustrates a shellac baseplate in which the border has been rolled, one-half of which has been smoothed, and the other half which has been left with no modification from the step seen in **Figure 9**. It is not always necessary to smooth the junction line in the shellac baseplate since it will be covered by wax from the occlusion rim. The only area in which the junction should be smooth is across the posterior border.

    Smoothing the junction is done by flaming the border area of the baseplate while it is on the cast with a Hanau torch. A light coat of Vaseline is then placed on the heated baseplate and the baseplate is rubbed briskly with a towel. This produces a smooth, shiny surface and hides the junction of the material.

Figure 5   After the material is softened, the baseplate is adapted to the surface of the cast. This is done by pressing the material firmly to place while it is soft. Shellac baseplate material retains heat and will burn the fingers unless the fingers are dampened or a light coat of petrolatum jelly is applied to the fingers.

Figure 6   After the preliminary adaptation is completed, the baseplate is removed from the cast and the border area heated over the Bunsen burner.

Figure 7   The excess material is trimmed from the border with scissors. Some people prefer to do this trimming while the baseplate remains on the cast. Trim the border so there will be a border of uniform thickness on the completed baseplate.

Figures 11 and 12   The completed shellac baseplates. Please note the smooth borders on these baseplates in **Figure 12**.

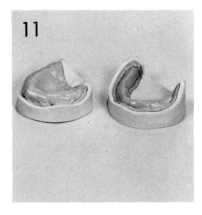
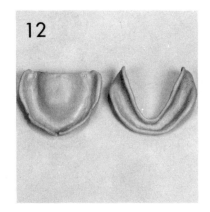
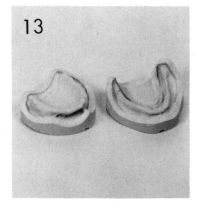
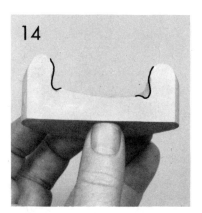

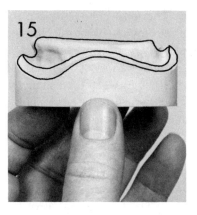
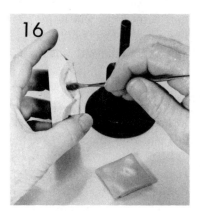

STABILIZED BASEPLATES

One of the disadvantages attributed to shellac and wax baseplates is the lack of detail present in the tissue surface. This fault can be overcome by making stabilized baseplates.

The technique for making stabilized baseplates is basically that of making a regular baseplate and then lining it with a material which accurately reproduces the surface and borders of the master cast. Several methods are employed to accomplish this. A regular shellac or wax baseplate may be lined with zinc oxide-eugenol impression material. When this procedure is used, the master cast is coated with Vaseline to avoid having the impression material adhere to the cast. Rubber base impression and similar materials have also been used to stabilize baseplates but they are not recommended as their resiliency often prevents their accurate return to the master cast.

Auto-polymerizing resins are the most widely used materials for stabilizing baseplates. These materials permit the production of a baseplate which is both accurate and stable. These baseplates maintain their accuracy for a period of one or two weeks before any noticeable warpage occurs. Two methods may be employed for making stabilized baseplates utilizing auto-polymerizing resin. The first method employs a matrix of wax or shellac baseplate material into which a mix of auto-polymerizing resin is poured and then placed on the cast. The second method is a sprinkle technique involving alternate applications of powder and liquid.

Because of the rigidity of the auto-polymerizing resin, the master cast *must* be relieved so that the completed baseplate can be removed

from the cast. All undercuts and sharp projections must be relieved conservatively. Excessive relief will cause a baseplate to fit inaccurately and may result in false illusions when determining proper lip contours.

MATRIX TYPE STABILIZED BASEPLATES

Figure 13 The master casts are ready to begin construction of the stabilized baseplates.

Figures 14 and 15 These illustrations demonstrate the presence of undercuts in the master casts. The common place for undercuts in maxillary casts is on the facial of the anterior ridge, sometimes in the

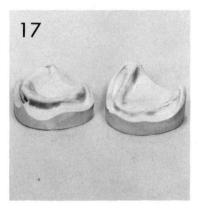
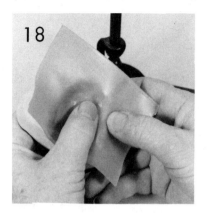
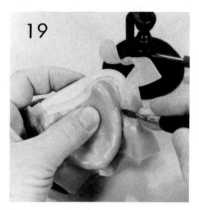
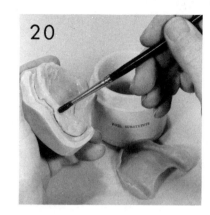

tuberosity areas and in the rugae areas. The most common place for undercuts in mandibular casts is in the retromylohyoid area. On both maxillary and mandibular casts undercuts may be present near the crest of the ridge. Extreme caution must be exercised in blocking out these ridge areas or the crest of the ridge may fracture when the completed baseplate is removed from the cast, which will usually necessitate a new final impression. This danger is minimized by proper procedures and attention to detail.

Figure 16   Baseplate wax is used to relieve the undercut areas in the master cast. This is applied in small amounts and is built up so that the undercuts are just barely relieved. The undercut on the facial of the anterior maxillary ridge need not always be completely eliminated as the completed baseplate may be removed in an anterior direction. You may estimate if the blockout is adequate by looking down on the cast in the direction that the baseplate will be removed from the cast.

Figure 17   The blockout has been completed on the maxillary and mandibular casts. Note that wax has been added on the rugae area, on the facial of the anterior ridge of the maxillary cast, and in the tuberosity area. The retromylohyoid area and two small areas on the facial of the ridge have been relieved on the mandibular cast.

Figures 18 and 19   A sheet of baseplate wax is softened and adapted to the cast. This wax is trimmed one to two millimeters short of the borders of the master cast. This wax matrix is well adapted as it forms a tray for carrying the auto-polymerizing resin to the cast.

Figure 20   A liberal coat of tinfoil substitute is applied to the cast. This should cover the complete cast including the land areas. Apply extra tinfoil substitute to the crest of the ridge; two or three coats of tinfoil substitute are advisable but not necessary.

Figure 21   The materials required for mixing the auto-polymerizing resin are a small spatula, graduates for measuring the powder and liquid, a container for mixing the resin, and the powder and liquid (monomer and polymer). A *thin* mix of resin is used in this technique. The proportions are two parts polymer (powder) to one part monomer (liquid). A mix of 15 cc. of powder and 7½ cc. liquid provides adequate resin for one baseplate. Depending upon your proficiency, you may wish to make separate mixes for the mandibular and maxillary baseplates or you may use one larger mix and make both baseplates simultaneously.

Figure 22   The polymer and monomer are mixed in a paper cup.

Figure 23   The paper cup is squeezed to make a pouring spout. As soon as the mixture reaches a creamy consistency, a small amount is poured into the border area of the cast, being careful not to trap any air bubbles. A small amount is also poured into the palatal area of the maxillary cast.

Figure 24   The remainder of the resin is poured into the wax matrix, filling the ridge areas.

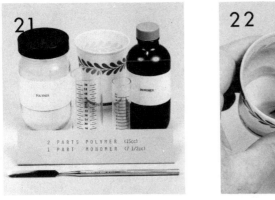
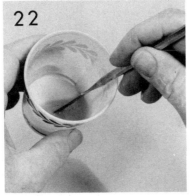
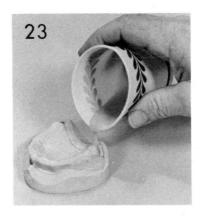
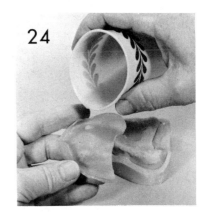

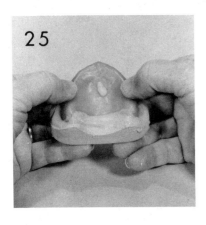
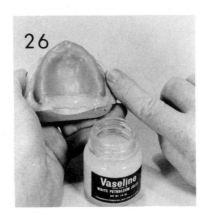
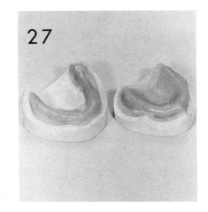
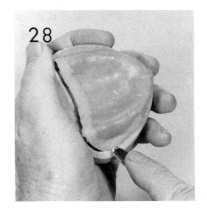

Figure 25 The wax matrix is placed on the master cast and is pressed firmly to place. Excess will exude around the edges of the wax.

Figure 26 ˙ A small amount of Vaseline should be rubbed on the finger tips. This prevents the resin from adhering to the fingers. The excess resin is then pressed down as is shown in this illustration around the edge of the cast. *Do not attempt to roll the excess resin over the wax matrix.* Press the resin down and use the sharp outside edge of the land area to trim off the excess resin. If resin is allowed to roll back on the wax matrix, difficulty will be encountered when the teeth are set in later stages of denture construction.

Figure 27 The master cast and the uncured resin baseplates are set aside to allow the resin to cure. The time for curing will vary depending upon the brand of resin used, the proportions of powder and liquid, and the temperature of the room. It is recommended that the baseplates *not* be placed in a pressure cooker to speed curing as this may cause some distortion.

Figure 28 The maxillary baseplate is removed by lifting the posterior edge with a knife. Do not exert too much pressure. If difficulty is encountered in removing the baseplate, soak the cast for a few minutes in warm water. Do not use water hot enough to melt the wax. Soaking the cast expands the separating medium and makes separation easier. The mandibular baseplate is removed from the cast by carefully lifting the anterior region and then slipping the baseplate off the cast. The direction in which removal is easiest will be determined by the placement of the wax blockout in previous steps.

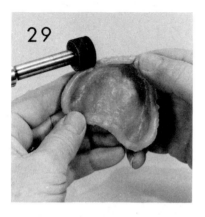 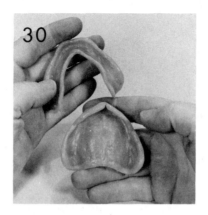 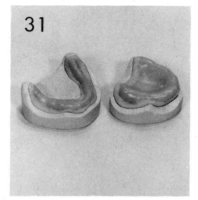 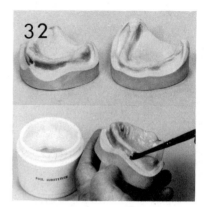

Figure 29   The excess resin is trimmed from the borders of the baseplate. Arbor bands on a lathe are the most efficient method for doing this. Polishing of these baseplates is not necessary as the wax from the occlusion rims will cover the areas which have been ground with the arbor band.

Figure 30   The completed baseplates showing the tissue surface. Please compare the detail on the tissue surface of these baseplates and the detail on the shellac baseplates. Even though the rugae area has been relieved, the detail in these baseplates is superior to shellac or wax baseplates.

Figure 31   The completed baseplates have been placed on the master casts. This technique produces a stabilized baseplate easily and quickly. The baseplate is thin and usually does not interfere when arranging teeth.

SPRINKLE METHOD STABILIZED BASEPLATES

Figure 32   The preparation of the master cast for the construction of a sprinkle method baseplate is identical to the preparation for the matrix method. The undercuts are conservatively relieved and the casts are painted with a tinfoil substitute.

Figure 33   The materials for making the sprinkle method baseplate are

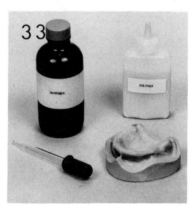 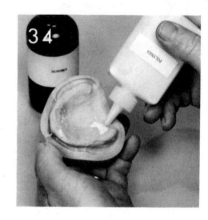

monomer (liquid), polymer (powder), a plastic squeeze bottle, and a small dropper. The polymer may be stored in the plastic squeeze bottle.

Figure 34   A small mound of polymer is sprinkled onto the prepared cast.

Figure 35   A medicine dropper is then used to carry the monomer to the polymer. The polymer is wetted with the monomer.

Figure 36   Alternate applications of polymer and monomer are made until the contour of the stabilized baseplate is achieved. Care must be exercised that the resin does not slump away from the crest of the ridge.

Figure 37   After the baseplate contour has been achieved, the cast is

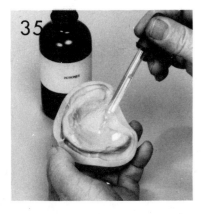

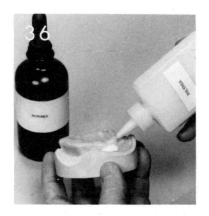

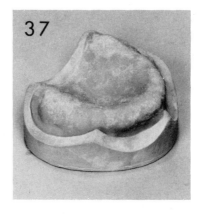

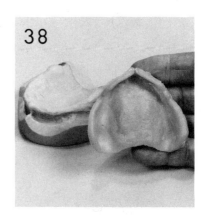

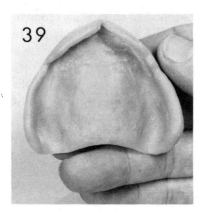

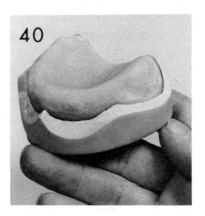

set aside to allow the resin to cure. The curing can be hastened by immersing the cast in a pan of warm water. This also prevents the monomer from evaporating and helps eliminate porosity.

Figure 38   After curing, the baseplate is removed from the cast in the same manner as the matrix baseplate was removed. The same precautions must be followed. This illustration shows the flash which is present around the borders of the baseplate.

Figures 39 and 40   The sprinkle method baseplate is completed. The same methods for trimming and completing this baseplate are followed as were done for the matrix baseplate.

Some dentists feel that the sprinkle method baseplate is more accurate than the matrix type. However, there are disadvantages to this

technique. It is more time consuming. The primary disadvantage is that it is difficult to control the thickness of this baseplate and more finishing time may be required. If too much bulk is allowed to remain on this baseplate, it will be difficult to set teeth in subsequent procedures.

SUMMARY

Three techniques have been presented for making baseplates. The technique which you use will be determined by the prescription which the dentist sends to the laboratory. All of these techniques are in general use and a competent dental technician should be proficient in all methods.

REVIEW QUESTIONS

1. List the areas on master casts which usually require relief before making stabilized baseplates.
2. What is the difference between a baseplate and a stabilized baseplate?
3. Describe the procedure for making a matrix type stabilized baseplate on a mandibular cast.
4. What are the disadvantages of shellac baseplates?
5. Why are stabilized resin baseplates not polished?

SECTION 6

Occlusion Rims

Wax blocks or rims mounted on baseplates are used to determine the contours needed to restore an edentulous patient's appearance. These occlusion rims are also used to determine the necessary amount of jaw separation and to record the proper relationship of the mandible to the maxillae.

An occlusion rim is "an occluding surface built on temporary or permanent denture bases for the purpose of making maxillomandibular (jaw) relation records and for arranging teeth." (CCDT) An occlusion rim is also known as a record rim. Some older technicians and dentists refer to occlusion rims as bite-blocks or bite-rims, but this terminology is nondescriptive and obsolete.

As commonly used, an occlusion rim is a horseshoe shaped block of wax which is attached to a baseplate. The facial surface of the occlusion rim will be contoured by the dentist to simulate natural facial contours and will later aid the dental technician in arranging the teeth. The occlusal surface of the occlusion rim will be altered by the dentist to indicate the proper occlusal plane. This determination of the occlusal plane is usually done on the maxillary occlusion rim, but may be done on the mandibular, the choice being that of the individual dentist.

Occlusion rims are also used to record maxillomandibular relationships or, as older practitioners might say, "take the bite." Some remove part of the occlusion rim opposing the one upon which the occlusal plane was established and substitute a wax which retains heat longer. These special waxes make the recording of the maxillomandibular relations more accurate. Some dentists use plaster instead of wax to record these relationships. With either method an index is carved in the occlusion rim which has been used to establish the occlusal plane. This aids in reassembling the occlusion rims when the casts are being mounted on the articulator. Instead of using the index method, some dentists will seal the maxillary and mandibular occlusion rims together with a hot spatula or will insert staples into the occlusion rims to hold them together in the proper relationship.

Properly contoured occlusion rims are essential for proper denture techniques. They restore facial contour, they establish the occlusal plane, and they aid in the recording of maxillomandibular relations. In order to fulfill these functions the occlusion rims must be located properly on the baseplate. They must not be placed over the crest of the ridge in the anterior region but should be placed so that the facial surface will simulate the natural contours. If there is any doubt as to the proper position of the occlusion rim, it should be placed farther facially. This enables the dentist to easily reduce the occlusion rim with a wax melting plate. This is much easier than to add wax to restore the proper contour. Therefore, *it is best to over-contour occlusion rims*.

The proper contour for occlusion rims is illustrated in **Figures A through F**. The composite cast shown in **Figures A** and **B** was developed from a cast made of a maxillary arch before extraction and a cast made of the same patient about three months after the teeth were extracted. This vividly illustrates the amount of facial tissue which has been lost subsequent to tooth loss. With time the amount of resorption will be greater. **Figure C** illustrates an occlusion rim made on the edentulous half of the composite cast. **Figure D** shows the facial contour on the same cast. **Figures E** and **F** show the inclination of the occlusion rim on

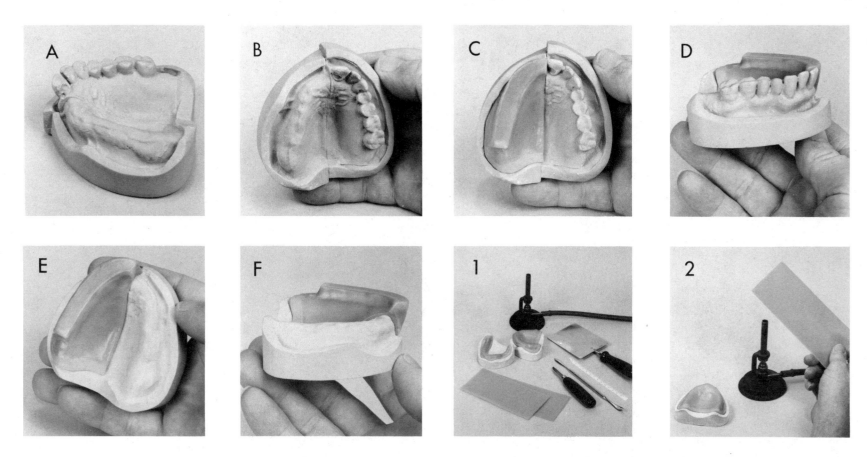

the edentulous cast. Note how the occlusion rim slants forward and reproduces the natural contour of the teeth. Reference to these illustrations will help you to make occlusion rims which will be contoured properly and which will produce better results for the dentist with less effort on his part.

The length of the occlusion rim is also important. The length should be slightly greater than the anticipated need to allow the dentist to adjust the occlusal plane to the proper level. The length of the maxillary occlusion rim should be 22 millimeters from the greatest depth of the facial (anterior) border to the surface of the occlusion rim. The mandibular occlusion rim should be 18 millimeters high, measured from the greatest depth of the mandibular facial (anterior) border.

Figure 1   The materials for making wax occlusion rims are two sheets of wax, maxillary and mandibular stabilized baseplates, a Bunsen burner, knife, hot plate, and a suitable spatula.

Figure 2   The baseplate wax is warmed over the Bunsen burner.

Figures 3 and 4   The wax is rolled after heating to make a square bar of wax. The wax is heated so that the surfaces will fuse to make a solid bar of wax without laminations. During this process the bar of wax will expand so that it will be longer than the width of the wax sheet and should be long enough to make an occlusion rim.

Figure 5   The wax bar is placed on the baseplate and shaped to the proper contour.

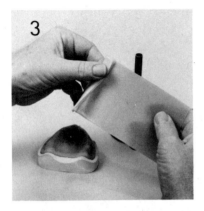
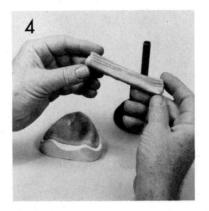
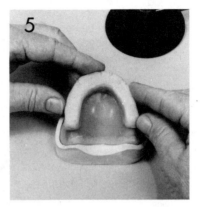
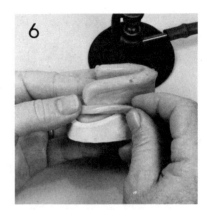

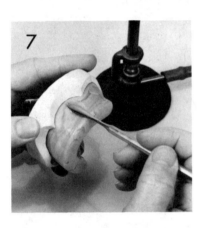
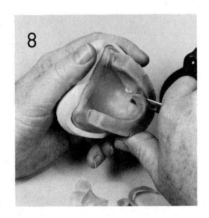
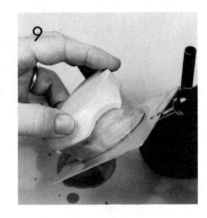
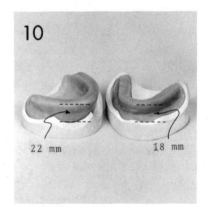

Figure 6   An additional piece of wax is softened and is adapted at the facial junction of the wax and the baseplate.

Figure 7   A hot spatula is used to make a smooth facial contour.

Figure 8   Excess wax is trimmed from the lingual surface to make the rim a uniform width.

Figure 9   The occlusal surface is reduced and smoothed using a hot plate. The same procedures are followed in making a mandibular occlusion rim.

Figure 10   The mandibular and maxillary occlusion rims have been completed. Note the height of the rims and the points from which the measurements are made.

REVIEW QUESTIONS

1. Define occlusion rim.
2. What is the purpose of occlusion rims?
3. Why is it best to over-contour occlusion rims?
4. What should be the length of the maxillary and mandibular occlusion rims at the greatest depth of the anterior facial borders?

SECTION 7

Articulators, Articulator Movement, and Mounting Casts

An articulator is an instrument which simulates movements of the mandible. The records made with occlusion rims are used to mount the master casts and to adjust the articulator. The type of articulator used is determined by the complexity of the restoration and the desires of the dentist.

An articulator is "a mechanical device that represents the temporomandibular joints and jaw members to which maxillary and mandibular casts may be attached." (CCDT) By definition it is evident that an articulator is any instrument which has a movable joint on which casts of maxillary and mandibular arches may be mounted. Articulators are available in many forms from the simplest hinge-type instruments to very complicated and expensive instruments.

For ease of description it is best to classify articulators. The simplest type of articulator is the *nonadjustable* or hinge-type articulator. This type accepts only centric relation maxillomandibular records for mounting casts and can be opened and closed only. This type articulator is illustrated in **Figure A**, Number 1. Another type of nonadjustable articulator is the articulator with a fixed condylar guide. Such articulators are illustrated in **Figure A**, Numbers 2 and 3. Number 2 is a Stephan articulator, and Number 3 is a Gysi Simplex articulator. These instruments also accept only centric relation records and the condylar guides cannot be adjusted in any manner. They do have the advantage of having the upper member movable so that a semblance of lateral excursions may be observed.

The second type is the *semi-adjustable* articulator. These articulators have adjustable horizontal condylar guides and accept both centric relation and protrusive maxillomandibular relation records. **Figure B**, Numbers 1 and 2, illustrates semi-adjustable articulators. Number 1 is a Hanau Model H articulator, and Number 2 is a Hanau Model H-2 articulator. These articulators are similar in design and use, the only difference being that the Model H-2 has longer posts and an orbital plane guide. The orbital plane guide allows the casts to be mounted in relation to the axis-orbital plane of the patient and orients the casts on the articulator in the same relationship to the bench top as the dental arches are in the patient.

The semi-adjustable type of articulator is the most widely used articulator in dental schools throughout the United States. By adjusting the condylar elements, better dentures and restorations can be constructed than are possible on simple, non-adjustable articulators. The Hanau Model H-2 articulator is the one which has been selected for the balance of illustrations in this manual. This articulator is relatively inexpensive, is sturdily constructed, and is widely used throughout the United States. An enlarged view of a Hanau Model H-2 articulator is shown in **Figure C**.

The third type of articulator is the *fully adjustable* articulator. These articulators accept not only centric relation maxillomandibular records, but also protrusive and right and left lateral maxillomandibular relation records. These articulators are more complex than the semi-adjustable articulators and are more expensive. The articulator in **Figure B**, Num-

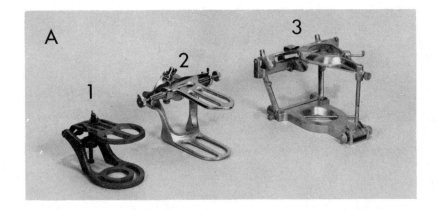

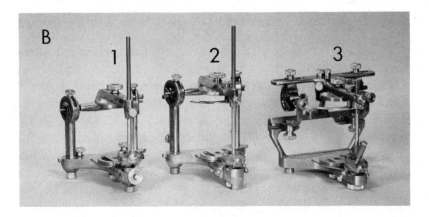

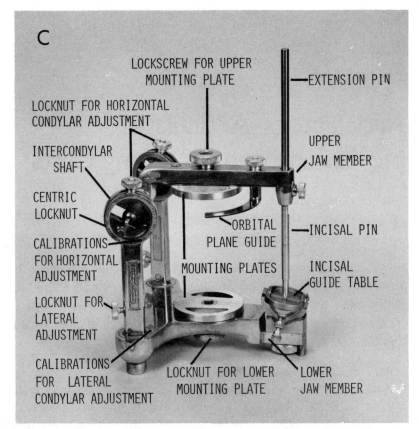

ber 3, is a Hanau Model 130-21, and was designed to be a fully adjustable articulator.

Figure D is a Gnatholator, a fully adjustable articulator, which is adjusted by means of a pantograph and is said to duplicate jaw movements. This type of articulator is used primarily in full mouth reconstruction when the occlusal surfaces of the natural teeth are to be restored.

The Stewart articulator is another fully adjustable articulator similar in appearance and use to the Gnatholator. The Whip-Mix articulator (**Figure E**) is a student model of the Stewart articulator. The Whip-Mix instrument is a semi-adjustable articulator in that it accepts centric and protrusive jaw relation records only. Lateral jaw relation records may be used but the arbitrary intercondylar distances will not permit accurate adjustment to all of these records.

Each type of articulator has its place in the dental laboratory. The nonadjustable articulators are used to make simple dental appliances, such as all plastic temporary partial dentures. Semi-adjustable articulators are used in many phases of dentistry, but are of particular importance in complete and partial denture construction. Some dentists use semi-adjustable instruments for crown and bridge procedures. The fully adjustable articulators are used by relatively few dentists and, as stated previously, are used primarily for full mouth reconstruction procedures. Additional training and experience beyond that offered in most dental schools is necessary before a dentist or technician can intelligently use one of the fully adjustable instruments.

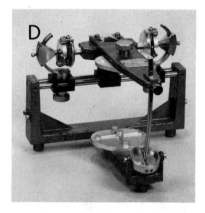
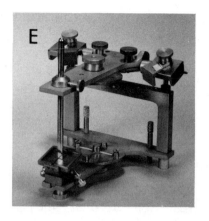

JAW AND ARTICULATOR MOVEMENTS

The complexity of an articulator determines the movements of which it is capable. A nonadjustable, fixed-hinge articulator can only open and close. A nonadjustable articulator with fixed condylar guides can make lateral movements, but these movements are dictated by the articulator.

Semi-adjustable articulators are designed to be adjusted so that the articulator movements will *simulate* the jaw movements of the patient. The word simulate is used because the condylar paths have a fixed contour which cannot be altered and the distance between the condyles cannot be varied. Even though semi-adjustable articulators cannot duplicate jaw movements, most prosthodontists consider these instruments satisfactory for the construction of removable dental appliances.

The movements a human mandible can make are infinite. Within certain boundaries, the mandible is capable of vertical, horizontal, and protrusive movements, as well as combinations of these movements. In most articulators, the concern is to record the border movements—those points which limit the movement of the mandible. When your head is held still, the mandible is limited in movement by the temporomandibular joint, the muscles, and the ligaments attached to the mandible. These limitations determine the border movements.

Theoretically, when border movements are recorded accurately, it is assumed that the articulator accepting these records will simulate the random movements of the mandible. Dental appliances and restorations constructed in harmony with the border movements should function effectively and comfortably for the patient.

A pantograph is an instrument which, when attached to the jaws, records all border movements. Advocates of fully adjustable gnathostatic articulators (examples are the Gnatholator and the Stewart articulator) believe that jaw movements can be duplicated on their articulators by using a pantograph.

All casts are mounted on articulators in centric relation (see definition below). Semi-adjustable and fully adjustable articulators are adjusted by using eccentric jaw (maxillomandibular) relationship records. Articulators with a fixed intercondylar distance, such as a Hanau H-2, accept only one eccentric jaw relationship record, a protrusive record. This is made by having the patient hold his jaw in a protruded relationship while a record is being made. This record is then used to adjust the horizontal condylar inclination (Section 8, **Figure 26**).

Articulators with a variable intercondylar distance will accept three eccentric jaw relationship records, a protrusive record and right and left lateral jaw relationship records. More accurate restorations are possible on these fully adjustable instruments.

DEFINITION OF TERMS

A technician must be familiar with several terms in order to use an articulator intelligently. An understanding of these terms will make communication easier between technician and dentist.

Centric Relation is "(1) the most posterior relation of the mandible to the maxillae at the established vertical dimension; (2) the relation of the mandible to the maxillae when the condyles are in their most posteriosuperior unstrained position in the glenoid fossae, from which unstrained lateral movements can be made at the occluding vertical relation normal for the individual. Centric relation is a relation that can exist at any degree of jaw separation." (CCDT) It is a designation of a horizontal relation.

The importance of centric relation in complete denture construction is that it is the one position which a patient is able to repeat. When a person loses all of his teeth, he loses most of the tactile sense which permits him to make repeated identical eccentric jaw closures. Thus, many edentulous individuals are unable to repeat any jaw position except centric relation. It is the dentist's responsibility to record centric relation and the technician's responsibility to maintain this relationship through careful laboratory procedures. If centric relation is recorded improperly, the completed dentures will not occlude or function correctly in the mouth.

Centric Occlusion is "the relation of opposing occlusal surfaces that provides the maximum planned contact and/or intercuspation. It should exist when the mandible is in centric relation to the maxillae." (CCDT) Centric occlusion is a "tooth to tooth" relationship while centric relation is a "bone to bone" relationship. In complete denture construction it is essential that *centric occlusion is in harmony with centric relation* even though this condition does not always occur in the natural dentition. Edentulous casts are mounted in centric relation and the artificial teeth are arranged in centric occlusion.

In correct dental terminology, centric is an adjective and should never be used alone. To speak of "recording centric" is incorrect since it is impossible to know if centric occlusion or centric relation has been recorded.

Vertical Dimension is "a vertical measurement of the face between any two arbitrarily selected points that are conveniently located one above and one below the mouth, usually in the midline." (CCDT)

There are two types of vertical dimension which are involved in restorative dentistry and in complete and partial denture prosthodontics. *Rest vertical dimension* is "the vertical dimension of the face with the jaws in rest relation." (CCDT) This is the position of the jaws when all the muscles are relaxed. *Occlusal vertical dimension* is "the vertical dimension of the face when the teeth or occlusion rims are in contact in centric occlusion." (CCDT) Occlusal vertical dimension is simply the vertical relation of the mandible to the maxillae when the teeth are in contact.

The *interocclusal distance* or *free-way space* is "the distance between the occluding surfaces of the maxillary and mandibular teeth when the mandible is in its physiologic rest position." (CCDT) Free-way space is the difference between rest vertical dimension and occlusal vertical dimension. Determining proper interocclusal distance is one of the most important clinical steps in complete denture construction. If the teeth and dentures are made too long, there will be insufficient interocclusal distance and the teeth will be constantly in contact. This produces pressure on the tissues underlying the denture bases with resultant soreness and ultimate resorption. The teeth will appear too long and may click when the patient speaks. On the other hand, too

great an interocclusal distance will lead to a denture deficient in appearance and efficiency.

In reviewing these terms, we find that centric relation is a horizontal relationship while vertical dimension is a vertical relationship. Both of these relationships are recorded simultaneously during denture construction, but are distinct entities. Proper recording of centric relation at the correct vertical dimension is essential to successful denture construction.

A *face-bow* is "a caliper-like device that is used to record the relationship of the maxillae to the temporomandibular joints (or opening axis of the mandible) and to orient the casts in this same relationship to the opening axis of the articulator." (CCDT) The use of the face-bow in complete denture construction assures proper placement of the casts on the articulator and makes the casts better simulate jaw movements when the articulator is moved into lateral excursions.

The *axis-orbital or Frankfort plane* is a theoretical plane which passes through the centers of rotation of the mandible (condyles) and the inferior border of the bony orbit (the bone surrounding the eye). This plane is relatively parallel to the floor when a patient stands erect. The orbital pointer on a face-bow permits the face-bow to be related to the axis-orbital plane (**Figure S**).

The orbital plane guide on a Hanau H-2 articulator is a semicircular element attached to the upper member of the articulator. This guide and the condylar elements form the equivalent of an axis-orbital plane on the articulator, a plane parallel to the bench top. Thus when casts are mounted with a face-bow and orbital pointer, the casts (and occlusal plane) will be in the same relation to the bench top as the patient's ridges (and occlusal plane) are to the floor. The advantage of using an orbital pointer is that teeth set on casts mounted with an orbital pointer have the same inclination on the articulator as they will have in the patient. The necks of teeth set on casts mounted with the occlusal plane parallel to the floor will appear protruded or the incisal edges will appear retruded when placed in the patient.

MANIPULATION OF THE HANAU H-2 ARTICULATOR

The adjustment of the condylar elements of an articulator is useless unless the articulator is manipulated correctly during construction of

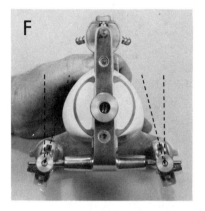

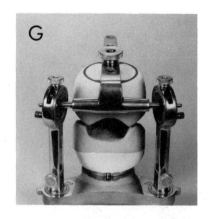

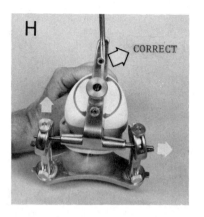

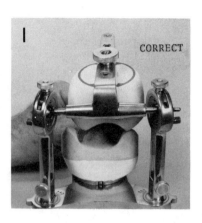

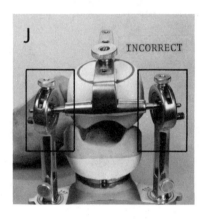

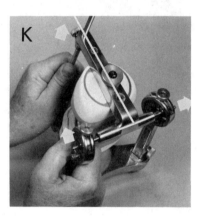

dental appliances and restorations. For example, in complete denture construction the teeth must be arranged to *follow* the movements of the articulator. Often the individual arranging the teeth allows the teeth to guide the articulator, which is not correct.

The Hanau H-2 articulator has two adjustments in the condylar region, the horizontal condylar inclination and the lateral condylar inclination. The inclination of the horizontal condylar guide simulates the contour of the mandibular fossa of the temporal bone (**Figures 7 and 9**, Section 1). The lateral condylar guide (**Figures F and G**) is the mechanical equivalent of the lateral shift of the mandible (Bennett movement).

According to the manufacturer, the lateral condylar inclination is determined by the formula $L = H/8 + 12$, where L is the lateral condylar inclination and H is the horizontal condylar inclination. Thus,

if the horizontal condylar inclination is 40 degrees, the lateral condylar inclination is 40/8 + 12, or 17 degrees. In practice, the lateral condylar inclination is often left on 15–18 degrees.

When an articulator is moved in a lateral excursion, one condyle slides posteriorly. Concurrently, the upper member must slide laterally to accomplish the Bennett movement. On a Hanau H-2 articulator, the working condyle is the one which remains against the anterior stop while the balancing condyle slides posteriorly. This is because this articulator is built with the condyles on the upper member which is the reverse of the natural condition.

Figure H illustrates the proper movement of the Hanau H-2 articulator. The working condyle is held against the anterior stop while the balancing condyle slides posteriorly and the upper member shifts toward the balancing side. The articulator will make these movements automatically when the incisal pin is pushed in the direction indicated by the large arrow.

Figure I is a posterior view showing an H-2 articulator in a correct lateral excursion. Note that the upper member has shifted to the balancing side and the condylar shaft is against the balancing condyle. **Figure J** is a similar view showing an incorrect articulator movement. The upper member has not shifted to the balancing side but has simply rotated. No Bennett movement has been incorporated in this excursion. Fixed or removable dental restorations made to interdigitate in such a rotary movement will not function harmoniously in the mouth.

Figure K shows the proper method to hold and move an articulator into lateral excursions. The importance of proper articulator movement cannot be overemphasized.

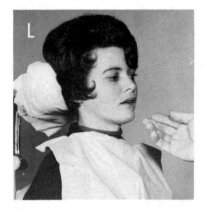
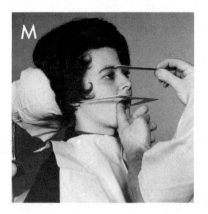
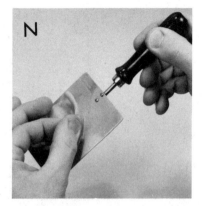
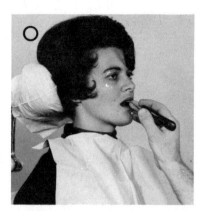

CLINICAL PROCEDURES FOR RECORDING MAXILLOMANDIBULAR RELATIONS

Figure L   The occlusion rims and baseplates (hereafter referred to simply as occlusion rims) are sent to the dentist. When the patient appears for the next appointment the occlusion rims are checked to see that they fit properly. The occlusion rims are then adjusted until proper lip contours are achieved.

Figure M   The occlusal plane is checked to see that it is in proper relation to cranial and facial landmarks.

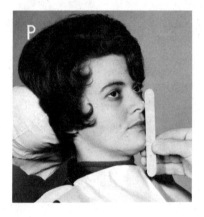
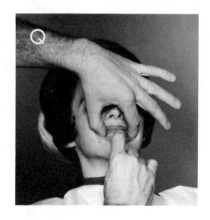

Figure N   Excess wax on the occlusion rim is removed by the dentist with a wax melting plate. It is used to remove wax from the occlusal and facial surfaces of the rim.

Figure O   The center line, high lip line and cuspid lines are placed on the maxillary occlusion rim after it is contoured. These lines will aid in selecting and arranging the teeth.

Figure P   The rest vertical dimension is then determined. This determination is made with the patient's head unsupported so that all of the muscles in the upper part of the body are in equilibrium. This illustration shows the dentist checking vertical dimension after the lower occlusion rim has been adjusted.

Figures Q and R   The dentist then records centric relation at the oc-

clusal vertical dimension. In these illustrations the dentist has removed a portion of the wax in the posterior part of the mandibular occlusion rim and has replaced this area with soft wax or plaster. The patient is then guided into proper closure. These figures illustrate two different methods for this procedure.

Figure S   The face-bow is attached to the occlusion rims and adjusted to the patient. The orbital pointer should touch the lower border of the bony orbit, the bone directly under the eye. The face-bow assembly and maxillary occlusion rim are then removed from the mouth.

Figure T   A shade is best selected before the natural teeth are removed. When this information is not available, a shade is selected to harmonize with the patient's skin tones.

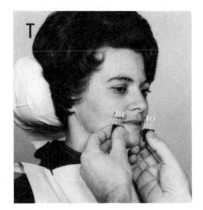

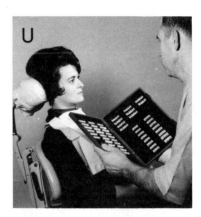

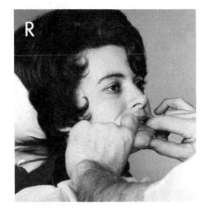

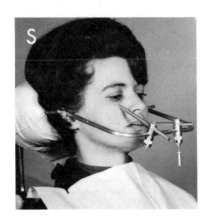

Figure U   An anterior mold is selected by the dentist which he feels will best suit the patient.

LABORATORY PROCEDURES
FOR MOUNTING CASTS ON AN ARTICULATOR

When the dentist has completed recording the maxillomandibular records and making the face-bow transfer, the occlusion rims, casts, face-bow and a prescription containing instructions, tooth shade and mold are sent to the laboratory.

Some precautions must be observed when mounting casts. The articulator *must* be checked to be sure it is adjusted correctly. The condylar elements *must* be locked in centric position. There must be no lateral "play" in the articulator. The mounting rings *must* be firmly attached. The casts *must* be seated completely in their respective occlusion rims. Failure to observe these precautions will result in having the casts mounted in an improper relationship.

Figure 1   The equipment required for mounting casts on a Hanau H-2 articulator is shown. Note the cast support directly behind the maxillary cast. This is attached to the articulator in place of the lower mounting ring to support the maxillary occlusion rim during mounting procedures.

Figure 2   The face-bow has been mounted and centered on the articulator. The condylar rods on the face-bow are adjusted so that they fit snugly on the condylar rod of the articulator but the face-bow is not distorted. Note that the mounting support has been placed on the articulator and that the jack screw on the assembly holding the bite fork has been lowered until the orbital indicator is on the same level as the orbital plane guide, the semicircular device attached to the upper member of the articulator.

Figure 3   The maxillary cast has been seated in the baseplate. It must be seated completely. Index grooves have been placed in the base of the cast. (See Section 4, **Figure 48**.) The articulator has been opened ready for application of plaster to the base of the maxillary cast.

Figure 4   A medium thin mix of impression plaster is prepared. The plaster is placed on the base of the cast and piled up until it extends above the level of the mounting plate.

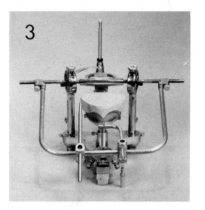
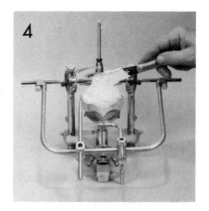
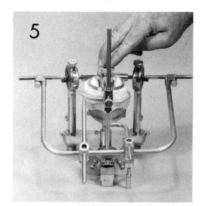
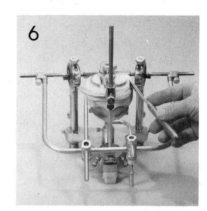

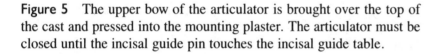

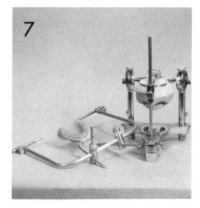
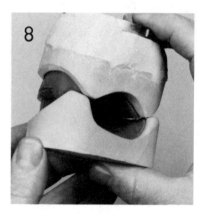

Figure 5   The upper bow of the articulator is brought over the top of the cast and pressed into the mounting plaster. The articulator must be closed until the incisal guide pin touches the incisal guide table.

Figure 6   The plaster is smoothed and the excess removed. A wet finger can be used to smooth the plaster after the excess is removed.

Figure 7   After the plaster has set, the face-bow is removed from the articulator. The bite fork is heated with a Hanau torch and removed from the occlusion rim. (The bite fork is the portion of the face-bow which attaches to the maxillary occlusion rim.) Care should be exercised so that the lines which have been placed by the dentist on the occlusion rim are not obliterated.

Figure 8   The maxillary cast and mounting ring are removed from the articulator. The maxillary and mandibular occlusion rims are placed on their respective casts and the casts are placed together to check clearance in the posterior region of the casts. As can be seen in this illustration there is interference in this region. This interference prevents the proper seating of the casts into their respective occlusion rims.

Figure 9   The interference is eliminated by carefully removing some of the nonanatomical portion of the cast. The anatomical portion or denture-bearing area of the cast is not altered.

Figure 10   The casts are again reassembled with the occlusion rims to assure that proper clearance is present in the posterior part of the casts.

Enough clearance must be provided so that a definite space is present when the casts are seated in their baseplates.

Figure 11   The maxillary and mandibular occlusion rims and casts are sealed together with wax. Any wax which will attach the mandibular and maxillary occlusion rims to each other and to the casts is satisfactory.

Figure 12   The maxillary cast and mounting are replaced on the articulator and the articulator inverted on a plastering stand. Any device which will support the articulator in this fashion is acceptable if a plastering stand is not available.

Figure 13   A mix of plaster is placed on the base of the mandibular cast

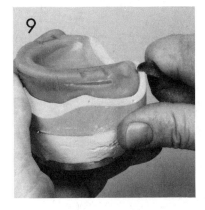
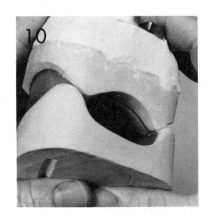
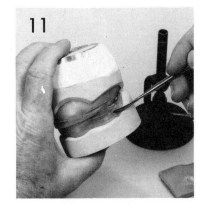
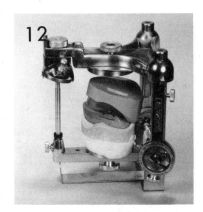

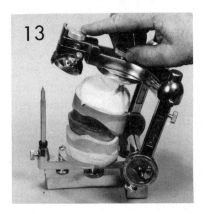
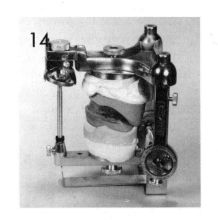
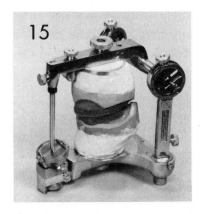
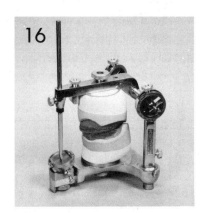

and the articulator closed on this plaster. Before closing the articulator, *some plaster must be pushed down into the spaces in the mounting ring adjacent to the bottom of the articulator*. Note that the mandibular cast has been wet to provide better adhesion of the mounting plaster to the cast.

Figure 14   The articulator is closed onto the mounting plaster so that the incisal pin touches the incisal guide table. The excess plaster is removed with a plaster spatula and the plaster smoothed with a wet finger.

Figure 15   The mounting of the mandibular cast is completed.

Figure 16   The mounting plaster is smoothed to produce a neat appear-

ance. The incisal guide pin extension has been replaced and the articulator is now ready for the arrangement of artificial teeth and/or the mounting of a central bearing device.

REVIEW QUESTIONS

1. Describe the three types of articulators.
2. Define centric relation.
3. Define centric occlusion.
4. Outline the method of adjusting the horizontal and lateral condylar guides on a Hanau H-2 articulator.
5. What four precautions must be observed when mounting casts?

SECTION 8

Central Bearing Devices

A central bearing device aids in recording maxillomandibular relationships by distributing forces evenly throughout the denture bases. The correct anteroposterior position of the mandible can be located graphically by a central bearing device.

In the previous section a method of recording maxillomandibular or jaw relationships was described which depended upon the tactile sense of the dentist. The importance of recording centric relation was emphasized. Central bearing devices provide a graphic means for verifying centric relation records. Their use is an optional step.

Theoretically, the application of a point of pressure to the center of a rigid flat surface distributes the pressure uniformly. This is the basis of the use of central bearing point devices and also explains why it is important to locate the point properly. Improper location of the point and/or inability of patients to follow instructions may induce errors.

The materials used for making jaw relation records must be uniformly soft when the record is made and then become hard at mouth temperature. These materials are waxes, impression compound, impression materials or plaster. All meet the foregoing requirements. Plaster is the material of choice for making jaw relationship records with central bearing devices.

A central bearing device theoretically distributes forces evenly throughout the supporting areas of the maxillary and mandibular bases when the device is properly located. Central bearing devices are not used when abnormal conditions exist which prevent the placement of the central bearing point in the center of the support area of the maxillary and mandibular denture bases. Another drawback of central bearing devices is that the patient may exert unequal or excessive force on the central bearing device and induce errors.

There are two basic types of central bearing devices, intra-oral devices and extra-oral devices. Each type produces an arrow-point tracing which is a graphic representation of centric relation. An intra-oral central bearing device produces an arrow-point tracing inside the mouth while the extra-oral devices produce arrow-point tracings on a plate which extends outside the mouth. Intra-oral tracers are generally simpler in design and simpler to use, while the extra-oral devices magnify the arrow-point tracing and allow the dentist to verify that the patient is maintaining the proper jaw relation while the recording substance (usually plaster) is setting. With intra-oral devices the dentist cannot check the accuracy of his record until after the material has set and the baseplates and the central bearing device have been removed from the mouth.

The use of a central bearing device may require an additional visit by the patient to the dentist. One method of avoiding an extra visit is to construct an extra set of base plates upon which the central bearing device is mounted. When this is done new records are made using the central bearing device at the same appointment that the tentative set-up of the teeth is checked.

TECHNIQUE FOR USING EXTRA-ORAL TRACER

There are several types of extra-oral central bearing devices, most of them similar in design and function. The one shown is the Hight Tracer. It is simple to use and is designed for use with Hanau articulators.

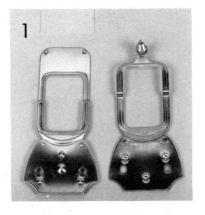
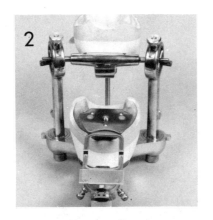
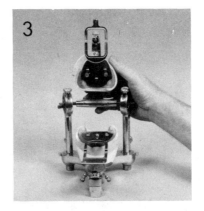
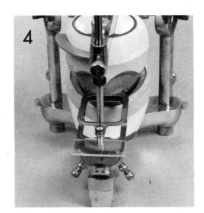
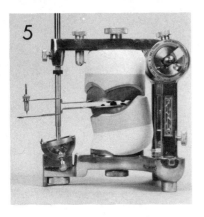
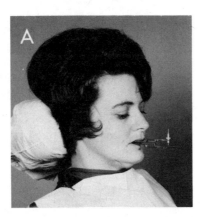
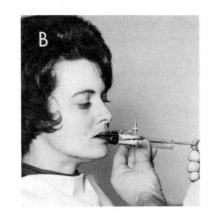
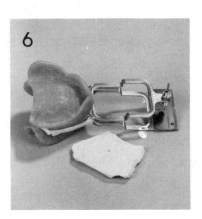

Figure 1   The Hight tracer consists of (a) a mandibular plate and (b) a maxillary plate to which extension arms are attached. The mandibular extension arm has a tracing plate containing two studs over which a plexiglass plate fits. The maxillary extension arm contains a spring-loaded stylus which is encased in a threaded collar. This allows the stylus to be raised and lowered at the discretion of the dentist.

Figure 2   The mandibular portion of the device is mounted so that it is as parallel as possible to the mandibular ridge and the central bearing point is centrally located. The proper location for the central bearing point is determined by drawing a line from each canine area to the opposite second molar area. The intersection of these lines usually indicates the proper location for the central bearing point.

Figures 3 and 4   The maxillary portion of the tracer is mounted parallel to the mandibular portion. Displacing forces will be induced when the device is placed in the patient's mouth if the two portions are not parallel.

Figure 5   The central bearing point is raised until it just contacts the maxillary plate. The central bearing point should touch at the same time the incisal guide pin of the articulator touches the incisal guide table. Any variation will induce a change in the vertical dimension. The dentist may wish to raise or lower the central bearing point to alter the vertical dimension, but this will cause a change in the parallelism of the plate and should be done only with the greatest caution. This illustration shows the threaded collar in which the stylus is located on the maxillary extension arm and also shows the lock nut which maintains the collar in position. A similar lock nut is present on the inferior surface of the mandibular plate, maintaining the central bearing point at

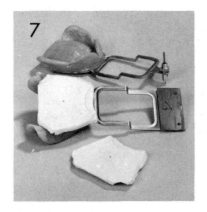
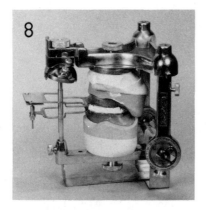
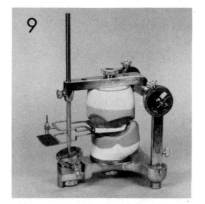
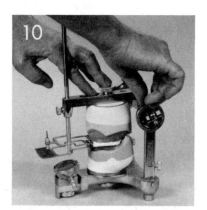

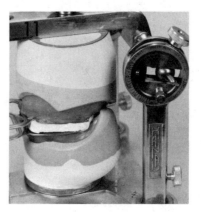
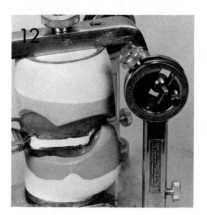

the proper height. At this stage the central bearing devices are returned to the dentist for making the maxillomandibular or jaw relation records.

Figure A The central bearing devices are inserted and the patient is trained in their use. The arrow-point tracing is scribed by lowering the tracing stylus and instrucing the patient to make the proper jaw movements.

Figure B The dentist makes jaw relation records by injecting plaster between the plates of the tracing device. In the Hanau technique a protrusive record is usually made first and is removed from the device. Subsequently a centric relation record is made. The extra-oral device allows the dentist to verify that the patient maintains the proper position while the plaster is setting.

Figure 6 The central bearing device with the new centric relation and protrusive records is returned to the laboratory.

Figure 7 The maxillary portion of the tracing device has been removed to show the arrow-point tracing. Not all arrow-point tracings will be as symmetrical as the one illustrated. Centric relation is the point of the arrow. This illustrates that centric relation is a point and not some diffuse area.

Figure 8 The mandibular cast is removed from the mounting plaster and is remounted on the articulator utilizing the centric relation record made with the central bearing device (the casts must not touch—see

Figure 23). Dentists using central bearing devices usually assume that the records made with these devices are correct and remount the mandibular cast to the new record.

Figure 9 The remounting of the mandibular cast is complete.

Figure 10 The horizontal condylar guides are adjusted. First the incisal pin is raised. Then the protrusive lock nut is loosened. The protrusive record is then placed between the plates of the central bearing device. The horizontal condylar guides are rotated until the maxillary and mandibular plates seat into the protrusive record. Note the position of the hands. The left hand holds the upper member of the articulator firmly in place while the right hand rotates the horizontal condylar guide.

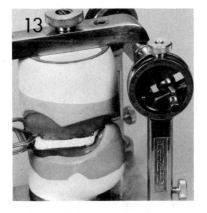

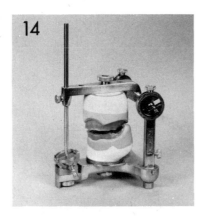

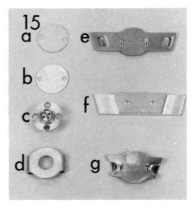

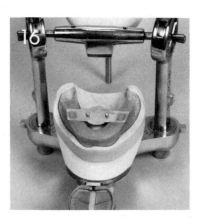

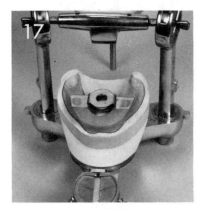

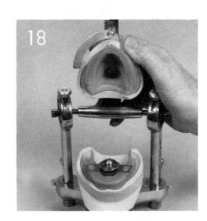

Figure 11　Separation between the plates of the central bearing device will occur in the anterior region when too great a negative inclination is placed on the horizontal condylar guide.

Figure 12　Separation in the posterior region occurs when too great a positive inclination of the horizontal condylar guide occurs.

Figure 13　This illustrates that the proper position of the horizontal condylar guide occurs when both plates of the central bearing device seat firmly in the protrusive record. Wiggling of the horizontal condylar guide as shown in **Figure 10** will produce this result. Both condylar guidances are adjusted in order to have the plates of the central bearing device contact throughout the protrusive record.

Figure 14　The central bearing device has been removed and the occlusion rims are ready to be built back to the proper occlusal plane and the teeth set. If extra baseplates have been made to make the arrow-point tracing, they are discarded and the baseplates containing the set-up are returned to the articulator for final adjustment of the teeth.

INTRA-ORAL CENTRAL BEARING DEVICES

Figure 15　The intra-oral central bearing device shown in **Figure 15** is a Coble Balancer. This simple central bearing device is used either with occlusion rims or complete dentures to facilitate remounting procedures (Sections 12 and 14). The Coble Balancer consists of seven parts: (a) a plastic disc which may be used to help maintain the central bearing point in place, (b) an aluminum marking plate, (c) a central bearing pin, (d) a mounting jig, (e) a bridge to be used with occlusion rims, (f) and (g) a mounting jig and bridge which are used to mount the device on completed dentures.

The plastic disc is not utilized by all people who use the Coble Balancer and was not utilized in this exercise. When used, it is mounted over the aluminum tracing plate and a hole is drilled through the plastic disc directly over the apex of the arrow-point tracing. This is done to help the patient maintain the proper position.

Figure 16　The bridge is mounted on the mandibular occlusion rim parallel to the occlusal plane and centered in the same manner as the Hight Tracer.

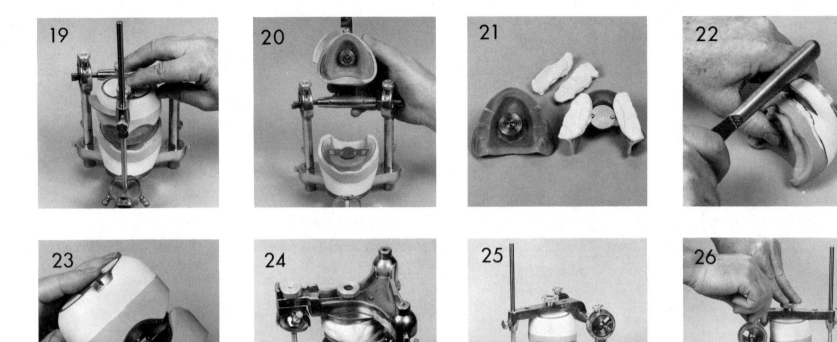

Figure 17   The mounting jig is then placed over the bridge.

Figure 18   The central bearing pin is placed into the mounting jig. The central bearing pin should be adjusted so that it does not touch the bridge. A ball of softened wax is placed in the palate of the maxillary occlusion rim.

Figure 19   The upper member of the articulator is closed so that the softened wax engages the top of the central bearing pin.

Figure 20   The central bearing pin is attached to the maxillary rim and the aluminum tracing plate is placed on the bridge. The central bearing pin is adjusted so that it touches the aluminum tracing plate at the same time that the incisal guide pin strikes the incisal guide table. At this

stage the occlusion rims with the mounted tracing device are returned to the dentist.

Note: Interocclusal records are made in the same manner as with the Hight Tracer. The only difference is that it is impossible for the dentist to verify that the patient is maintaining centric relation while the plaster is injected. This verification must occur after the lower cast has been remounted or may be done in the dental office by using a small piece of articulating paper between the central bearing pin and the tracing plate.

Figure 21   The occlusion rims and the central bearing device are returned to the laboratory after the dentist has made his protrusive and centric relation records. The protrusive records are next to the occlusion rims. Note the fine arrow-point tracing which was made by the patient. Ordinarily arrow-point tracings made with intra-oral tracing devices or intra-oral central bearing devices are not this distinct but do have a sharp apex which indicates centric relation.

Figure 22   The mandibular cast is removed from the mounting plaster. The cast and mount must be soaked in water before separation.

Figure 23   The casts are checked to ascertain that adequate clearance occurs in the posterior regions of the casts.

Figure 24   The mandibular cast is remounted utilizing the new centric relation record.

Figure 25   The mounting has been smoothed and is now complete.

Figure 26   The condyles are set with the protrusive record in the same manner as with the Hight Tracer. *Whenever adjusting the horizontal condylar guidances the incisal pin must not touch the incisal guide table but must be raised.* (See **Figure 10**.)

REVIEW QUESTIONS

1. What is the primary difference between intra-oral and extra-oral central bearing devices?
2. What is the purpose of a central bearing device?
3. In mounting the mandibular portion of an extra-oral central bearing device, how is the proper location of the central bearing point located?
4. Which cast is remounted when the occlusion rims and the central bearing device are returned to the laboratory after the dentist made the appropriate recordings?

SECTION 9

Artificial Tooth Arrangement

Appearance and function cannot be restored with artificial teeth unless they are placed in the position of the natural teeth. Proper arrangement of artificial teeth makes a removable dental appliance attractive and functional.

The guides used for arranging artificial teeth are the occlusion rims which were discussed in Section 7. The occlusion rims, alone or in conjunction with central bearing devices, are used to make five determinations: (1) proper lip contours, (2) proper placement of the occlusal plane, (3) correct vertical dimension of occlusion, (4) recording of centric relation at the vertical dimension of occlusion, and (5) placement of lines on the occlusion rim to aid in the selection and arrangement of teeth. In complete denture construction, occlusion rims are used with a face-bow to transfer the relationship of the maxillae to the condyles to the articulator.

Most dentists do not stock their own artificial teeth, but have mold and shade guides available in their offices which enable them to select teeth. (Section 7, **Figures T–U**) Teeth are usually stocked in the dental laboratory, or are purchased by the laboratory from the local dental supply dealer. A description of the methods for selecting teeth is included here to give the dental technician a better idea of the procedures used in the dental office for selecting teeth.

The selection of teeth is done in two parts: anterior tooth selection and posterior tooth selection. In *anterior tooth selection* there are three steps to be followed: (1) determination of the proper shade, (2) determination of the proper size of the tooth, and (3) determination of the

proper shape of the tooth. The best way to select teeth is to match the artificial teeth to the natural teeth. The use of pre-extraction casts and shade determinations is the best way to select teeth. When these are not available, other aids must be used, including snapshots, portrait photographs, X-rays of the teeth before extraction and any other material which may be of assistance. When these are not available, a systematic procedure can be followed to select teeth which will harmonize with the patient's facial characteristics.

The shade is selected to harmonize with the patient's skin tones. Selection of shade is influenced by age, sex, and ethnic background. The determination of shade *without* pre-extraction records is entirely subjective.

The size of the tooth is determined by using several guides. It is generally agreed that a maxillary central incisor is one-sixteenth the bizygomatic width; that is, the distance between the cheek bones measured just in front of the ears. Some simple devices are available from tooth manufacturers for making this determination, or a caliper may be used to measure this distance, which is then divided by sixteen. A face-bow may be used as a caliper to make this determination. An additional guide to the size of the maxillary anterior teeth is the size of the patient's mouth and other facial features. The dentist, using these guides, marks "canine lines" on the occlusion rim. The measurement of the distance between these lines helps to select teeth which will esthetically fill this space. The length of teeth can also be determined by use of the sixteen-to-one ratio, or may be guided by the use of the high lip line which is marked on the occlusion rim when the patient smiles. With the measurements thus obtained (the size of the central incisor and the canine to canine width), the dentist is able to narrow the choice of teeth to the molds which fulfill the size requirements.

The final determining characteristic is the shape of the tooth, which is selected to harmonize with the patient's face. If the patient has a long tapering face, a long tapering tooth is usually indicated. An ovoid face usually requires an ovoid tooth, while a square-shaped face will require a tooth of a similar shape. The correlation of tooth form with face forms is not always accurate, but it does serve as a guide when pre-extraction records are not available.

The selection of posterior teeth is more empirical than selection of anterior teeth. The selection of posterior teeth is determined primarily by the preference of the dentist. Certain fundamentals should be followed when selecting posterior teeth, regardless of the occlusal pattern on these teeth. The lower teeth should not extend posterior to the mesial border of the retromolar pad. Posterior teeth should have a small faciolingual diameter to keep forces on the basal or tissue surface of the denture to a minimum. Many prosthodontists believe narrow teeth are more efficient. When in doubt about two molds of posterior teeth, choose the smaller one.

There are three basic occlusal patterns available in posterior teeth: anatomical teeth, nonanatomical teeth, and semi-anatomical teeth. The anatomical teeth are those which have been carved to simulate natural teeth. Dentists using anatomical teeth usually believe in balanced occlusion; that is, teeth on both sides of the arch should be in contact when the jaw makes excursive movements. These dentists also feel that natural occlusal forms are most efficient. Examples of artificial anatomical teeth are Thirty-Three Degree Teeth, and Pilkington-Turner Teeth.

Nonanatomical teeth have flat occlusal surfaces. There are no cusps on these teeth, although there are usually some grooves and/or mechanical pattern present to improve appearance and efficiency. Dentists using this type of tooth generally do not believe in balanced occlusion, but feel that uniform contact of the teeth in centric relation is all that is required in dentures. These dentists also feel that nonanatomical teeth transmit less destructive force to the tissue. Examples of nonanatomical artificial teeth are Rational Teeth and Bio-Mechanical Teeth.

Semi-anatomical teeth are a hybrid between anatomical and nonanatomical teeth. The designers of these teeth felt that the good attributes of both types could be found in a tooth with shallow cusps and a semi-mechanical occlusal surface. Semi-anatomical teeth have low cusps and contain various geometric occlusal carvings purported to improve the efficiency of these teeth. Some are arranged as anatomical teeth, others are arranged like nonanatomical teeth, while some can be arranged either way. Examples of semi-anatomical teeth are Twenty Degree Teeth, Functional Posteriors, NIC Posteriors, and French's Posteriors.

Some guides have been set forth in the dental literature concerning the selection of posterior teeth. The age of the patient, the condition of the mouth, and other factors have been advanced as ways to help determine the choice of posterior tooth form. Basically, the choice of posterior teeth is a personal matter on the part of the dentist.

The prescription sent to the laboratory will indicate the anterior mold, the posterior tooth form and whether resin or porcelain teeth are to be used. The choice of resin or porcelain teeth is primarily a matter of personal preference on the part of the dentist, influenced by conditions present in the individual patient. Various combinations of resin and porcelain teeth may be used, such as resin anterior teeth and porcelain posterior teeth. One such combination should *never* be used: porcelain anterior teeth should never be used in conjunction with resin posterior teeth. Resin posterior teeth will wear more rapidly than the porcelain anterior teeth, resulting in anterior occlusal discrepancies, which in turn cause destruction of the underlying tissue.

TERMINOLOGY

Cusp height is defined as "the shortest distance between the deepest part of the central fossa of a posterior tooth and a line connecting the points of the cusps of the tooth." (CCDT) The cusp height on artificial posterior teeth and the angulation of the cusps are determined by the settings of the articulator upon which the teeth were carved. Thus a Thirty-Three Degree Tooth does not necessarily have thirty-three degree cuspal angulations, but refers to the condylar inclinations and the incisal guidance which was present on the articulator when these teeth were carved.

Condylar guidance is "the mechanical device on an articulator; intended to produce guidance in articulator movement similar to that produced by the paths of the condyles in the temporomandibular joints." (CCDT)

The *incisal guidance angle* (**Figure 29**) is "the angle formed with the occlusal plane by drawing a line in the sagittal plane between the incisal edges of the maxillary and mandibular central incisors when the teeth are in centric occlusion." (CCDT) The *incisal guide* is "the part of an articulator that maintains the incisal guide angle." (CCDT) In a natural dentition the incisal guidance is determined by the position of the maxillary and mandibular central incisors. The only way the incisal guidance angle may be altered in a natural dentition is by grinding the incisal edges of these teeth. In an artificial dentition the incisal guidance angle is determined by the position in which the mandibular and maxillary incisors are set. The incisal guide is a mechanical equivalent of the incisal guidance angle.

The *occlusal plane* is "an imaginary surface that is related anatomically to the cranium and that theoretically touches the incisal edges of the incisors and the tips of the occluding surfaces of the posterior teeth. It is not a plane in the true sense of the word, but represents the mean of the curvature of the surface." (CCDT) In an artificial dentition the occlusal plane may be flat, but ordinarily it is curved as in the natural dentition.

The *compensating curve* is "the curvature of alignment of the occlusal surfaces of the teeth that is developed to compensate for the paths of the condyles as the mandible moves from centric to eccentric positions. A means for maintaining posterior tooth contacts on the molar teeth and providing balancing contacts on dentures when the mandible is protruded. Corresponds to the curve of Spee in natural teeth." (CCDT) The compensating curve may be altered in an artificial dentition to help achieve balanced occlusion.

FACTORS OF OCCLUSION

There are five factors of occlusion which influence the arrangement of teeth, particularly anatomical teeth arranged to achieve bilateral balance. These factors are: (1) condylar guidance, (2) cusp height, (3) incisal guidance, (4) the compensating curve, and (5) the orientation of the occlusal plane between the edentulous casts.

Four of the five factors of occlusion are under the control of the person arranging artificial teeth. Condylar guidance is recorded from the patient and is the only factor of occlusion which cannot be altered

while setting teeth. An arbitrary alteration of the condylar guidance will result in dentures which do not function in the mouth the same way as they occlude on the articulator.

All the factors of occlusion are interrelated. Variation of any one produces effects in all of the others. For example, increasing the cusp height of the posterior teeth must be compensated for by a decrease in the compensating curve, a reorientation of the occlusal plane or an increase in the incisal guidance. An increase in the condylar guidance as recorded from the patient will require an increased cusp height, a reduction in the incisal guidance, an increase in the compensating curve, a reorientation of the occlusal plane or a combination of all these factors.

GUIDES FOR ARRANGING ARTIFICIAL TEETH

The guide for arranging the anterior teeth is the facial surfaces of the maxillary and mandibular occlusion rims. This surface is contoured by the dentist to simulate the position of the natural teeth. The occlusion rim not only indicates the faciolingual position and inclination of the anterior teeth, but also indicates the proper position of the incisal edges.

Posterior teeth are generally placed to enhance the stability of the mandibular denture. This is done by arranging the teeth so that the mandibular posterior teeth are over, or slightly lingual to, the crest of the mandibular residual ridge. This procedure usually results in having the posterior teeth near the position of the natural teeth. Wherever possible, it is important to maintain natural tooth positions and arch form to achieve good speech and esthetics.

SEQUENCE OF ARRANGING TEETH

The sequence in which artificial teeth are arranged is not as important as the end result. Theoretically, the arrangement of artificial teeth could begin with the second molar. Practically, that is unwise. However, there are many acceptable methods for arranging artificial teeth.

Most acceptable methods for arranging artificial teeth begin with the arrangement of the maxillary central incisors. These teeth maintain the center line as indicated by the dentist. Most sequences require the arrangement of all the maxillary anteriors first, although some methods alternate between the maxillary and mandibular teeth; i.e., maxillary incisors, mandibular incisors, maxillary lateral incisors, mandibular lateral incisors, etc.

In the sequence advocated by most manufacturers of artificial teeth the maxillary teeth are set first. The mandibular posterior teeth are then set, followed by the mandibular anterior teeth. The first premolar is the last tooth which is set, and essentially acts as a space filler between the mandibular anterior and posterior teeth. The primary disadvantage of this method is that it is difficult to set maxillary posterior teeth in the proper faciolingual relationship as determined by the position of the mandibular residual ridge. There is also a tendency to set the mandibular anterior teeth in a stereotyped manner.

Many technicians and dentists set the maxillary and mandibular anterior teeth first. While this allows esthetic factors to be introduced earlier, the position of the posterior teeth must be considered concurrently with the placement of the anterior teeth.

The sequence of setting the posterior teeth when all of the anterior teeth are set first can also vary. Some people will set all of the mandibular posterior teeth and then set the maxillary posterior teeth. Others will reverse the procedure and set the maxillary posterior teeth first. Others will alternate, usually setting the maxillary first and second premolars, then the mandibular second premolar, the maxillary first molar, mandibular first molar, maxillary second molar and mandibular second molar. The mandibular first premolar is usually adjusted to fill the space between the canine and second premolar.

Regardless of the sequence used to set posterior teeth, one should always complete one side and not jump back and forth from one side to the other. For example, the right side should be completely set in centric occlusion, and in lateral and protrusive excursions, before the left side is set. It is permissible, and usually encouraged, to make minor alterations in the occlusal surface of the posterior teeth in order to achieve good excursive movements and to maintain good centric occlusion.

Most dentists who set the mandibular posterior teeth before setting the maxillary posterior teeth feel that this method places the mandibular teeth in the proper position relative to the mandibular residual ridge and avoids resetting teeth as often as otherwise might be necessary. In some odd jaw relationships, it is almost essential to set the mandibular posteriors first and then alter the occlusal surface of the posterior teeth to achieve good occlusion.

The sequence of arranging teeth illustrated in this manual was selected because it was felt that this method is the simplest for beginning technicians. It is an accepted procedure and will produce good results. With experience, each person who routinely sets teeth will make individual variations in the sequence, all of which are acceptable if the end result is satisfactory.

When the teeth are "set for try-in" it is not necessary or advisable to set the teeth into all excursive movements. Often, rearrangement of the anterior teeth for esthetics at try-in will require that the posterior teeth be re-set. If a central bearing device has not been used, the condylar inclination will not be set until the time of the try-in; this, too, may require some rearrangement of the posterior teeth. *Remember, for try-in, set the teeth in tight centric occlusion, then rearrange the posterior teeth for excursive movements* after *the try-in.*

TECHNIQUE

The occlusion rims are prepared to arrange the teeth after the casts have been mounted. The wax or plaster used to make the centric relation record is removed and the space is filled with baseplate wax. The occlusal plane should be determined by the dentist, but an adjustment in the occlusal plane is permissible at this stage. The occlusal plane may be determined by three points: The anterior portion of the maxillary occlusion rim and the junction of the middle and upper thirds of each retromolar pad on the mandibular cast. The occlusal plane must be oriented properly before the arrangement of teeth is begun.

The incisal pin has been removed from the articulator in most of the following illustrations. This was done to improve the clarity of the photographs. Usually the incisal pin is left in place while teeth are being arranged, although some technicians will remove the pin while arranging anterior teeth.

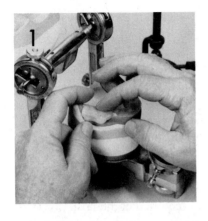
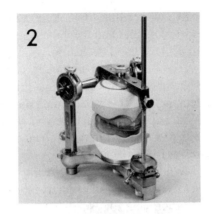
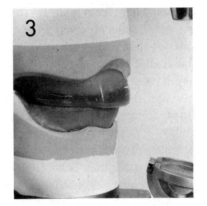
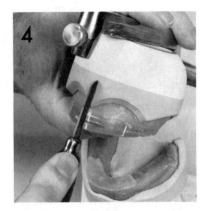

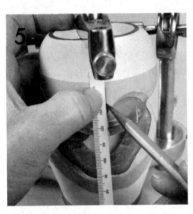
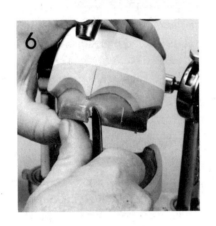
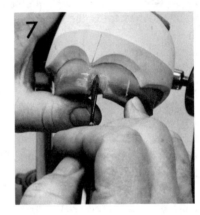
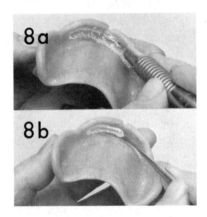

PREPARATION FOR ARRANGING TEETH

Figure 1   The mandibular occlusion rim is built up with baseplate wax after the material used for making the interocclusal jaw relation record is removed.

Figures 2 and 3   The occlusion rims have been rebuilt with baseplate wax and are ready for the arrangement of teeth. Note the horizontal overlap.

Figure 4   Note the position of the center line, the canine line and the high lip line. These are the lines which the dentist uses to select teeth for his patient. The center line is transferred from the occlusion rim to the maxillary cast as a permanent reference.

Figure 5   The center line may first be marked with a pencil to insure its proper placement.

Figure 6   A block of wax corresponding to the position of the maxillary left central incisor is removed from the occlusion rim.

Figure 7   The wax surrounding this area is softened with a hot spatula.

Figure 8   Sometimes the baseplate may interfere with proper placement of the teeth. When this occurs a portion of the baseplate is removed. The section is first cut on the tissue surface with a fissure bur (a) and is then lifted out with an instrument (b). The cast opposite the alteration should be lightly coated with Vaseline.

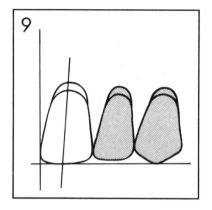
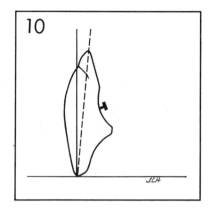
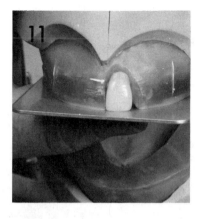
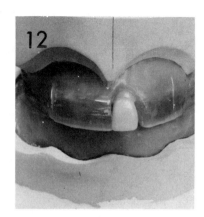
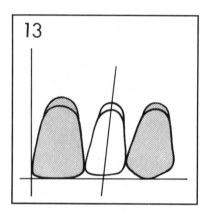
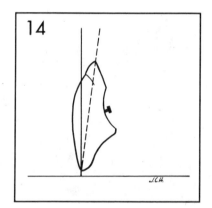
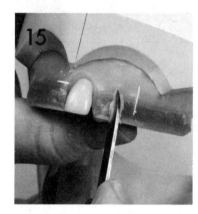
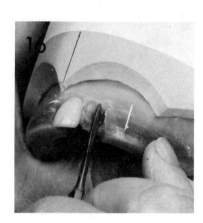

ARRANGING THE MAXILLARY ANTERIOR TEETH

Figure 9　The maxillary central incisor is placed so that the long axis shows a *slight* distal inclination to the perpendicular. The incisal edge is on the occlusal plane.

Figure 10　The neck of the tooth should be slightly depressed. However, the facial surface of the tooth is nearly perpendicular to the occlusal plane. Avoid over-depressing the neck of this tooth or the tooth will not be in a natural position when viewed in the mouth.

Figure 11　The maxillary left central incisor is placed in the molten wax to conform to the position shown in **Figures 9 and 10**. The incisal edge is on the occlusal plane. An aluminum plate may be used to orient the teeth to the occlusal plane.

Figure 12　The maxillary left central incisor is in proper position. A small amount of wax has been flowed around the tooth to insure its retention in the wax.

Figure 13　The maxillary lateral incisor has slightly more distal inclination than the central incisor. The incisal edge is usually ½ to 1 mm. above the occlusal plane.

Figure 14　The neck of the maxillary lateral incisor is depressed more than the central incisor, although the facial surface will be nearly in line with the central incisor.

Figure 15　A block of wax is removed in the left lateral incisor area.

Figure 16　The wax is softened with a hot wax spatula.

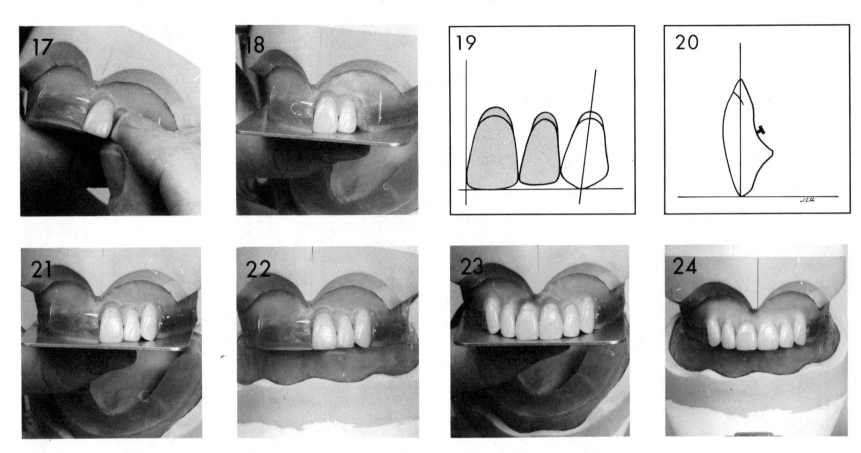

Figure 17   The lateral incisor is placed in position in the softened wax.

Figure 18   The maxillary left lateral incisor is placed to conform to the position shown in **Figures 13 and 14**. Note that the incisal edge is slightly above the occlusal plane and that the neck is *slightly* depressed.

Figure 19   The maxillary canine is placed so that the long axis is almost vertical. It may have a slight distal inclination but should not lean mesially. The incisal tip is on the occlusal plane.

Figure 20   The neck of the maxillary canine is prominent.

Figures 21 and 22   The maxillary left canine is placed in position using the same technique previously used for the central and lateral incisors. The canine tooth is an important tooth in any tooth arrangement be-

cause it forms the corner of the dental arch. The maxillary canine has two planes on the facial surface; the mesial plane should follow the contour of the anterior teeth while the distal plane will be in line with the posterior teeth. The neck of the tooth is prominent as it supports the corner of the patient's mouth.

Figure 23   The maxillary right anterior teeth are set in a similar fashion. Note the relation of the incisal edges to the occlusal plane. Note also the prominence of the gingival third of the maxillary central incisors and canines. The gingival third of anterior teeth is primarily responsible for lip support. Depressing the gingival third causes the upper lip to have a flaccid appearance. (The proper angulation of the maxillary anterior teeth may be judged by imagining that the artificial tooth has grown a root. By judging the amount of resorption—using the position of the incisive papilla as a guide—this imaginary root should

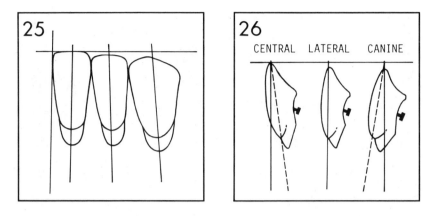

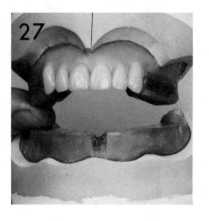

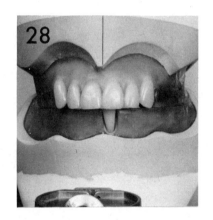

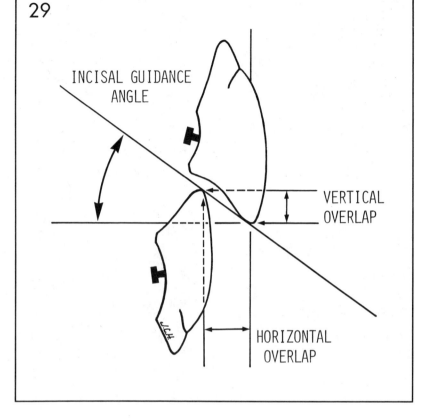

assume a natural position in the dental arch. Utilization of this image will result in having the maxillary incisor teeth in a natural and correct angulation.)

Figure 24 The arrangement of the maxillary anterior teeth has been completed and the wax smoothed around the teeth.

ARRANGING THE MANDIBULAR ANTERIOR TEETH

Figures 25 and 26 The *mandibular central incisors* are set with the long axis perpendicular to the occlusal plane with the neck depressed. The *mandibular lateral incisors* are set with a slight distal inclination and with the facial surface at a right angle to the occlusal plane. The

mandibular canines have more distal inclination than the lateral incisors and the neck is set prominently.

Figures 27 and 28 A block of wax is removed from the mandibular occlusion rim, the wax softened and the mandibular central incisor placed in position.

Figure 29 The incisal guidance angle is the angle formed by a line drawn through the incisal edges of the maxillary and mandibular incisors and the horizontal plane. (The incisal guide table is the mechanical equivalent of the incisal guidance angle.) The person arranging artificial teeth determines the incisal guidance angle by the level at which he sets the mandibular and maxillary incisors. In denture construction, the mandibular incisors should *never* touch the maxillary incisors in centric occlusion and the incisal guide angle should be kept as low as possible

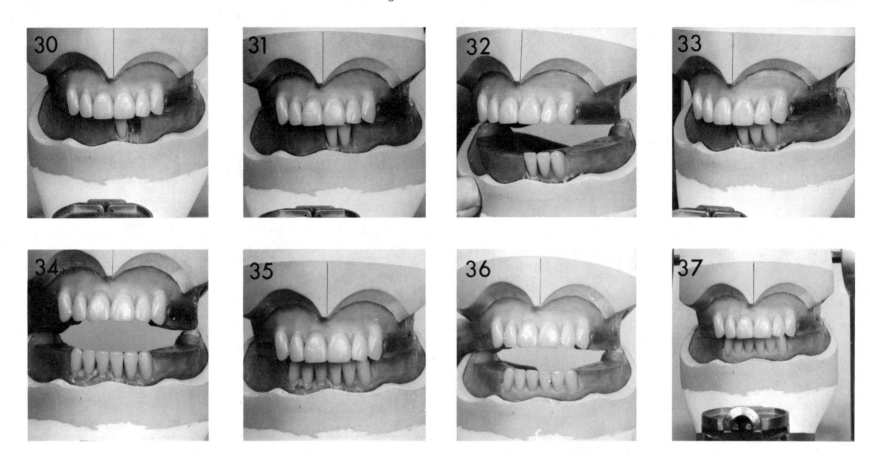

to enhance free movement of the teeth in protrusive and lateral excursions. These objectives can usually be realized and still achieve good esthetics.

Figures 30 and 31   The same procedure is used to set the mandibular left lateral incisor in proper position.

Figures 32 and 33   The mandibular left canine is set in position as indicated by the facial surface of the occlusion rim and the inclinations shown in **Figures 25 and 26**.

Figure 34   The mandibular right anterior teeth are arranged in a similar manner.

Figure 35   Note the vertical and horizontal overlap.

Figures 36 and 37   Wax has been added and roughly contoured around the anterior teeth. Excess wax should be removed from the surface of the teeth.

Figure 38   The anterior teeth should be examined from the occlusal aspect to insure that the facial surfaces of the teeth follow the original contours of the occlusion rim.

Figure 39   Artificial teeth should not be arranged in a stereotyped manner. Some variations, without losing natural inclinations, will make artificial teeth appear more natural. These variations may be laps, rotations, differences in the level of incisal edges, or esthetic spacing. These deviations should be placed in the teeth by the dentist at the time of the try-in, or by the technician upon prescription by the dentist.

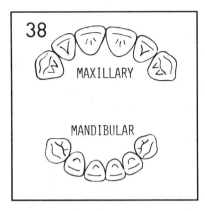
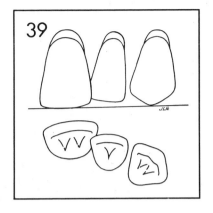
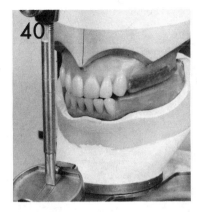
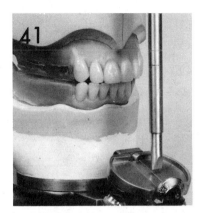

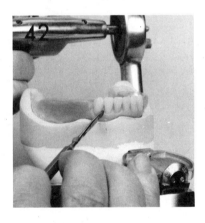
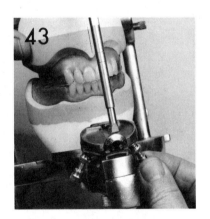
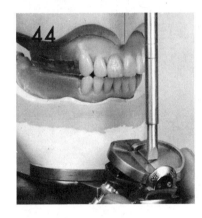
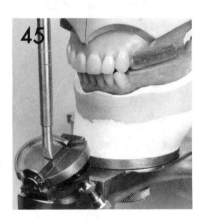

Figure 40   The arrangement of the anterior teeth is not complete until they have been checked in protrusive and lateral excursions. Here they are being checked in protrusive. Note that the teeth touch and that the incisal pin is contacting the incisal guide table. To insure proper contact, each mandibular anterior tooth may be checked for excursive movements while it is being set.

Figure 41   The right lateral movement is checked. Note that the pin is above the incisal guide table.

Figure 42   The mandibular right canine and lateral incisor are lowered slightly to provide better contact and lower the incisal guide plane.

Figure 43   The lateral wing of the incisal guide table is raised until it contacts the incisal pin. The extent to which the lateral wings may be

raised is determined to some extent by the type of posterior teeth to be used; the higher the cusps, the steeper the lateral guides may be set. However, free articulation is improved by keeping the wings as low as possible.

Figures 44 and 45   Right and left lateral excursions are checked after adjusting the lateral wings.

PREPARATION FOR ARRANGING THE POSTERIOR TEETH

Figure 46   The mandibular occlusion rim is removed and a dot placed on the crest of the residual ridge in the first premolar areas and on the mesial of the retromolar pads.

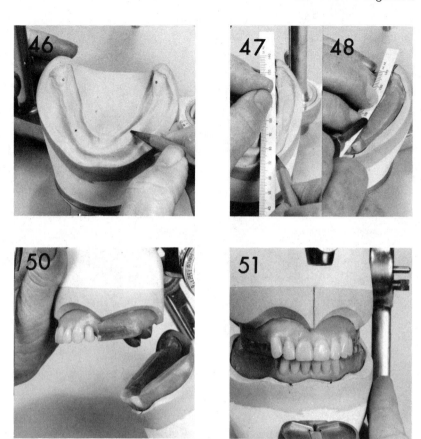

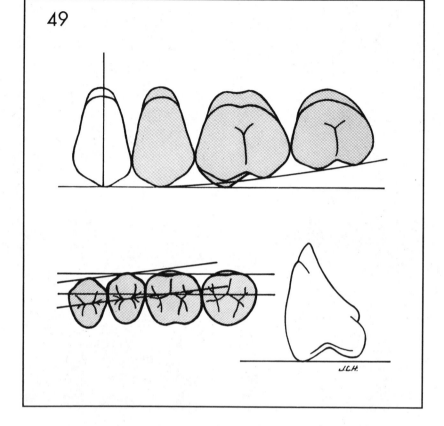

Figure 47   A straightedge is laid over the dots on each side and a mark is placed on the land area of the cast, anteriorly and posteriorly.

Figure 48   The mandibular occlusion rim is replaced. A straightedge is used to connect the two marks on the land areas and a line indicating the crest of the ridge is scribed on the occlusion rim.

ARRANGING THE MAXILLARY POSTERIOR TEETH

The most difficult posterior teeth to arrange are anatomical posteriors. The angulations must be precise and marginal ridge discrepancies minimal. The opposing teeth must occlude precisely and be in the correct mesiodistal relationship in order to prevent lateral interferences.

The illustrations which follow are based on Thirty-Three Degree Posterior Teeth. They are "classic" in that the same basic procedures used here are used in arranging all anatomic posterior teeth.

Figure 49   The inclinations of the maxillary first premolar are shown.

Figure 50   A portion of wax is removed, the wax softened and the maxillary left first premolar is placed in position.

Figure 51   The facial surface of the maxillary first premolar must harmonize with the canine.

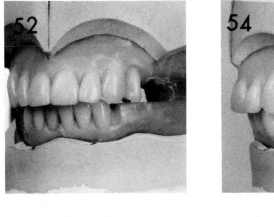
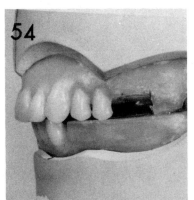
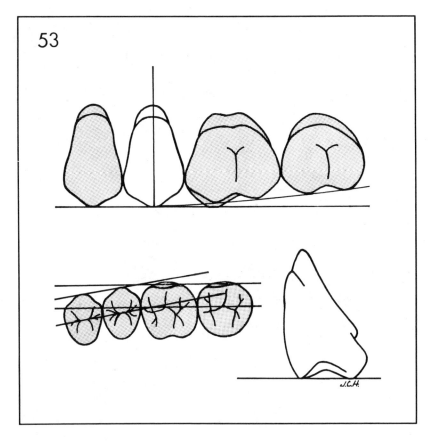
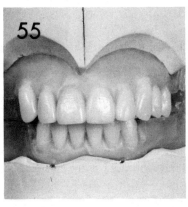
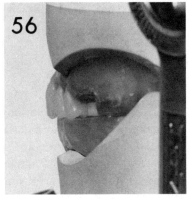
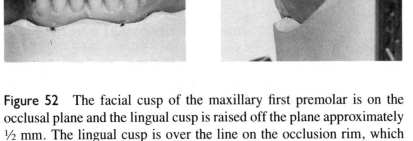

Figure 52 The facial cusp of the maxillary first premolar is on the occlusal plane and the lingual cusp is raised off the plane approximately ½ mm. The lingual cusp is over the line on the occlusion rim, which represents the crest of the mandibular ridge.

Figure 53 The inclinations of the maxillary second premolar are shown.

Figures 54 and 55 The maxillary left second premolar is set and checked.

Figure 56 The facial and lingual cusps of the maxillary second premolar touch the occlusal plane. The lingual cusp is over the crest of the ridge.

Figure 57 The inclinations for the maxillary first molar are shown. Note that only the mesiolingual cusp touches the occlusal plane.

Figures 58, 59 and 60 The maxillary left first molar has been set and checked from all directions. The mesiolingual cusp touches the occlusal plane and the lingual cusps are over the crest of the mandibular ridge.

Figure 61 The inclinations of the maxillary second molar are shown. No cusp touches the occlusal plane. Note how the facial cusps of the maxillary teeth form a gentle curve, while the lingual cusps form a similar curve about ½ mm. below the facial cusps. This is the compensating curve defined earlier in this section.

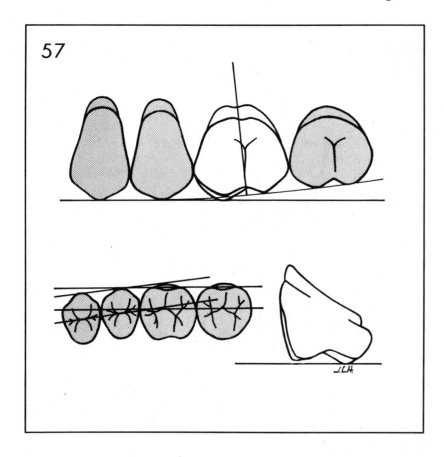

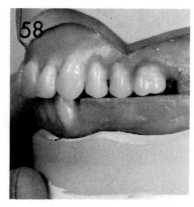

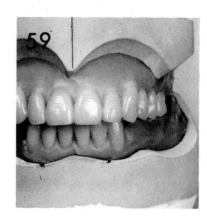

Figures 62, 63 and 64   The maxillary left second molars have been set and checked. The left maxillary posterior teeth are checked. Note how all the teeth are in a pleasing alignment, harmonizing with the anterior teeth. All the lingual cusps are over the crest of the mandibular ridge.

Figure 65   The maxillary right posterior teeth are arranged in the same manner as was the left side.

Figure 66   The mandibular occlusion rim has been removed and a piece of baseplate wax erected over the crest of the mandibular ridge. This illustrates that the lingual cusps of the maxillary posterior teeth are over the crest of the mandibular ridge. Note that the facial cusps are in line as are the lingual cusps. The adjacent marginal ridges are level and the central fossae form a continuous groove.

"BALANCING" POSTERIOR TEETH

As indicated earlier in the text, different dentists have different theories of occlusion for artificial posterior teeth. Sometimes it appears that these differences are geographical due to the influence of regional dental schools. Some understanding of these differences may help to better meet the needs of various dentists.

Anatomical teeth, those that closely resemble natural teeth, are used by dentists who believe artificial teeth should be "balanced." This means that when teeth are moved in lateral working excursions (**Figures 68 and 69**) there is planned simultaneous contact on the opposite side. When moved into protrusive excursions (**Figure 70**) there is planned simultaneous contact on posterior teeth. Proponents of balanced occlusion contend that this scheme adds to the stability of the completed dentures.

Others believe that uniform contact in centric occlusion is all that is necessary and balancing contacts are superfluous. This group tends to favor flat teeth (also termed monoplane, 0°, etc.) and tends to arrange them flat, with no compensating curve (**Figures 95–99**).

Then there is a middle group who favor low cusp heights and some balance. The teeth used by this group are "semi-anatomical"; they have low cusps with more "mechanical" occlusal anatomy. Generally, the principles of arranging anatomical posteriors are followed with these teeth. However, specialized teeth such as Centrimatic Posteriors use a different technique; follow instructions from the manufacturer and/or the dentist in arranging such teeth.

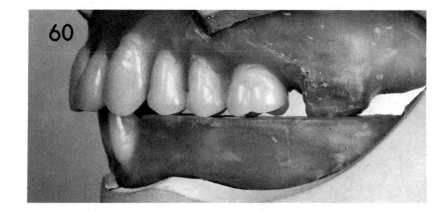

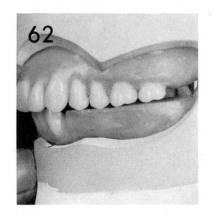

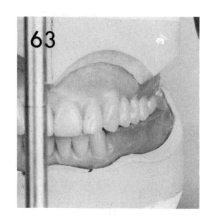

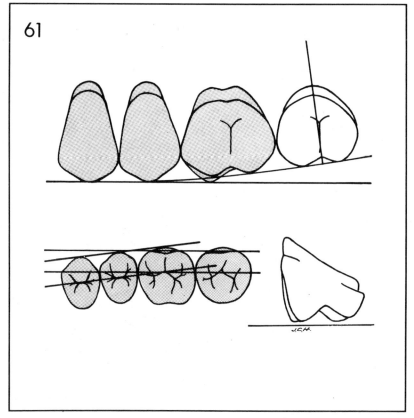

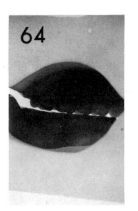

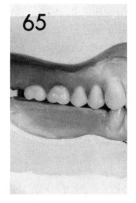

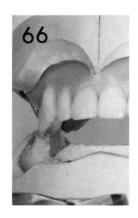

ARRANGING THE MANDIBULAR POSTERIOR TEETH

The placement of the mandibular posterior teeth determines how well the teeth occlude, both in centric occlusion and in lateral and protrusive excursions. When difficulty is encountered either in setting the mandibular posterior teeth or achieving proper function, check the maxillary teeth for proper placement. Often, errors in arranging the maxillary teeth do not become evident until the mandibular teeth are set.

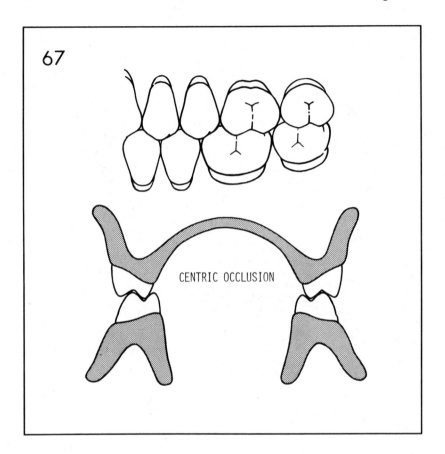

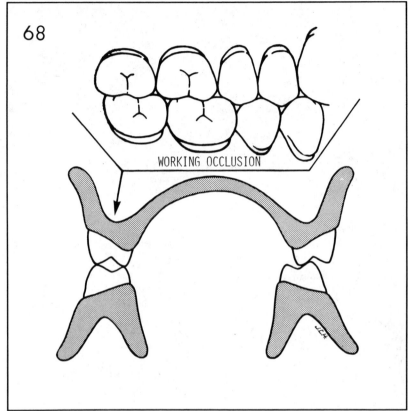

Figure 67 In centric occlusion, the facial cusps of the mandibular teeth contact the central fossae of the maxillary teeth while the lingual cusps of the maxillary teeth fit into the central fossae of the mandibular teeth. Note how the facial cusps of the maxillary teeth extend beyond the facial surfaces of the mandibular teeth. This facial overlap prevents cheek-biting when the dentures are completed.

Figure 68 Working or functional occlusion occurs when the facial cusps of the maxillary teeth meet the facial cusps of the mandibular teeth and the lingual cusps of the maxillary teeth meet the lingual cusps of the mandibular teeth. The relationship is not cusp tip to cusp tip, but cusp tip into cusp "valley" with each maxillary cusp distal to the corresponding mandibular cusp. Working occlusion enables a person to hold and crush food.

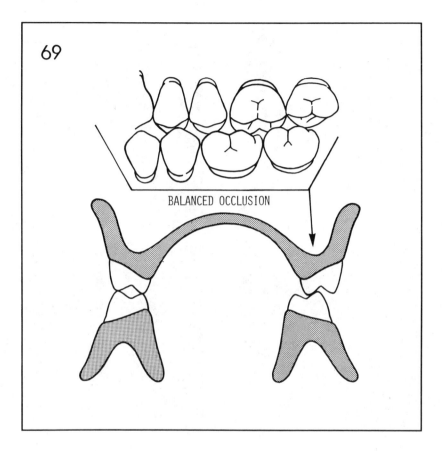

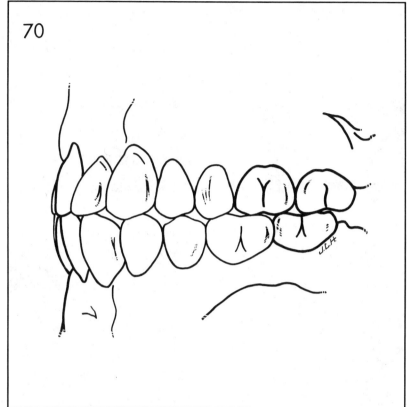

Figure 69   Balancing occlusion occurs simultaneously on the opposite side from working occlusion. Balancing occlusion functions to maintain the dentures in position during lateral excursive movements. In balancing occlusion, the lingual cusps of the maxillary teeth contact the facial cusps of the mandibular teeth. In many techniques, balancing contacts are necessary only on the second molars.

Figure 70   Balancing contacts in protrusive excursions permit the posterior teeth to touch when the anterior teeth are in contact. This helps maintain denture stability. In protrusive balance, the distal inclines of the maxillary facial cusps contact the mesial inclines of the mandibular facial cusps. Protrusive balancing contacts may also occur on the lingual cusps.

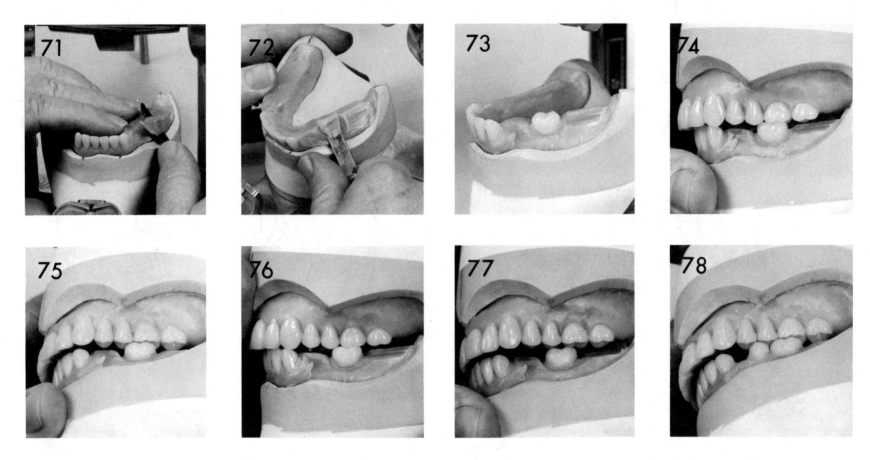

Figure 71   The mandibular occlusion rim is reduced preparatory to arranging the mandibular posterior teeth.

Figure 72   A section of the mandibular rim is removed to make room for the mandibular left first molar. The wax is softened to permit placement of the tooth.

Figure 73   The mandibular left first molar is placed in position.

Figures 74 and 75   The mandibular left first molar is first set into centric occlusion and checked carefully. Note that the facial cusps of the mandibular tooth fit into the fossae of the maxillary teeth. The mesiolingual cusp of the maxillary first molar fits into the central fossa of the mandibular first molar. Proper placement of the mandibular first molar is essential to insure proper placement of the remaining mandibular posterior teeth.

Figure 76   The mandibular left first molar is checked in working occlusion. Be sure to move the articulator properly. (See Section 7, **Figures H–K.**)

Figure 77   The mandibular first molar is checked in balancing occlusion.

Figure 78, 79 and 80   The mandibular left second premolar is set and similarly checked in centric, working and balancing occlusion.

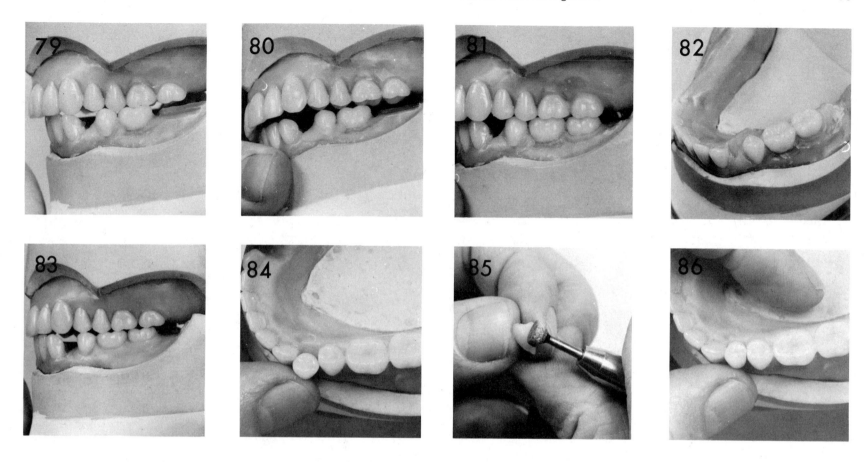

Figure 81 The mandibular left second molar is set in position and is checked in centric, working and balancing occlusion.

Figure 82 Note how the mandibular teeth are aligned. Faulty alignment should be corrected at this point. Poor alignment may be a reflection of improperly set maxillary teeth.

Figure 83 The teeth are checked for protrusive balance. Note the cuspal relations of the posterior teeth.

Figure 84 The mandibular left first premolar is placed to position. Here, as often happens, the tooth is too large for the space.

Figure 85 The tooth is reduced mesially and distally. The ground surface is polished before the tooth is waxed to position.

Figures 86 and 87 The mandibular left first premolar now fits the space and is waxed to position.

Figure 88 The mandibular left posterior teeth are now in proper position and have been checked in centric occlusion and in excursive movements. Note: The incisal guide pin must remain on the incisal guide table and the teeth must contact during all excursions. Interference in excursive movements may be removed by grinding the occlusal surfaces of the teeth. The rules for occlusal correction in Section 12 must be followed.

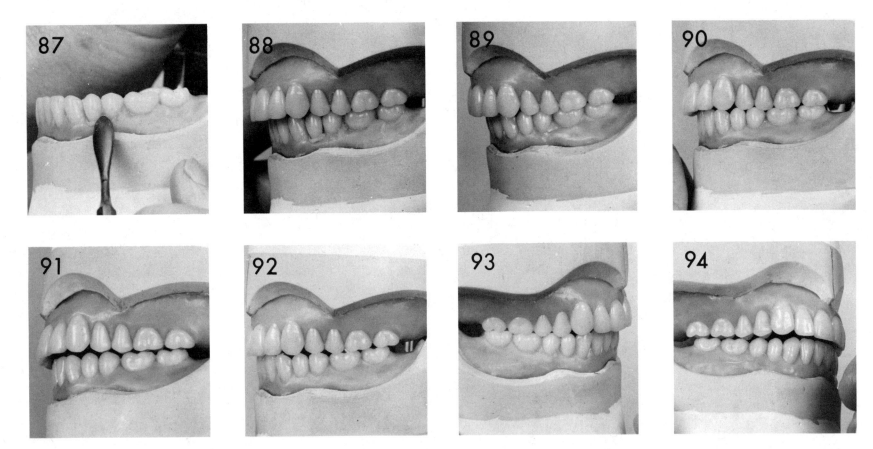

Figure 89   The mandibular left posterior teeth are now set. (Remember: arranging teeth for function is simpler if one side is set and checked for excursive movements before the opposite side is set.) The completed arrangement is shown in centric occlusion.

Figure 90   The teeth are shown in working occlusion on the left side.

Figure 91   The teeth are shown in balancing occlusion on the left side.

Figure 92   The left side is shown in protrusive balance.

Figures 93 and 94   The teeth are shown in working and balancing occlusion on the right side. The arrangement of the teeth is now complete.

As mentioned earlier in this section, the teeth are not generally set with this precision until after the teeth have been checked for esthetics in the patient's mouth and the jaw relationships verified. The teeth are checked in the patient's mouth and, after the dentist makes the necessary alterations, the patient is given an opportunity to approve the arrangement (**Figure A**). Usually, the patient will force an unnatural smile and must be instructed on how to observe the teeth in a natural manner. Often this is done by giving the patient a prepared poem or paragraph to read.

At this appointment, the fourth or fifth depending on whether a central bearing device was used, the dentist also checks the jaw relationships and, if a central bearing device was not used, makes a protrusive record and adjusts the condyles as was shown in Section 8, **Figures 10 through 13**. The teeth are then rearranged to harmonize with the new

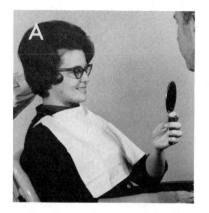
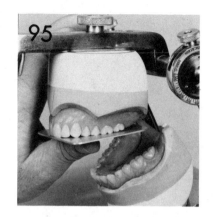
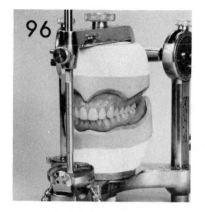
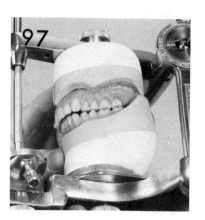

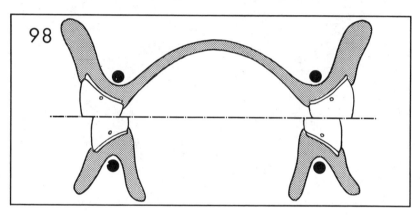
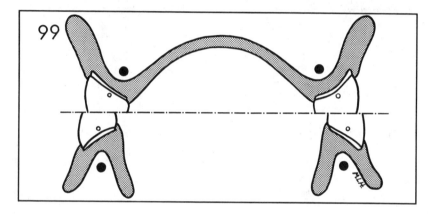

jaw relationship and/or condylar guidance. The teeth must be arranged as accurately as possible before the bases are waxed to the proper contours (festooned) and the dentures processed.

ARRANGEMENT OF
NONANATOMICAL POSTERIOR TEETH

Nonanatomical teeth have a flat occlusal surface; therefore, interdigitation of cusps and correct mesiodistal relationship is not a problem when arranging these teeth. Otherwise, principles for arranging nonanatomical posterior teeth are essentially the same as for arranging anatomical teeth. The teeth should be set in a natural position and the

facial overlap should be sufficient to prevent cheek-biting. The mesiodistal position of the teeth is not as critical as with anatomical teeth.

Nonanatomical teeth are set with a plane contact; i.e., the maxillary and mandibular teeth must contact each other throughout their occlusal surface. Precaution should be taken to insure that the mandibular teeth are not inclined so that only the facioocclusal angle contacts the maxillary teeth.

There are two basic methods for arranging nonanatomical posterior teeth. The first method uses a balancing ramp. This is done by tilting the second molars so that they contact when the anterior teeth contact. The second molars may be tilted so that they also balance working contacts on the opposite side. The second method requires all the teeth to be flat and does not utilize balancing ramps. The illustrations which follow show the arrangement of nonanatomical teeth with a balancing

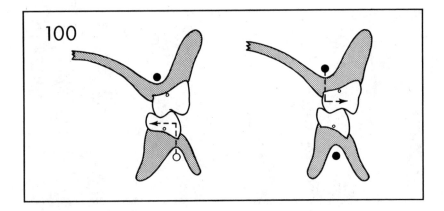

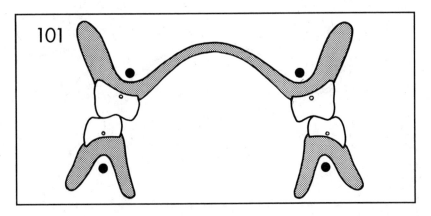

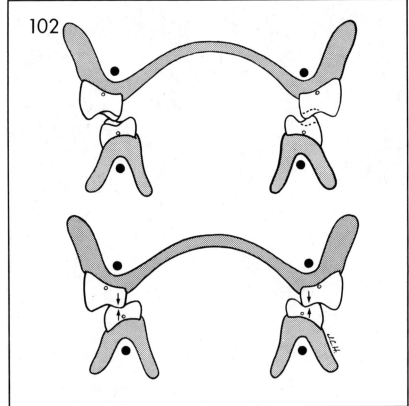

ramp. If the dentist selects not to use a balancing ramp, the only variation required is that the second molars be set on the occlusal plane.

Figure 95 The maxillary teeth have been set with all of the teeth on the occlusal plane. An aluminum plate may be used to insure that the full surface of the tooth is on the occlusal plane.

Figures 96 and 97 The set-up has been completed with the mandibular teeth contacting the maxillary teeth. Note how the occlusal surface of the mandibular teeth contacts the occlusal surface of the maxillary teeth. Note that a facial overlap has also been produced in this set-up.

Figure 98 When arranging nonanatomical posterior teeth, the teeth may be set over the residual ridges in the most advantageous mechani-

cal manner. The facial overlap may be increased if this enhances the ridge-tooth relationship.

Figure 99 Nonanatomical teeth lend themselves to odd jaw relationships. It is a simple matter to set nonanatomical teeth in a crossbite relationship if the mandibular arch is wider than the maxillary arch.

ABNORMAL JAW RELATIONSHIPS AND CUSP TEETH

Cusp teeth may be modified to achieve balanced occlusion when abnormal jaw relationships are encountered. In a crossbite situation, where the mandible is larger than the maxillae, some techniques require that the mandibular right teeth be set in the maxillary left arch and the mandibular left teeth be set in the maxillary right arch. Then the maxillary right teeth are set in the mandibular left arch, etc. Briefly, the posterior teeth are "X'd." This technique is satisfactory except that the inclination of the teeth produces a poor esthetic result. A better solution is to modify the occlusal surfaces of the teeth.

Figure 100   If a "normal" arrangement is attempted when a crossbite is indicated, the maxillary teeth will fall outside the base of the maxillary denture or the mandibular teeth will fall too far lingual to the crest of the mandibular ridge and overhang the tongue. This induces a displacing factor, as the tongue will tend to dislodge the denture when the teeth are set too far lingually.

Figure 101   In a crossbite relationship, cusp teeth may be modified in order to achieve proper interdigitation. The modification will vary according to the extent of the crossbite and the position of the tooth in the dental arch. For example, the molars may be in a crossbite, the first premolars in a normal relationship and the second premolars in an "end-to-end" relationship. Occlusal correction is needed to achieve smooth lateral and protrusive excursions.

Figure 102   In a Class II jaw relationship, the mandible is smaller than the maxillae. In these situations, the teeth must be modified to provide for an increased facial over-jet. This is done as diagramed in this illustration. Usually the molars will be in a normal relationship with the greatest modification being needed in the premolar region.

It may be easier in Class II jaw relationships to first set the teeth in working occlusion and then modify the teeth to achieve centric occlusion.

REVIEW QUESTIONS

1. What are the three basic patterns available in posterior artificial teeth?
2. What combination of porcelain and resin teeth should never be used?
3. What is the compensating curve on a complete denture?
4. Describe the positioning of the maxillary central incisors, lateral incisors and canines in the original set-up for complete dentures.
5. What preparations are made on the mandibular cast for arranging the posterior teeth?

SECTION 10

Festooning

The gingival portion of a complete denture is carved to simulate natural gingival contours. These carvings are made in wax after the teeth have been arranged. The term "festooning" is used to differentiate waxing a denture base from making wax patterns for cast metal restorations.

Festooning is the process of carving the denture base to simulate the contour of the natural tissues which are being replaced by the denture.

When festooning a denture for the first time, a cast of a natural dentition with healthy gingiva should be used as a model (**Figure A**). Carving a denture base to simulate natural gingiva is much simpler than attempting to induce contours which some people believe look natural but which may detract from the appearance of the denture. Outlandish gingival carvings not only detract from appearance, but make a denture more difficult to keep clean.

One of the most common errors in festooning is to make the interdental papilla nonexistent, or too small. This provides a space between the teeth into which food tends to pack, and also makes the denture difficult to polish. There are times when it is proper to simulate gingival recession, such as occurs in periodontal disease, but this can usually be done without creating food traps between the teeth.

Another common error is to place grooves on the denture base between each tooth. This practice is a hold-over from earlier days and results from misconceptions regarding normal gingival contours.

When the teeth have been set for a try-in, the denture base must be contoured so that the teeth and base look natural. The proper amount of

tooth must be exposed and the wax must be neat. However, fine details need not be incorporated in a wax-up for a try-in.

PROCEDURE FOR FESTOONING COMPLETE DENTURES

Figure 1   The materials required for festooning a denture are the casts and baseplates upon which the artificial teeth have been arranged, baseplate wax, suitable wax spatulas and carvers, a Bunsen burner, and a Hanau torch. Final festooning should not be attempted until arrangement of teeth has been completed. Once a denture has been festooned in detail, time will be lost if it is necessary to reset any teeth.

Figure 2   The casts and mounts are removed from the articulator.

Figures 3 and 4   A portion of a sheet of baseplate wax is softened and rolled into a wax stick a little larger than the diameter of a lead pencil. The wax stick is heated in the Bunsen burner flame and then the molten wax on the end of the stick is dripped onto the denture base. The wax may be built up around the teeth and the borders by this method. Another method is to use a medicine dropper to place molten wax on the denture base. Do not allow the wax to drip between the wax denture base and the cast as the wax denture will be removed from the cast in later stages. A light coat of Vaseline on the cast will assure that the wax denture can be easily removed.

Another method of adding wax is to use an electric wax melting pot. These are advantageous in commercial situations.

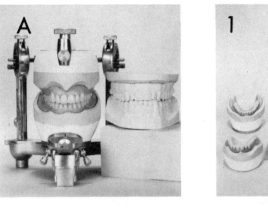
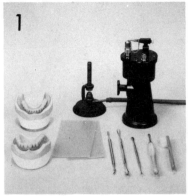
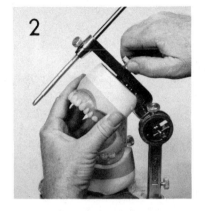
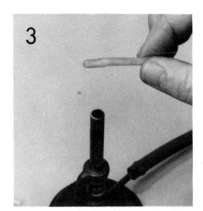

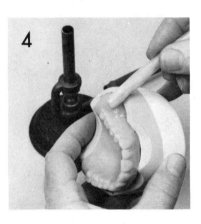
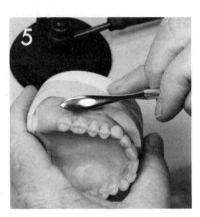
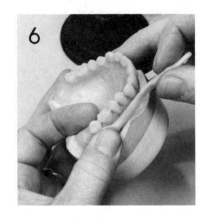
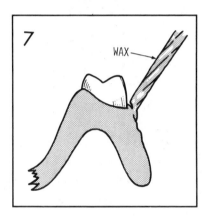

Figure 5   The wax is flowed into position with a warm spatula after the wax has been dripped onto the denture base.

Figure 6   An alternate method of placing wax on the denture base is to soften the entire stick of baseplate wax and to mold this into place with your fingers. Some people believe that this method causes less distortion than the "drip-on" method.

Figure 7   This drawing illustrates the addition of wax to the denture base. The *objective* of either the "drip-on" or "press-on" method is to add a sufficient bulk of wax to the denture base which can then be carved to the proper contours.

Figure 8   These cross-sections illustrate the proper shape of a denture base. The objective is to reproduce natural contours and to aid retention. The cross-sections are arranged in the same order as indicated on the casts in the upper left line drawings.

The anterior portion of the maxillary denture base replaces tissue lost through resorption (**Figure 8, t**). This portion of the denture base is not heavy unless there has been extensive bone loss. Excessive thickness or "plumpers," usually indicates improper placement of the anterior teeth. "Plumpers" are indicated in some instances such as paralysis of the lip resulting from disease or surgery.

The maxillary denture is shaped so that the borders are rounded. The wax is contoured so that the width of the borders as recorded in the impression is preserved in the denture (**Figures 8, u, v**).

The contours of the mandibular denture aid in its retention. In the anterior region (**Figure 8, w**), the facial surface is relatively straight.

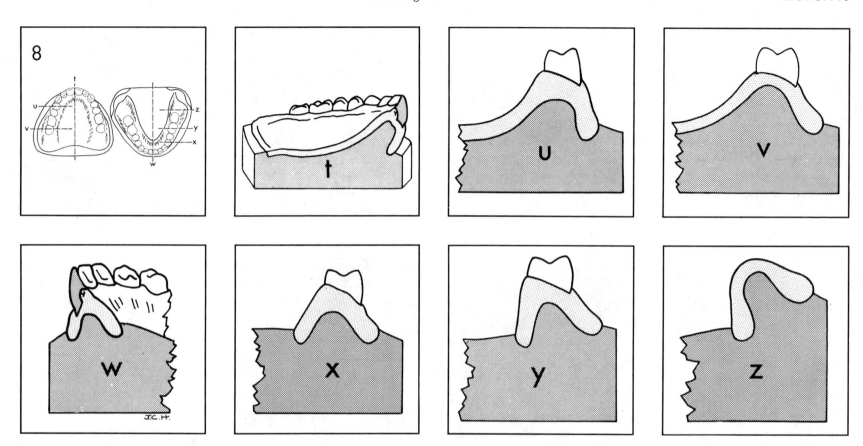

The lingual surface slopes to the lingual border and is relatively straight.

In the posterior region, the facial surface faces upward and outward. This contour allows the buccinator muscle to lie against the denture (**Figures 8, x, y, z**). The lingual surface in the premolar and molar region is a straight surface from the gingival cuff to the lingual border (**Figures 8, x, y**). (A concave surface in this area provides a space for the tongue to "catch" and lift the denture unintentionally.)

The lingual surface posterior to the second molar dips into the retromylohyoid region and faces downward and inward. This area is contoured so that it dips under the base of the tongue and is thinned so that it does not interfere with normal tongue movements (**Figure 8, z**).

STEPS TO BE FOLLOWED IN CONTOURING WAX DENTURE BASES

Figure 9   A sharp instrument, such as a Roach carver, is used to cut the wax back around the teeth. The wax is cut back to the cervical line on the artificial tooth, or, if gingival recession is to be simulated, a little beyond the cervical line. Failure to cut the wax to the cervical line will result in the teeth appearing too short and will also result in having the teeth fall out of the flask when the wax is eliminated after flasking.

Figure 10   This illustrates the proper angle at which the instrument must be held when carving the wax to the cervical line. Holding the instrument in this position will prevent a "ditch" being formed around the tooth. It will also maintain the proper convex contours of the

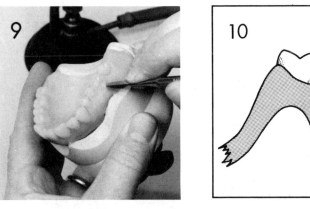
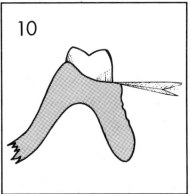
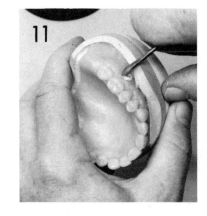
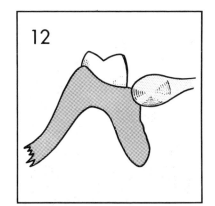

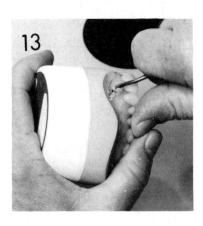
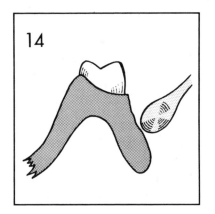
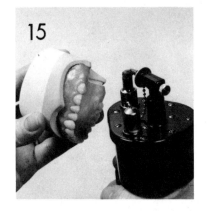
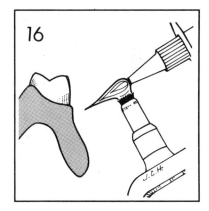

interdental papillae. Define the gingival line on the entire arch before proceeding.

Figures 11 and 12   A Kingsley scraper, or other suitable instrument, is then used to reduce the ledge formed around the tooth in the previous step to a width of one to one-and-one-half millimeters. The narrow ledge carved around the teeth extends around the entire dental arch. The combination of proper instrument angulation (**Figure 9**) and narrowing of the ledge produces interdental papillae of the proper contour.

Figures 13 and 14   The remainder of the denture base is contoured with a Kingsley scraper. A sharp instrument with a spoon-shaped end is the best type of instrument to use for contouring a denture base. The contours should follow those shown in **Figure 8**.

Figures 15 and 16   A Hanau torch is used to smooth the facial contours of the denture base. Note the distance at which the torch is being held from the denture base to avoid melting the wax. Hanau and other types of waxing torches are used to smooth wax, not to contour wax, and only seldom to flow wax.

When the denture base has been properly carved and contoured, as shown in the preceding steps, flaming will round the marginal gingival area, the interdental papillae, and form a natural gingival cuff. If the ledge (**Figure 10**) has been left too wide, a ditch will be left around the tooth. If the ledge is too narrow, wax will flow onto the denture tooth leaving no gingival cuff.

Figures 17 and 18   Sometimes a little wax will flow onto the tooth while the denture base is being flamed. This little flash is removed with

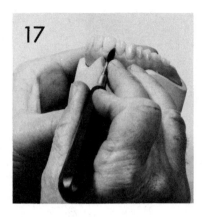
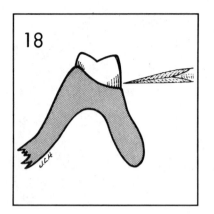
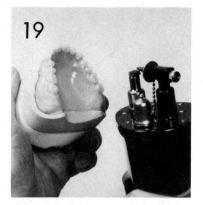
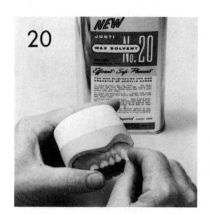

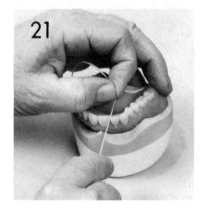
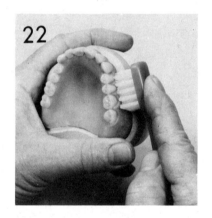

a sharp instrument to redefine the gingival cuff. During this final trimming only the wax which has flowed onto the tooth is removed. Do not attempt to recontour the denture or to reflame after this final trimming around the teeth.

Figure 19 Gingival carvings to simulate the lingual gingiva are placed in the same manner as they were on the facial surface of the denture. The palatal surface is then smoothed with a Hanau torch.

Figures 20 and 21 Wax solvent is used to clean any wax film from the surface of the teeth. This is done by moistening a small piece of cotton with wax solvent and wiping the excess wax off the teeth. Care should be exercised to keep excess wax solvent from contacting the wax around the gingival portion of the tooth for any protracted period.

Prolonged contact of the wax solvent with the wax may result in loosening the teeth in the wax denture base. A piece of dental floss may be used to clean the wax from between the anterior teeth. After the wax solvent has been used to clean the teeth and the dental floss passed through the interproximal areas, the teeth should be washed with cool water and soap on a piece of cotton. This will remove the wax solvent and prevent any deleterious effect on the wax.

When using resin artificial teeth, it is of the utmost importance to remove all wax from the teeth, facially, interproximally and lingually. Otherwise, denture base material will adhere to the teeth causing a poor esthetic result, and making finishing procedures difficult.

Figure 22 A denture base with a stippled effect simulates natural gingiva and prevents light being reflected from the denture base.

Stippling in the wax denture base is done by *first lightly flaming* the surface of the wax. The wax base is then struck repeatedly with a stiff toothbrush. The bristles, being held in a vertical direction, produce many small indentations in the wax.

Figure 23 The wax base is then flamed in a light and fleeting manner with a Hanau torch to smooth out the gross roughness caused by the toothbrush. The result is a stippled surface, which, when transferred to the completed denture, produces a pleasing appearance in a patient's mouth.

The denture base should be stippled only where the base will show when the patient talks and smiles. This area should be indicated by the dentist. A stippled denture base is not as hygienic as a polished base,

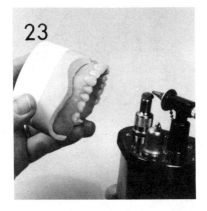 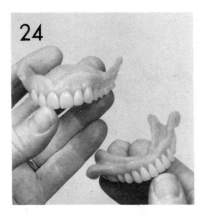 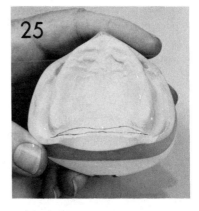 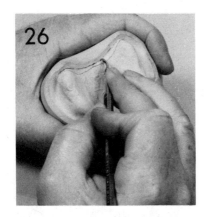

and therefore should be avoided when not necessary or if the patient does not have good oral hygiene habits.

Figure 24 The wax denture bases are removed from the casts and the contours checked. Removal at this time enables the technician to see the dentures as they will be when they are completed. This gives him an opportunity to check the border areas and the thickness of the palate before the dentures are processed. The palate should be one and a half to two millimeters thick.

Note the lingual contours of the mandibular wax denture. The lingual surface of a mandibular denture extends in a straight line from the lingual surface of the teeth to the lingual border. The only exception is in the posterior portion where the retromylohyoid area is contoured to allow more tongue room. Undercuts in other than the retromylohyoid area will catch the tongue and cause displacement of the denture.

Figure 25 The posterior palatal relief, sometimes called the post-dam, is carved in the cast at this time if it has not been done previously. The posterior palatal relief is a depression carved in the cast which improves retention of the maxillary denture. The placement of this relief is the responsibility of the dentist and if not carved in the cast by the dentist, its placement should be indicated by him. It is carved just forward to the posterior border of the denture. There are several types of posterior palatal seals, the most common of which is the so-called "butterfly." The butterfly is so termed because it is wider in the glandular areas of the palate and narrow across the mid-line, giving it a butterfly configuration.

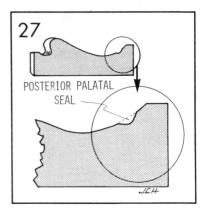

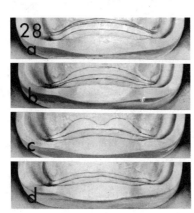

Figure 26 A sharp instrument, such as the spoon-shaped end of a Roach carver, may be used to form the posterior palatal relief.

Figure 27 This drawing illustrates the proper shape of a butterfly post-dam in cross-section. Note how it feathers toward the anterior portion of the cast.

Figure 28 Various other types of posterior palatal reliefs are widely used. "a" is a posterior palatal relief which has been placed two to three millimeters anterior to the posterior border of the denture. This type of relief results in a ridge on the tissue surface of the denture which has the tissue surface of the denture in its natural position both anterior and posterior to it. This type of posterior palatal relief can be adjusted more accurately if soreness develops in this region. "b" is a similar type of

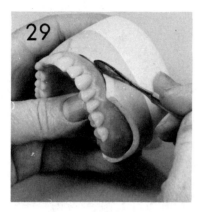 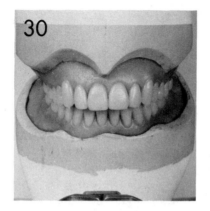 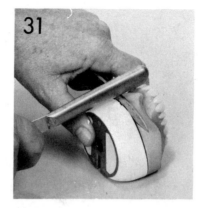 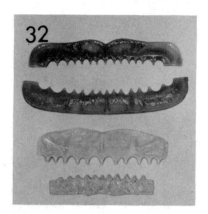

posterior palatal relief. It is carved with its posterior edge on the posterior border of the denture. The main difference is that the posterior edge of the relief is at the level of the tissue and is not depressed as is done in the butterfly type. "c" is the butterfly type. "d" is carved in a similar manner to the butterfly variety but does not extend forward into the glandular areas.

Figure 29   The wax dentures are returned to the casts and sealed into position. Both maxillary and mandibular dentures are sealed to the casts throughout their circumference. This prevents any stone from working under the wax base during flasking procedures.

Figure 30   The casts and their mounts are returned to the articulator and the occlusion checked. Check the teeth to be certain that none has shifted position during the waxing procedures.

Figure 31   The casts are removed from their plaster mountings by placing a knife at the junction of the plaster base and cast and tapping with a handle of a plaster spatula. *Warning:* The cast and plaster mount must be soaked for five minutes before attempting to split the mount from the cast unless a mounting plate has been used. Failure to soak the cast and mount may result in the cast being broken.

The maxillary and mandibular casts and their respective wax dentures are now ready to be flasked. It can now be seen that the wax denture base is a pattern which will be reproduced in the resin denture

base material. The more accurate the wax pattern, the easier it will be to complete the dentures after they have been processed. *Five extra minutes spent in properly waxing a denture will save more time and produce better results than attempting to contour a denture base after it has been processed.*

Figure 32   There are patterns which simulate gingival contours and which may be used in lieu of contouring the denture base in wax. These plastic patterns properly used produce good results. However, they have serious drawbacks, among which are the extra time consumed in applying the patterns, an inadequate number of sizes to fit all situations, and a tendency to over-contour the denture base, which results in an unsatisfactory esthetic result.

REVIEW QUESTIONS

1. What is the most common error in festooning a denture base?
2. What results when the wax is not cut back to the cervical line?
3. Why is it important to remove all wax from the clinical surfaces of resin artificial teeth?
4. Describe four types of posterior palatal relief.
5. Describe how stippling is done on the wax denture base and where it is done on the wax denture base.

SECTION 11

Flasking, Packing, Processing, and Recovery

The festooned wax denture base must be converted to resin to make a denture. This is done by using the wax denture as a pattern to make a mold into which denture base resin is inserted and cured.

The wax denture base which was contoured in the last section forms a pattern for the completed denture. The wax denture base is invested and then the wax is eliminated, forming a mold into which methyl methacrylate resin is packed. After the resin is cured, the denture is removed from the flask. Thus, in this section we will see how the wax denture is converted into a resin denture.

The method of flasking and packing described in this section is known as the "open-pack" method. There are many other methods of flasking and packing dentures, some of which use an injection procedure in which uncured denture material is kept in a reservoir under pressure while the dentures are curing. Injection methods are more complicated, but the results of tests conducted at the United States Bureau of Standards indicate that dentures made by the "open-pack" method are as accurate as dentures made by the injection method.

Other methods of producing dentures are introduced from time to time. None has stood the "test of time" as well as the conventional methods shown in this section. A thorough understanding of these procedures and competence in them will allow an individual to intelligently evaluate and use some of these innovative methods as they appear.

If the procedures described in this section are not carried out correctly, all of the work which has preceded this step will be lost. No step in denture construction can be ignored or glossed over lightly.

Figure 1 The master casts have been removed from the plaster mounts and are soaked in room temperature water until the casts are thoroughly wet. This will take about five minutes. Do not leave the casts soaking for too long a period of time or the surface becomes etched.

Figure 2 The casts with the wax dentures are placed in the flask. This is done to insure that the flask and the casts are of a compatible size. Note that the flask consists of four pieces: (1) the base, which contains the cast under which is (2) a round, knock-out plate (see **Figure 3**), (3) the top half of the flask and (4) the lid.

Figure 3 The inside surface of the flask is coated *lightly* with Vaseline.

Figure 4 The base of the cast is coated with a plaster separating medium. This is particularly important if a mounting plate has not been used. The plaster separating medium may be any one of the commercial products sold for this purpose, waterglass (sodium silicate), or a green soap solution.

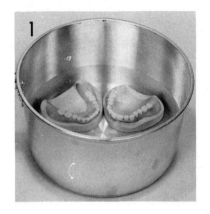
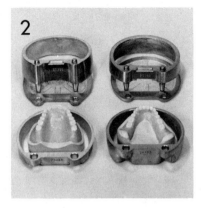
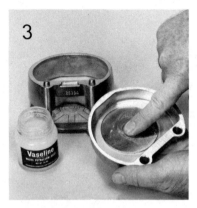
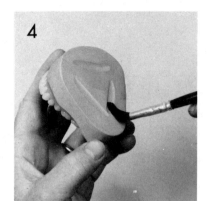

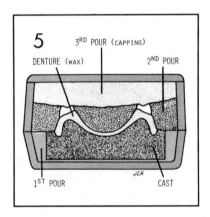
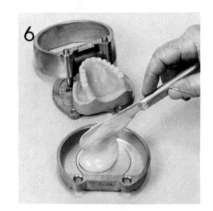
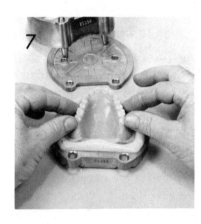
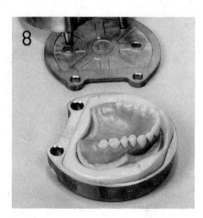

Figure 5 Flasking is done in three steps. In the first step the cast is secured to the base of the flask with stone. No undercuts should exist on the surface of this first stage. In the second stage the upper half of the flask is put in place and stone is poured to the occlusal surfaces of the teeth. The final stage is accomplished when the top portion or capping of the flask is poured and the lid placed on the flask.

The best results are obtained when all three sections are made in stone. Some laboratories pour the first two stages in plaster and the capping in stone to prevent the teeth from being displaced during packing. This method is satisfactory but better results are obtained when all three pours are made of stone.

Figure 6 Stone is mixed and placed in the base of the flask.

Figure 7 The maxillary cast is pushed to place until the bottom of the cast touches the base of the flask. The only exception is when the base of the cast is uneven; then the cast is leveled to permit easy separation and good access in later stages.

Figure 8 Note that the posterior portion of the cast is level with the edge of the flask.

Figure 9 The stone is smoothed even with the base of the cast and is contoured so that no undercuts will be present when the stone is set.

Figure 10 The flask is set aside until the stone reaches its initial set.

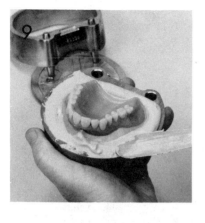
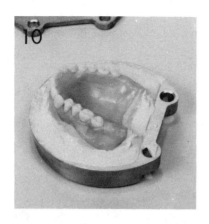
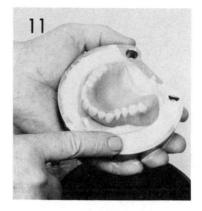
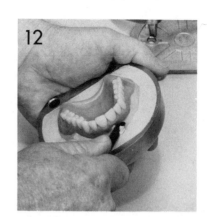

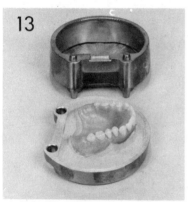
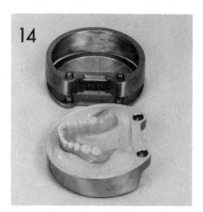
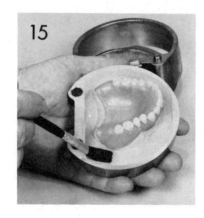
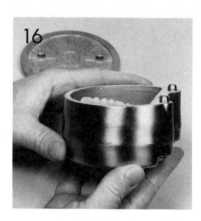

Figure II   When the stone reaches its initial set, a finger moistened with water is used to complete smoothing the lower portion of the flask.

Figure 12   If any small undercut areas exist, they should be trimmed with a knife after the stone has set.

Figure 13   The lower half of the flasking of the maxillary denture is completed.

Figure 14   Similar procedures are followed with the mandibular cast. Note that the posterior portion of the base of the lower flask is higher to accommodate the mandibular cast. The cast has been pushed to the base of the flask and the stone has been brought up around the posterior portion of the cast. No undercuts are present.

Figure 15   A plaster separator is painted on the first stage stone.

Figure 16   The upper half of the flask is put into place and the flask is checked to be sure that the teeth do not protrude above the top of the flask.

Figure 17   The second mix of stone is flowed to place. The flask is resting on a vibrator to be sure that the stone reaches all crevices around the teeth. There will be less likelihood of bubbles forming if the wax denture is first painted with a surface tension-reducing agent.

Figure 18   The stone is vibrated until the teeth are covered.

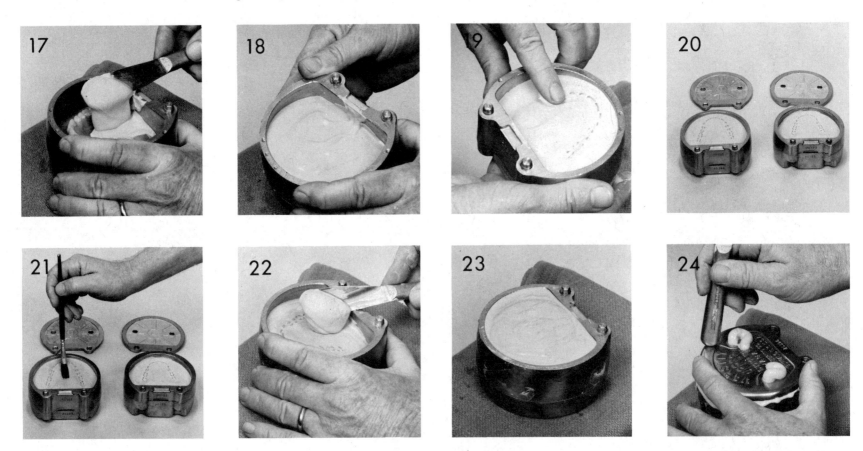

Figure 19   The stone is wiped off the occlusal surface of the teeth leaving the teeth exposed. The stone is allowed to set.

Figure 20   The second stage of the flasking has been completed for the maxillary and mandibular dentures.

Figure 21   A plaster separating medium is painted on the surface of the second stage stone.

Figure 22   A mix of stone is placed in the top half of the flask. This is referred to as the capping.

Figure 23   The flask is slightly over-filled.

Figure 24   The lid is placed on the flask and is tapped firmly to place. Excess stone will exude through the holes in the lid and around the edges. This stone is not removed until it has set.

Figure 25   The flasking of the maxillary and mandibular dentures is complete.

Now that the dentures have been flasked, the wax must be eliminated to form a mold into which resin may be packed. This is done by placing the flask in hot water, which softens the wax. The flask is then opened and the wax is flushed out. This is not done until the flasking stone has set.

Figure 26   This is a typical boil-out tank. A good boil-out tank is

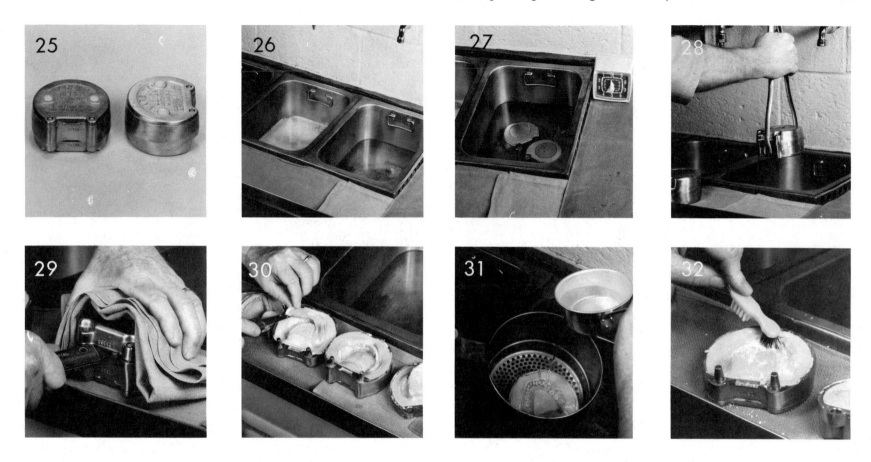

constructed so that at least one tank contains clean boiling water at all times.

Figure 27   The time required for melting wax in a flask depends upon the size of the flask and the temperature of the water. If the water is at a rolling boil, four minutes is sufficient time to soften wax in an average sized flask. Some boil-out tanks have a tank in which the water is maintained at 135°F. which softens but does not melt the wax. With this type of equipment, the flask may be left in the 135°F. water indefinitely without melting the wax.

Figure 28   After four minutes the flasks are removed from the boiling water.

Figure 29   The blunt end of a plaster knife is used to separate the flask. It is placed in the slot in the posterior portion of the flask and the flask is gently pried apart.

Figure 30   The flasks are opened and the baseplates and softened wax are peeled from the mold.

Figure 31   A dipper with a hole cut in the bottom is used to flush the mold. By having a hole in the bottom of the dipper, clean water is allowed to run over the flask. If some wax is present, it will remain on the top of the water and not contaminate the mold.

Figure 32   A detergent or wax solvent is used to scrub the mold. The

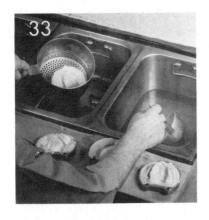
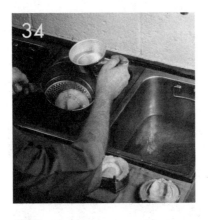
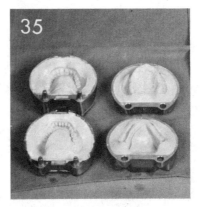
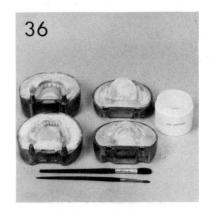

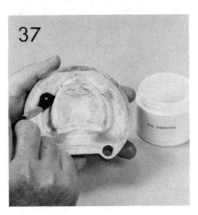
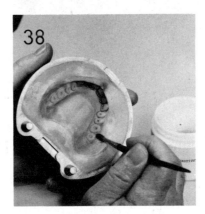
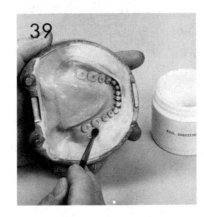
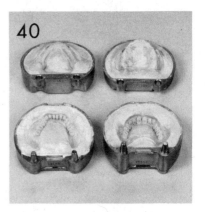

mold should be thoroughly scrubbed with a brush which reaches into all the recesses of the mold.

Figures 33 and 34   Water is taken from the clean tank to flush the mold. Note that the water is being allowed to run into the second tank containing the dirty water.

Figure 35   The maxillary and mandibular molds are clean and ready to be coated with tinfoil substitute.

Figure 36   Tinfoil substitute must be painted over the complete mold surface to prevent the resin from adhering to the stone. A large brush may be used to cover the cast and the open areas of the upper half of the flask. A small brush is used to carry the tinfoil substitute around the

teeth. Avoid covering the teeth or a small void will be present around the teeth in the completed denture. The void will stain in the mouth and result in a black line around the teeth.

Figure 37   The tinfoil substitute is applied to the maxillary cast.

Figure 38   A smaller brush is used to apply the tinfoil substitute around the teeth.

Figure 39   Similar procedures are followed on the mandibular mold.

Figure 40   The maxillary and mandibular molds have been coated with tinfoil substitute and are now ready for packing the denture resin.

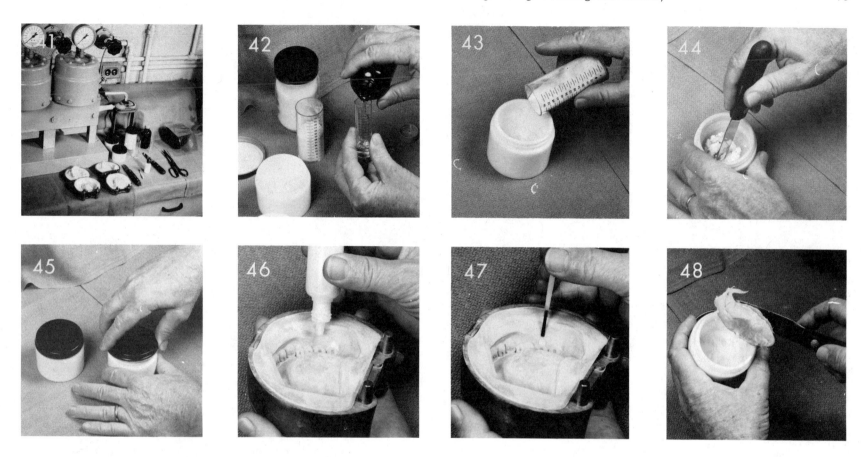

Figure 41   This is a typical packing bench in a dental laboratory. The largest item of equipment is a pneumatic press. The materials and equipment for packing are laid on the bench ready for use.

Figure 42   The monomer and polymer are measured in graduates following the manufacturer's instructions.

Figure 43   The monomer is placed in a mixing jar and the polymer is then sprinkled into it to insure that each particle of the polymer is wet with the monomer.

Figure 44   The mixture is then spatulated for a few seconds to insure that there are no clumps of powder which have not been wet with the monomer.

Figure 45   The mixing jars are covered to prevent evaporation of the monomer.

Figure 46   One method of characterizing, or making denture bases look more lifelike, is to place a little light colored acrylic made for this purpose over the neck of each tooth. This results in a lighted area of the gingiva which gives a pleasing appearance to the denture.

Figure 47   These small mounds of white polymer are then wet with monomer. This procedure does not have to be done over every tooth as too much uniformity will give the denture an artificial appearance.

Figure 48   Most denture resins reach proper packing consistency in two or three minutes. Proper consistency is usually indicated when the resin separates with a "snap" when pulled apart. However, read the

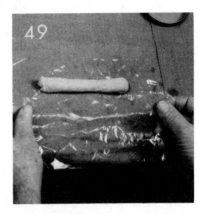 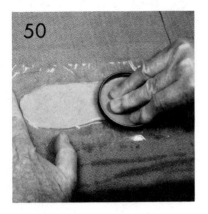 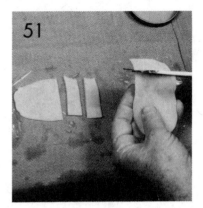 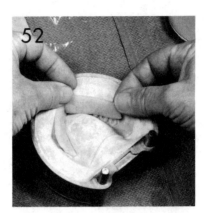

instructions accompanying the resin material to check mixing and packing procedures.

Precautions must be taken to avoid excessive skin contact with methyl methacrylate monomer or uncured resin mixtures. An allergy or contact dermatitis may develop which may be severe enough to prevent a technician from handling these materials. The cured material or polymer does not have the potential for causing these conditions.

Figure 49   Another way to make a denture base more lifelike is to be sure that all the fibers in a fibered material run in one direction. The fibers are aligned by rolling the denture material into a sausage shaped roll.

Figure 50   The roll is then placed between two sheets of wet cellophane and is flattened.

Figure 51   The flattened denture material is cut into pieces of a suitable size for packing.

Figure 52   The pieces of denture resin are placed in the flask in such a way that the fibers in the material run in the same direction as the long axes of the teeth. Additional pieces of resin are placed in the palatal area of the mold.

There are two basic methods of packing dentures. One is to initially underpack the mold and then apply increments of resin until the mold is filled. The flask is pressed or "test-packed" after each addition. In the

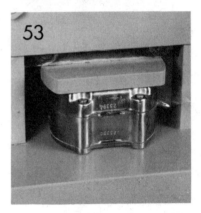 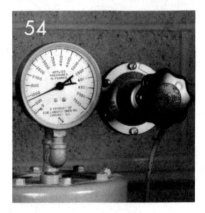

second method, the mold is overfilled. The excess is removed after each pressing of the flask until no more excess is evident.

A piece of wet cellophane or a dry polyethylene sheet is placed over the resin before the flask is assembled. This allows the flask to be reopened for inspection and resin can be added or removed without having the cast adhere to the tissue surface of the uncured resin.

Figure 53   The assembled flask is placed in the pneumatic press. Note the polyethylene sheet extending between the two halves of the flask.

Figure 54   When a pneumatic press is used, eight hundred pounds of pressure is sufficient for packing a denture. The pressure should never exceed two thousand pounds. Pressure should be applied gradually to allow the resin to flow within the mold.

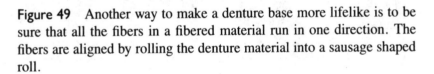

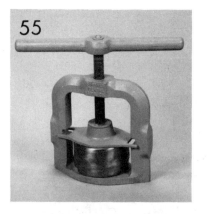

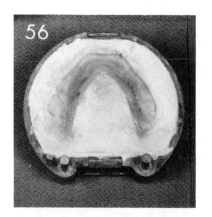

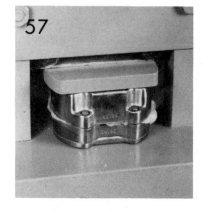

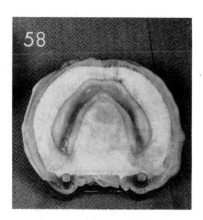

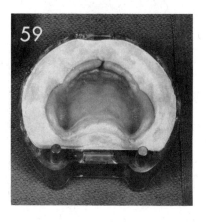

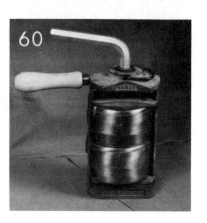

Figure 55   When a pneumatic press is not available, a hand bench press is satisfactory. When packing with a press of this variety, do not exert too much pressure. Light pressure at the ends of the handles is sufficient. Over ten thousand pounds per square inch can be exerted by a press of this type if it is tightened too much.

Figure 56   This mold was underfilled during the first trial pack. Note the appearance of the resin. Small increments of resin are added and trial packed until the mold is filled.

Figure 57   This flask was overfilled at the first trial pack. Note the excess exuding around the edges of the flask.

Figure 58   The flask is opened. Excess resin extends from the edge of

the flask. This excess must be trimmed so that no resin is beyond the border of the denture. This is done by using a sharp knife to make a cut next to the denture base and then removing the flash.

Often a technician overfilling a flask assumes that the mold is completely filled after the first trial pack. This is not always true. If the flask is closed too rapidly in the press, the cellophane or plastic sheet which is interposed between the cast and the upper half of the flask may prevent the denture resin from adapting to the cast surface. Proper inspection is necessary to be sure that the flask is filled properly.

Figure 59   The maxillary mold has been filled completely with denture resin and the excess removed. Note the fine detail present on the surface of the resin. A properly filled mold will be an exact negative of the cast and the resin will have a dense appearance. Several test closures are necessary to reach this stage. Failure to properly fill the mold will result in a porous denture which will require a remake.

Figure 60   After the mold is filled, the flask is re-assembled and pressed in the pneumatic press. Then the flasks are placed in a processing clamp and held in place by turning the hexagonal handle to close the clamp tightly. The wooden handle is used to hold the clamp while it is being tightened.

Figure 61   The flask-clamp assembly is then placed in a curing unit for processing. This is a Hanau Three-Stage Curing Unit which permits a three-temperature curing cycle to be used. Each stage is thermostatically controlled and timed automatically.

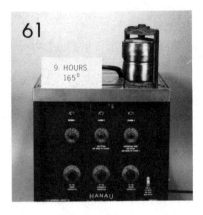
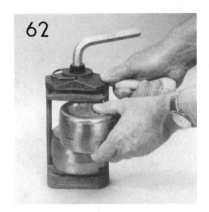
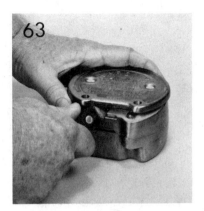
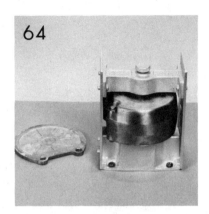

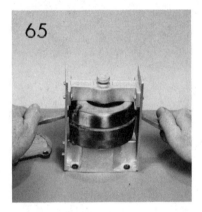
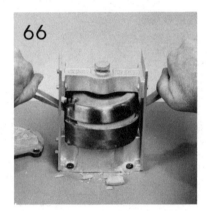

Most denture resins are cured by one of two methods, neither of which requires a three-stage cure. The preferred method is to cure the resin for nine hours at 165°F. No boiling is required. The second method requires that the resin be cured at 165°F. for one hour, and then boiled for half an hour. This alternate method may induce greater dimensional changes in the dentures than the slow-cure method. Check the manufacturer's instructions for curing times and temperatures.

Figure 62   After the dentures are cured, the flasks must cool to room temperature before they are removed from the clamp. They must cool slowly as rapid cooling induces dimensional changes in the denture base. When they have cooled, they are removed by loosening the clamp screw.

Figure 63   The lid of the flask is removed using a plaster knife.

Figure 64   The flask is placed into a flask ejector for removal of the flask. The screw on the top of the ejector is tightened to hold the flask in place.

Figure 65   The chisel-shaped ejecting tools are placed through the proper slots on the side of the ejector into the slots in the flask and pressed down. This lifts the bottom of the flask from the flask contents.

Figure 66   Reversing this procedure removes the top half of the flask.

Figure 67   The flask and its contents are removed from the ejector.

Note the raised base of the ejector which permits both parts of the flask to be removed without repositioning the flask.

Figure 68   An alternate method for removing the flask is to remove the lid and then to use a rawhide mallet to strike the knock-out plate on the bottom of the flask. The flask must be held in this manner when the rawhide mallet is used.

Figure 69   After the base of the flask is removed, the top half of the flask is removed.

Figure 70   The gypsum mold is now removed from the cured dentures and their casts. This is done carefully to avoid breaking any teeth. First the capping is removed using a plaster knife.

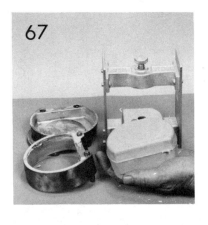
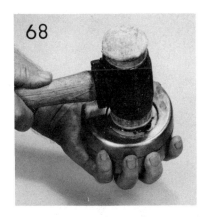
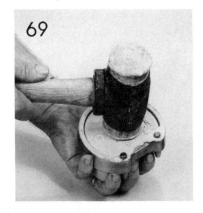
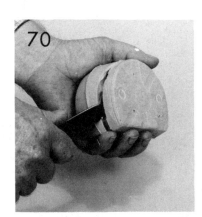

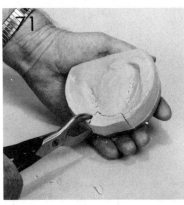
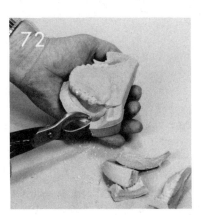
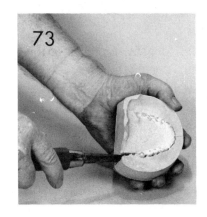
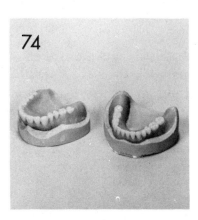

Figures 71 and 72 The stone around the denture is removed using a knife or a pair of plaster "nippers." This instrument conserves considerable time in deflasking, but must be used with care to avoid fracturing the cast. Note how the outline of the denture is shown by the position of the teeth. The easy removal of the capping makes deflasking much simpler.

Figure 73 An alternate method uses a pneumatic air hammer to remove the flasking. This instrument will speed the deflasking process, but *extreme* care must be used to avoid nicking the denture base or chipping teeth.

Figure 74 The cured dentures and their casts have been removed from the mold. Special care must be taken to insure that the casts are not

broken. They will be remounted on the articulator to remove the occlusal errors caused by dimensional changes of materials during flasking and curing. This remount procedure cannot be done in the laboratory if the casts are broken.

REVIEW QUESTIONS

1. What are the two basic methods of packing dentures?
2. List the four pieces of most denture flasks.
3. What are the three steps in flasking a denture?
4. During flasking, where is a plaster separator painted?
5. Describe two methods of packing dentures by the "open pack" method.

SECTION 12

Selective Grinding and Milling

Artificial teeth move about to a minor degree during festooning and while the wax denture base is being converted into resin. This tooth movement is due primarily to dimensional changes in the wax denture base, in the investing materials, and in the resin denture base during curing. Occlusal discrepancies caused by these dimensional changes ordinarily are removed before the dentures are polished.

Investing, packing and curing induce errors in the cured dentures. The setting expansion of the stone used to invest the dentures, slight movement of the teeth due to pressure during packing, and dimensional changes in the denture base resin during processing cause these errors. These processing errors, usually very small in magnitude, are removed before the dentures are delivered to the dentist.

The dentures and their casts are remounted on the articulator by means of the original plaster mounts and the indexes or mounting plates on the base of the casts. This procedure is called a laboratory remount. The processing errors are then removed by selective grinding.

Some dentists prefer a clinical remount. This is done after the dentures are polished, and uses new jaw relationship records made on the completed dentures. Clinical remounts are described in Section 14.

Selective grinding is defined as "modification of the occlusal forms of the teeth by grinding at selected places to improve function." (CCDT) A plan must be followed so that the portions of the teeth maintaining centric occlusion will not be destroyed. In selective grind-

ing, one cannot simply "grind the blue spots," but you must know which spots to grind, and in what sequence.

The amount of selective grinding which will be required to achieve good centric occlusion and free excursive movements depends upon the care which has been taken during the arrangement of teeth, and during investing and packing. Sloppy technique in any of these stages will result in excessive grinding which destroys the occlusal forms of the teeth.

After the teeth are selectively ground, there are some small rough areas which are removed by a process called "milling." Milling is "the procedure of refining or perfecting the occlusion of removable partial or complete dentures by placing abrasives between their occluding surfaces while the dentures make contact in the various excursions on the articulator." (CCDT) The cusps maintaining centric occlusion, the maxillary lingual and mandibular facial cusps, contact twice as much as the other cusps during the milling procedure. Milling must be limited to avoid reducing these cusps.

Milling paste used for porcelain teeth is a composition of glycerin and fine Carborundum. This formula does not work well with plastic teeth, and special milling pastes containing different abrasives are available for plastic teeth.

Figures 1 and 2 The casts which have been removed from the investment are cleaned and returned to the plaster mounts. If mounting plates have not been used, extreme care must be observed to be certain that

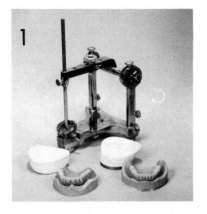
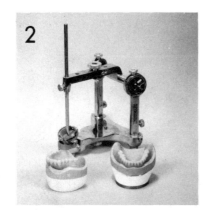
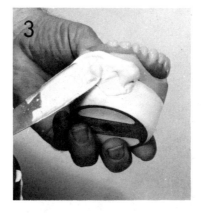
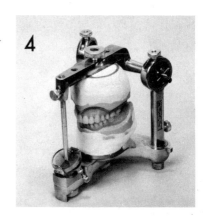

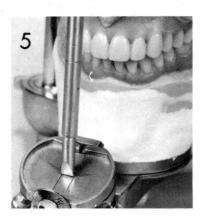
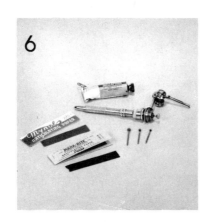
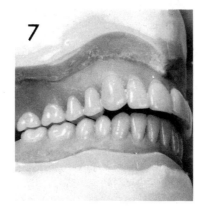
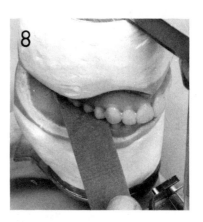

the casts fit the plaster mounts accurately. Inaccuracy at this stage will result in errors when the dentures are inserted in the patient's mouth.

Figure 3 The casts are attached to the plaster mounts by placing impression plaster around the junction between the cast and the plaster mount. Impression plaster maintains a better bond and is quicker and easier to use than sticky wax.

Figure 4 The casts and their plaster mounts are returned to the articulator. Use the same articulator as each articulator may have small variations.

Figure 5 The incisal pin of the articulator does not contact the incisal guide table when the dentures are remounted. Usually there will be 1 to

1½ mm. of pin opening if the proper techniques have been followed throughout the investing and packing procedures. Excessive pin opening is an indication that the flasks were not closed before the dentures were processed. If the pin touches, the dentures may have been underpacked.

Figure 6 The materials required for selective grinding are a dental handpiece, suitable stones, articulating paper (preferably red and blue), and milling paste.

Figure 7 The teeth are checked visually before articulating paper is inserted between them.

Figure 8 A piece of red articulating paper is inserted between the teeth

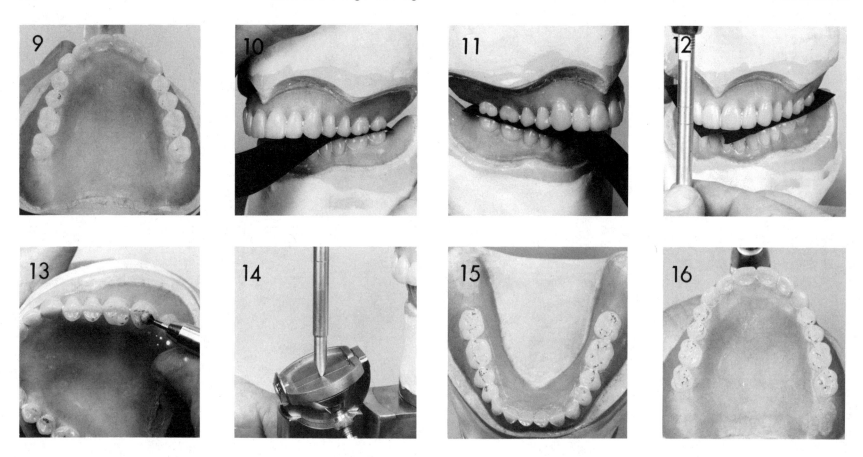

and they are tapped together gently but firmly. This is repeated on both sides.

At this time it must be emphasized that the articulator has to be handled correctly to insure that the teeth will follow the movements of the articulator. While checking for centric occlusion, the articulator must be locked in the centric position. When moving the articulator in subsequent steps, it must be handled as shown in the illustrations in Section 7.

Figure 9   This illustrates that the first contact occurs on the maxillary right second premolar and the maxillary left second molar. It must now be determined whether or not the maxillary or mandibular teeth will be ground.

Figures 10, 11 and 12   Blue articulating paper is next inserted between the teeth and the teeth are moved in lateral and protrusive excursions. It must now be determined whether the cusp or the opposing fossa should be relieved.

It is a relatively simple matter to make the foregoing determination. *If a cusp is high in centric and also in excursive movements, the cusp is ground. If the cusp is high in centric occlusion but is not high in excursive movements, then the opposing fossa must be ground.* It is particularly important to check balancing and protrusive movements before grinding is begun.

Figure 13   In this denture, the maxillary interferences are reduced, as these points are "high" in centric and excursive positions.

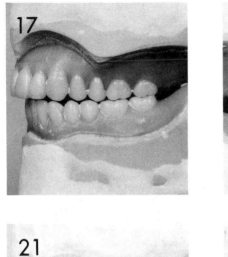
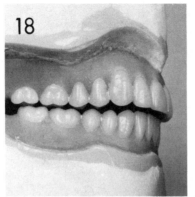
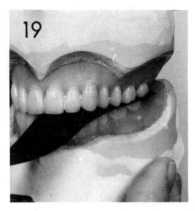
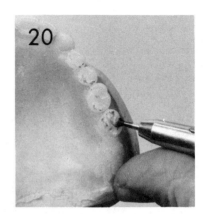
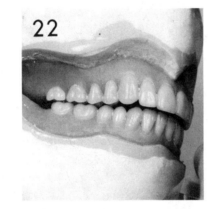
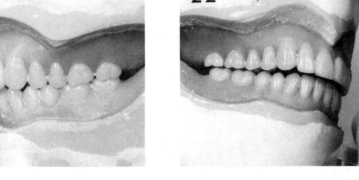

Figure 14 Centric occlusion is refined as described above until the pin touches the incisal guide table and the posterior teeth touch uniformly.

Figures 15 and 16 This illustrates the distribution of the markings which occur on the teeth after centric occlusion has been refined through selective grinding procedures. Note that the marks are distributed evenly throughout the teeth. This is the general pattern which is desired after centric occlusion has been refined.

Figures 17 and 18 When refining *excursive* movements by selective grinding, one excursion should be completed before proceeding to the next excursion. These two illustrations show that the left working (17) and right balancing (18) occlusions are checked simultaneously. You

can see that the teeth do not interdigitate as well on the working side as they did when the teeth were set. It must now be determined if premature contacts are present on the working side, the balancing side, or both. This is done visually and/or with articulating paper. On this denture it was determined visually that the first contact is on the working side.

Figure 19 Blue articulating paper is placed between the teeth and the articulator is moved as shown in Section 7. Be sure that the full lateral shift is incorporated into the movement of the articulator.

Figure 20 The blue spots which appear indicate premature contacts on the working side. The red marks remaining from the perfection of centric occlusion are still present so that these may be maintained during the grinding procedures.

In grinding *working occlusion*, the facial cusps of the maxillary teeth and the lingual cusps of the mandibular teeth may be ground without affecting centric occlusion.

In grinding the *balancing side*, a groove or sluiceway should be ground exactly where the balancing mark is made and is usually done on the mandibular tooth. This is shown in **Figure 26**.

Figures 21 and 22 The left working occlusion and right balancing occlusion have been selectively ground until the teeth contact properly. You can see that the teeth contact in much the same manner as they did when they were originally arranged.

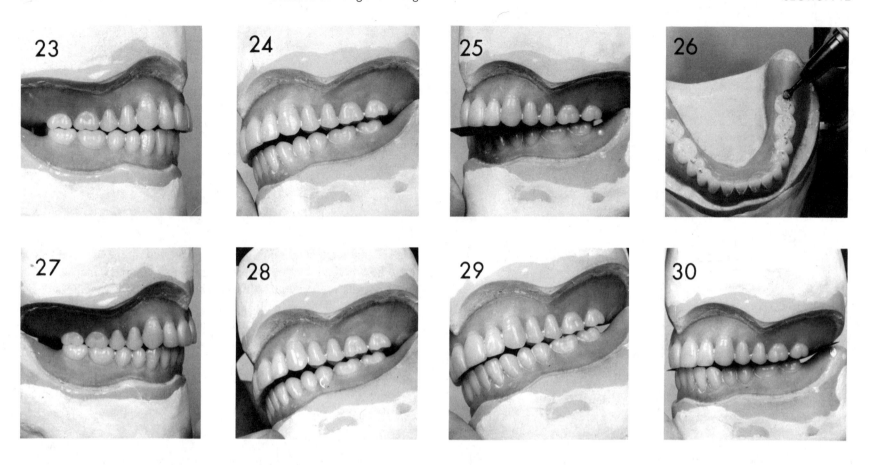

Figures 23 and 24 The same procedure is followed for perfecting the right working (**23**) and the left balancing (**24**) occlusion. On this denture visual inspection reveals that there is a premature balancing contact on the left second molars.

Figure 25 A piece of blue articulating paper is placed between the teeth and the articulator moved to mark the premature contact.

Figure 26 The premature contact is removed by grinding the mandibular tooth exactly where the prematurity is marked. When relieving for a balancing contact, the mark only must be relieved. Grinding of the surrounding tooth surface may result in loss of centric occlusion. By grinding the mandibular tooth only, centric occlusion will be maintained by the lingual cusp of the maxillary second molar. *When prema-*

ture contacts exist on both working and balancing sides, they are reduced concurrently.

Figures 27 and 28 *Smooth lateral excursive movements have been achieved in both lateral excursions.*

Figure 29 Next, the *protrusive relationship* is examined visually before placing articulating paper between the teeth. Visual inspection often reveals an excessive prematurity which may be relieved before using articulating paper.

Figure 30 Articulating paper is placed between the teeth and the articulator is moved in protrusive.

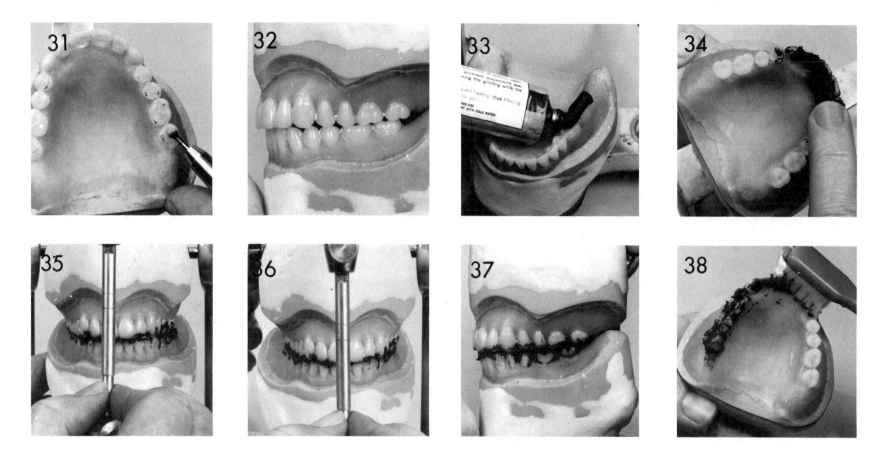

Figure 31 The premature contacts are removed. Care must be taken not to destroy centric occlusion or any of the cusps which maintain the lateral excursive movements. Usually the grinding for protrusive will take place on the distal incline of the upper facial cusps and a mesial incline of the mandibular lingual cusps.

Figure 32 The protrusive excursion is selectively ground until free movement is present.

Figure 33 Abrasive milling paste is spread on the occlusal and incisal surfaces of the teeth preparatory to milling. A good milling paste may be made from fine Carborundum grit and glycerin. These materials are available at hardware stores.

Figure 34 Additional milling paste is placed on the lingual surface of the maxillary incisors. A little water added to the surface of the milling paste makes milling easier.

Figures 35, 36 and 37 The movement of the articulator is important during milling. The teeth are placed in centric occlusion and moved into the excursive position. The upper member of the articulator is raised and brought back to the centric position. Thus, milling is done only from centric occlusion to the lateral or protrusive position, *not* on the return movement. The pin is raised from the incisal guide table during milling.

The articulator must be held firmly and the incisal pin moved so that the full lateral shift occurs in the condylar mechanism. (See Section 7) Milling is limited to 15 or 20 strokes in each excursive movement.

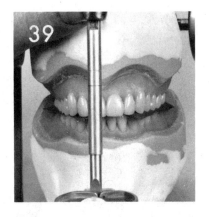

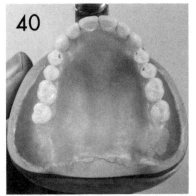

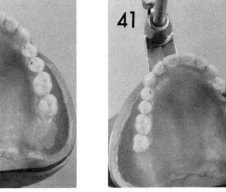

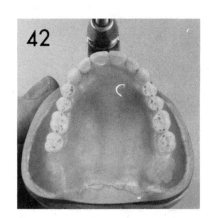

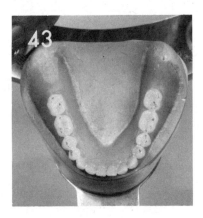

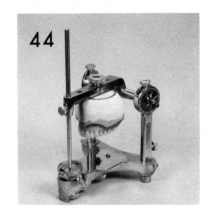

Figures 42 and 43   A minimum amount of grinding has restored good centric occlusion markings.

Selective grinding and milling are often neglected during the fabrication of complete dentures. Although no step may be ignored, the elimination of this step may lead to failure of the denture.

In Section 14 you will see how the dentures are remounted using new jaw relationship records from the patient's mouth. The procedure for selective grinding after a clinical remount is identical to that shown here, and reference should be made to this section after completing Section 14.

Figure 44   After the selective grinding is completed, an occlusal index is made. The purpose of this occlusal index is to preserve the face-bow mounting if and when a clinical remount is necessary.

The lower cast and plaster mount are removed from the articulator.

Figures 45 and 46   A remounting jig is mounted on the articulator in place of the mandibular cast. A mix of quick-set plaster is placed on the remounting jig.

Figure 47   The plaster is smoothed and the articulator, locked in centric position, is closed into the plaster. All that is necessary is a record of the occlusal surfaces of the teeth. If deeper indentations are made, it will be difficult to remove the upper denture from the occlusal record.

Figure 48   The plaster is allowed to set and the articulator is opened.

Milling is completed in one excursion before proceeding to the next; i.e., right lateral, left lateral, and then protrusive.

Figure 38   The milling paste is scrubbed off the teeth.

Figure 39   Even with minimum milling, some of the centric occlusion contacts may be lost. Therefore, the teeth are dried and centric occlusion is checked before the dentures are removed from the articulator.

Figure 40   Here it can be seen that the only spots touching are the areas on the premolars.

Figure 41   These spots are reduced *very lightly*. Usually a very slight relief will result in the return of all the centric occlusion markings.

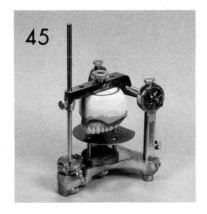 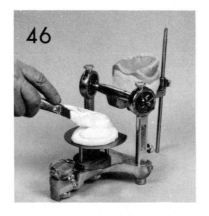 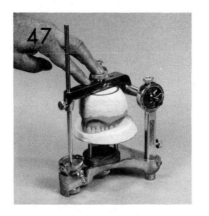 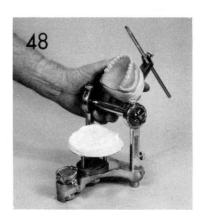

The dentures are now ready to be removed from their casts and polished.

REVIEW QUESTIONS

1. Why is selective grinding necessary after investing and packing dentures?
2. What is milling and how is it accomplished?
3. What determines whether a cusp or fossa is ground in selective grinding?
4. What is the purpose of an occlusal index and how is it made?
5. Where is selective grinding usually done to relieve premature contacts in protrusive relationship?

SECTION 13

Polishing

All dental restorations must be smooth to promote comfort and cleanliness. Polishing resin denture bases imparts a smooth surface without removing a significant amount of material.

After the selective grinding and milling are completed and the occlusal index is made, the casts are removed from the dentures which are then finished. Removing casts from dentures varies in difficulty depending upon the amount of undercut present. Usually the cast must be removed piece by piece from the denture. The dentures are then trimmed and polished.

POLISHING APPLIANCES WITH RESIN TEETH

Polishing a denture with resin teeth requires some precautions not necessary with porcelain teeth. Resin teeth have approximately the same hardness as the denture base. One slip with a pumice wheel may destroy resin teeth esthetically, functionally, or both. When resin teeth are used the wax denture base must be an *exact* duplicate of the completed denture. In addition, *all* wax must be removed from the teeth before they are flasked. When polishing, only the denture base, and not the teeth, is polished. Adhesive or electrician's tape may be placed over the teeth to prevent accidental mutilation of the teeth during polishing. (See Section 19, **Figure 69**.)

These precautions when using resin teeth will result in a more lifelike denture with retention of the anatomical carvings in the teeth.

REMOVING THE CAST FROM THE DENTURES

Figures 1 and 2   Strategic saw cuts are made in the cast with a plaster saw. They are placed so that the cast may be removed from the denture without breaking the denture or causing distortion.

Figure 3   A plaster knife is placed into the saw cut and the cast is gently fractured along the saw cut.

Figure 4   As the procedure continues, the cast is removed.

Figures 5 and 6   An alternate method is to use a pneumatic air hammer to remove the cast from the denture. This is a time saving device, but may be dangerous if it is not handled correctly. The cast must be removed in small pieces and care must be taken not to fracture the denture. Fracture may occur through the labial frenum. The last bit of stone in the labial area is removed carefully, either with the air hammer or with a knife.

Figure 7   The casts have been removed from the dentures and they are ready for finishing. Please note that the dentures at this stage are nearly the shape of the completed dentures. This illustrates the point made in Section 10 that a good wax-up saves time in finishing.

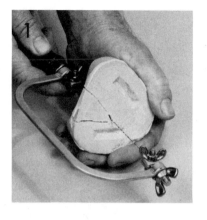
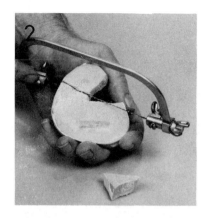
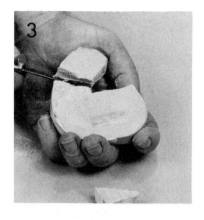
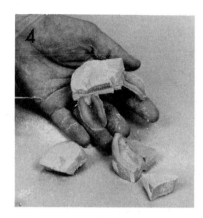

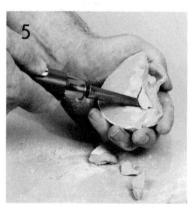
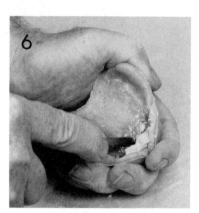
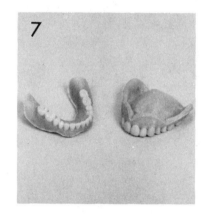
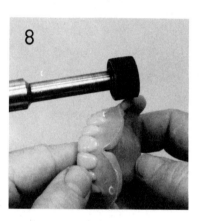

FINISHING AND POLISHING RESIN DENTURE BASES

Figure 8 The flash around the borders of the denture is removed with an arbor band on a lathe.

Figure 9 An alternate but less satisfactory method is to use a stone in a dental handpiece. A smaller stone, either in a lathe or handpiece is used to remove the flash from the lingual portion of the mandibular denture. A large acrylic bur may be used; however, bur marks are more difficult to remove during polishing than marks left by abrasive instruments.

Figure 10 Excess resin around the teeth is removed with a sharp instrument. This step is not necessary if *all* wax was removed from the teeth before processing. The instrument shown here is a carbide bur which has been sharpened to a chisel edge and is held in an instrument holder.

Figure 11 The flash has been removed from the borders of the dentures. The posterior area of the palate has been thinned to its proper thickness and the dentures are now ready for polishing.

Some technicians stone the entire surface of the denture before polishing. This is necessary if the surface of the investment was porous and blebs are present over the surface of the denture. It is not necessary if the dentures have a smooth surface.

Figure 12 Polishing is a process of removing scratches with finer scratches. The first step in polishing is to use pumice and a revolving wheel. Pumice is used as a wet slurry which is placed on the denture. In

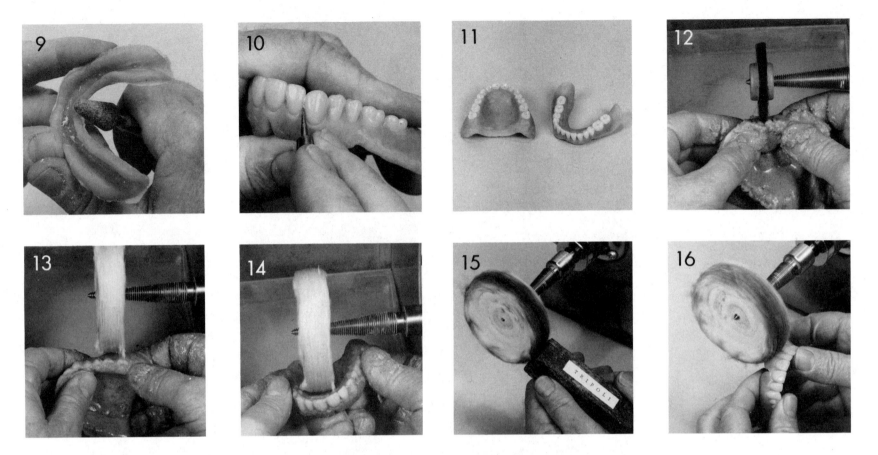

this illustration a brush wheel is being used to polish the interproximal areas between the teeth.

The tissue surface of a denture is never polished. Polishing destroys the details necessary for good fit and retention. The polished surface extends just over the borders, but the borders are not reduced in height or width during polishing.

Figures 13 and 14 A wet muslin buffing wheel is used to polish the border, lateral, and palatal surfaces of the denture. A similar procedure is followed with the mandibular denture. Felt cones or small buff wheels may be used to polish the palate. The choice of wheels or cones is dependent on the shape of the surface to be polished.

Care must be exercised when using pumice, as this material is very abrasive and may obliterate the details placed in the denture when they

were festooned. A well waxed denture will have a smooth surface and require little pumicing.

The denture is washed, dried and inspected to see that all scratches have been removed and the surface has a uniform appearance. Since each polishing agent consists of a different abrasive, different wheels must be used with each agent to prevent mixing of grit size on the same wheel.

Figures 15 and 16 The next stage in polishing is the use of tripoli. This material is applied to a dry muslin buffing wheel. This differs in that the polishing compound is applied to the wheel and not, as with pumice, to the piece of work being polished.

Figure 17 After the denture is completely polished with tripoli, it is

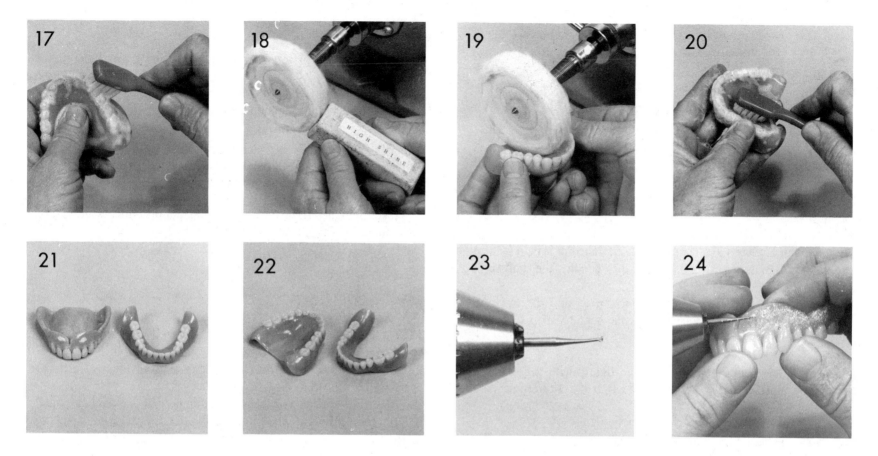

thoroughly scrubbed with soap or a detergent. Tripoli is a somewhat greasy material and must be removed from the denture before the final polishing.

After each stage of polishing the denture should be dried and inspected to make certain that all areas of the denture are polished completely to that particular stage.

Figures 18 and 19   Final polish is placed on the denture with a "high shine" material. There are numerous such materials on the market. They are basically materials composed of fine particles which impart a glossy surface to the work being polished. It is applied to a rag wheel in a similar manner as tripoli.

You will note that a different wheel is used for each polishing agent. A set of polishing wheels must be kept for each material to be polished

as well as each agent. There will be a set of wheels for use on resin denture base materials, and a set of wheels for gold. If base metal alloys are used, a third separate set of wheels must be maintained.

Figure 20   The denture is scrubbed and inspected.

Figures 21 and 22   The completed dentures. Note that the tissue surface of the dentures has not been polished or touched in any manner. The polished surface extends just over the border but not onto the tissue surface.

Figure 23   In Section 10 a method was described to stipple the wax denture base before investing. Sometimes it is necessary to stipple a resin denture base instead of doing it in the wax-up.

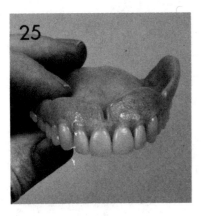 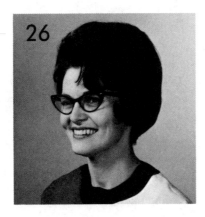

A bent bur is placed in a chuck on a lathe. The bur is bent by heating it red hot in a Bunsen burner flame and then bending the shaft slightly.

Figure 24 The lathe is rotated at slow speed and the bur is then allowed to "chatter" over the surface of the denture. This is done only in the areas specified by the dentist.

Figure 25 The denture is then polished lightly with tripoli and high shine. The stippled surface prevents reflection of light from the denture base.

Figure 26 Patient with completed dentures.

SUMMARY

The techniques which have been discussed in this and the previous twelve sections produce good dentures. The primary responsibility for pleasing the patient lies with the dentist, but it can be seen that the technician plays an important role in delivering a good product for the dentist to use in his treatment.

There are many variations in the techniques which have been shown. Some variations may be equal or superior to the techniques shown in this manual. However, shortcuts should be avoided which will diminish the quality of the end product. Quality workmanship and quality products result in better service for the dentist and his patients and enhance the reputation of the dental laboratory technician.

REVIEW QUESTIONS

1. State one procedure for protecting resin teeth during polishing of a denture.
2. Outline the steps in removing a denture from the cast after processing.
3. What is the sequence of agents used in polishing a denture base?
4. Why must different wheels be used with each polishing agent?
5. How can a denture base be stippled after the resin has been processed?

SECTION 14

Clinical Remounts

Occlusal errors may be removed by making corrections while the dentures are in the patient's mouth or by making new maxillomandibular relation records and replacing the dentures on an articulator. The latter method is more accurate because the dentures are seated on rigid bases, the errors are more easily seen and soft tissues and saliva do not interfere with selective grinding.

Often a dentist will wish to improve the occlusal relationships of his dentures after they are completed. This is done through the use of a clinical remount.

A clinical remount involves making new jaw relationship records, remounting the dentures on the articulator by use of the records, and selectively grinding the teeth so that they harmonize with the correct jaw relationship.

Occlusal errors in new dentures result from clinical errors and/or laboratory errors. Clinical errors usually involve incorrect jaw relationship records. Laboratory errors are associated with mounting procedures; the casts may not be seated in the baseplates, the articulator may not be locked in centric position, the rings may be loose or the jaw relationship record may be distorted. Regardless of origin, minor errors may be removed by selective grinding after the dentures are remounted using new records. Larger errors may require the resetting of some teeth after the dentures are remounted.

Many dentists believe that dentures are significantly improved by a clinical remount at the time of delivery. The completed denture bases are more accurate than baseplates so that more accurate jaw relationship records are possible. Dentists who follow this philosophy may request that selective grinding not be done after processing but be delayed until the dentures are clinically remounted.

Figure 1 The dentures are returned to the laboratory with new interocclusal records. The centric relation record is interposed between the dentures and the protrusive record, used for adjusting the articulator, is set to one side. The records shown are made of plaster, but some dentists use the waxes available for this purpose.

Figure 2 The undercuts on the maxillary denture are blocked out using wet asbestos. Block out only the undercuts. Excessive blockout will result in the denture falling off the cast unnecessarily.

Figure 3 The maxillary denture is set into the occlusal index which was made before the dentures were polished. (See Section 12.) The articulator is locked in centric position and the rings are secured firmly to the articulator.

Figures 4 and 5 A mix of quick-set plaster is made and placed in the denture. The denture is attached to the upper bow of the articulator.

Figure 6 The undercuts in the mandibular denture are blocked out in a similar manner as shown in **Figure 2**. The mandibular denture is then set onto a patty of impression plaster so that a cast of the lower denture is made.

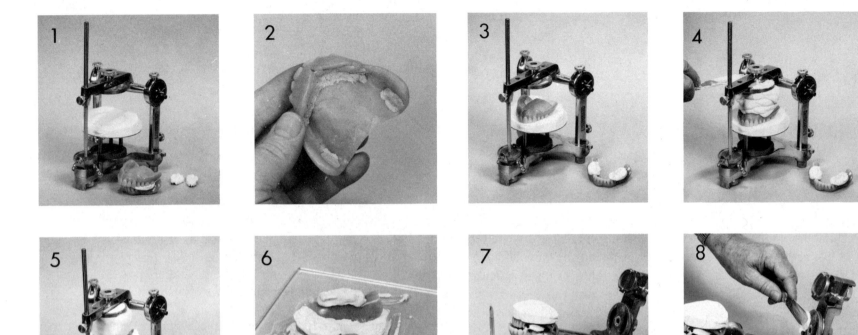

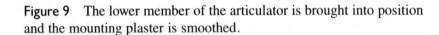

When using impression plaster to remount dentures, the whole procedure takes a short time. Usually the dentures can be replaced on the articulator as shown in this sequence of illustrations in less than ten minutes.

Figure 7 The maxillary and mandibular dentures, the mandibular with its own cast, are assembled on the articulator using the new centric relation record. They are held in position by small dabs of sticky wax. The upper bow of the articulator is supported in a Hanau plastering stand. *Be certain* that the articulator is locked in centric position and that the mounting rings are firmly attached.

Figure 8 Plaster is placed into the slots in the mounting ring and on the base of the mandibular cast.

Figure 9 The lower member of the articulator is brought into position and the mounting plaster is smoothed.

Figure 10 The mounting is complete.

Figure 11 The centric relation records are removed and the protrusive records are placed into position. Note that the pin is raised from the incisal guide table.

Figures 12 and 13 The condyles are adjusted to accept the protrusive record in the same manner as shown in Section 8, **Figures 10–13**. The mounting has been completed and the articulator adjusted to the new interocclusal records. The teeth are now ready to be selectively ground in exactly the same manner as shown in Section 12.

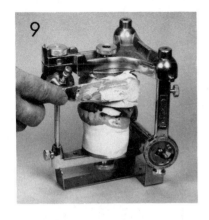
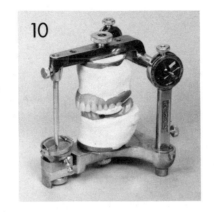
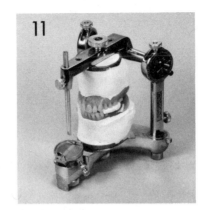
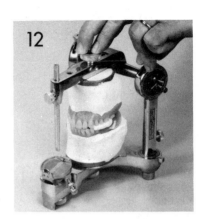

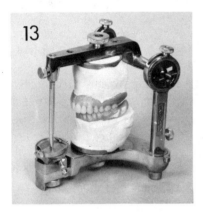

REVIEW QUESTIONS

1. What does a clinical remount involve and when is it accomplished?
2. Describe the procedure for a clinical remount in the laboratory.
3. What may cause occlusal errors in complete dentures?

SECTION 15

Vacuum and Pressure Forming Machines

Many uses have been found in the dental laboratory for air pressure and vacuum-forming machines which are similar to those widely used in the packaging industry. Impression trays, baseplates, surgical templates and mouth protectors for athletes are quickly made on these machines.

A group of machines are available which are used to make baseplates, custom trays, surgical templates (for immediate dentures), and mouth protectors for athletes. All machines in this category use preformed blanks of material, the type depending upon the use for which the appliance is intended. The blank or sheet of material is first heated in the machine and is then formed around the cast by either vacuum, air pressure, or a combination of both.

The machine shown in this section is a vacuum-forming machine. The use of this machine to make custom trays and baseplates is illustrated in this section. A similar procedure is followed for making mouth protectors and surgical templates. The only difference when making these appliances is the material used in the machine.

VACUUM-FORMED CUSTOM TRAYS

Figure 1 The cast is first prepared by blocking out any gross undercuts. The rugae area is also blocked out. Because of the heat to which the cast will be subjected, a special material must be used for block-out procedures with pressure and vacuum-forming machines.

Figure 2 A piece of clear plastic is attached to the crest of the ridge in the anterior region. This is a pattern for the handle of the tray.

Figure 3 This is a vacuum-forming machine and the material used to form the custom tray.

Figure 4 The material is placed in the holder. The blanks of material are of a uniform size and are supplied by the manufacturer of the machine.

Figure 5 This shows the structure of a vacuum-forming machine. The base of the machine holds a vacuum pump, the outlet of which is in the area of the cast. The back of the machine contains a heating unit which softens the material before the vacuum-forming is begun. In this illustration the sheet of material is being placed in the heating unit.

Other machines are much different in appearance but really are quite similar. They all consist of a material holder, a heater, and a vacuum pump.

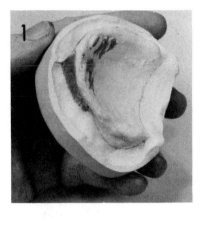 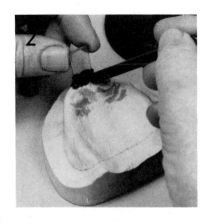 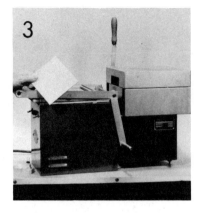 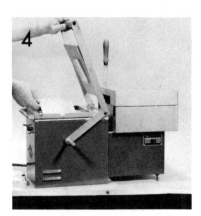

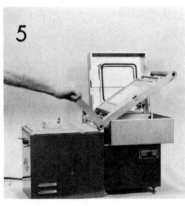 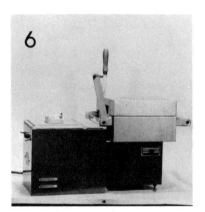 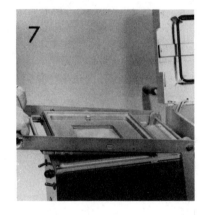 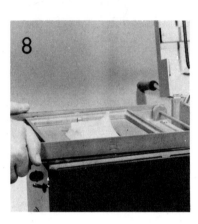

Figure 6   The material is heated for a specified period of time.

Figure 7   After the material is softened the heating unit is opened and the material in its holder is rotated toward the cast on the front of the machine. The vacuum pump is started just prior to this step so that a vacuum will be formed between the cast and the softened material as they come together.

Figure 8   The rack holding the soft material is pressed firmly to place to insure that a vacuum is developed between the cast and the softened material.

Figure 9   The vacuum pulls the material into close apposition with the

cast. The material is allowed to cool before it is removed from the machine to minimize distortion.

Figure 10   A coarse stone is used to cut the material around the edge of the cast. The excess is removed, and then the tray is removed from the cast.

Figure 11   The outline is marked on the tray.

Figure 12   The tray is trimmed to the outline. Refining the edge with an arbor band as shown in Section 13, **Figure 8** will produce a smooth border.

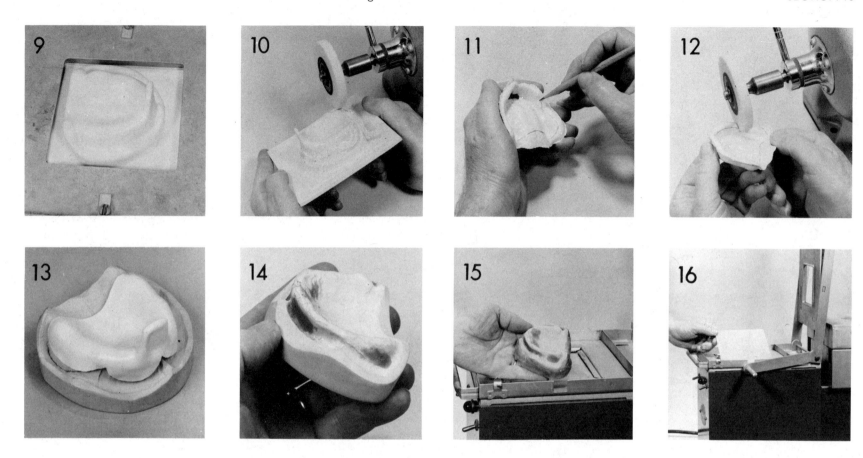

Figure 13   The completed tray is replaced on the cast. This technique works well for those dentists who do not require a spacer in their trays. A spacer may be made of wet asbestos but must be removed before delivery to the dentist.

VACUUM-FORMED BASEPLATES

Figure 14   In the previous section the preliminary cast was relieved for construction of a custom tray. When making baseplates the master cast must be relieved carefully but conservatively. Relief is provided as shown using heat resistant material.

Figure 15   The base of the cast is relieved to permit its removal from the excess resin baseplate material. This relief should extend at an angle so the base is not undercut.

Figure 16   The baseplate material is placed in the machine and heated.

Figure 17   After heating the material is rotated out of the heating unit.

Figure 18   The soft material is pressed down so that a vacuum forms between the cast and the baseplate material.

Figure 19   The vacuum pulls the material into close apposition with the cast.

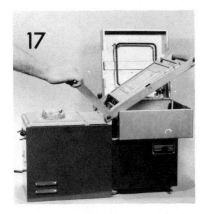
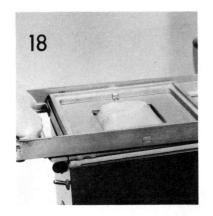
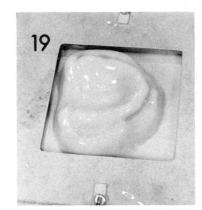
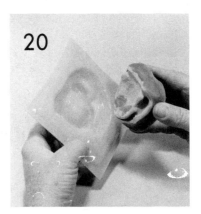

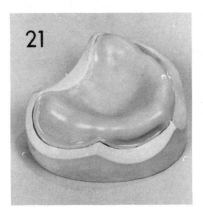

Figure 20   After the material has hardened the cast is withdrawn from the baseplate material. This illustrates the necessity for producing a flared base on the master cast.

Figure 21   The excess is cut from the baseplate and the edges are polished. This technique produces a stable baseplate, and is particularly adaptable to those casts which do not have deep undercuts. Maxillary and mandibular baseplates are made in the same manner. When mandibular baseplates or trays are being made, the vacuum may be increased by drilling a hole in the tongue space of the mandibular cast. More detail is achieved when the casts are no greater than ½ inch thick and are dry.

REVIEW QUESTIONS

1. Name four dental items that can be produced through the use of a vacuum-forming machine.
2. How is a cast prepared for use in a vacuum-forming machine?
3. Why is the plastic tray material allowed to cool in the machine before it is removed?

SECTION 16

Refitting Complete Dentures

Dentures become loose because the supporting structures change shape or shrink. Refitting is an economical method of restoring retention, stability and function to otherwise satisfactory dentures.

The tissues which support complete dentures are not as stable as the dentures themselves. The changes occurring in the soft and hard tissues eventually reach a point where dentures must be remade or refitted. Some dentists use a self-curing resin material within the denture. Most dentists prefer to make new impressions within the dentures and then have the dentures reprocessed. This results in a more permanent and hygienic result. Self-curing relines usually weaken the denture, while a processed reline does not affect its strength.

There are two basic procedures which may be followed in a dental laboratory when a refitting procedure is done. A *rebase* is "a process of refitting a denture by replacement of the denture base material without changing the occlusal relations of the teeth." (CCDT) A *reline* is the resurfacing of the "tissue side of a denture with new base material so that it will fit more accurately." (CCDT) In some places, the terms rebase and reline are used interchangeably, but rebase means replacing the entire base material, while reline implies an addition to the denture to correct the tissue surface.

The clinical procedure for either a rebase or a reline is essentially the same. The undercuts are removed from the denture base and new impressions are made while maintaining proper occlusal relationships. Some dentists do not relieve the undercuts when making impressions to

refit dentures. For this reason it is of primary importance for the technician to be informed of the impression technique which the dentist has used. If the undercuts are not removed by the dentist, it will be impossible to flask a denture directly for a reline.

LABORATORY PROCEDURES

The simplest method for relining a denture is to take the denture as it comes from the dental office, trim the excess impression material from the polished surface, and flask it directly. This procedure has the advantage of saving time. The disadvantages far outweigh the advantages. The procedure is messy, especially when zinc oxide impression material is used, and may only be done when all undercuts have been removed from the denture base before the impression is made. If undercuts are present, the cast will fracture when the flask is separated. The denture base will distort because of the heat necessary to soften the impression material within the flask. (The best way to warp a denture is to confine it, as in a flask, and then to raise its temperature above 165°F. This is exactly what must be done when a denture is flasked directly for a reline.)

A better method, the one shown in this section, is to pour a cast in the impression within the denture. The cast and denture are then mounted on a rigid jig to preserve the tooth-tissue relationships. The denture is then separated from the cast, the impression material removed, and the denture base altered as necessary. This gives the technician a great deal

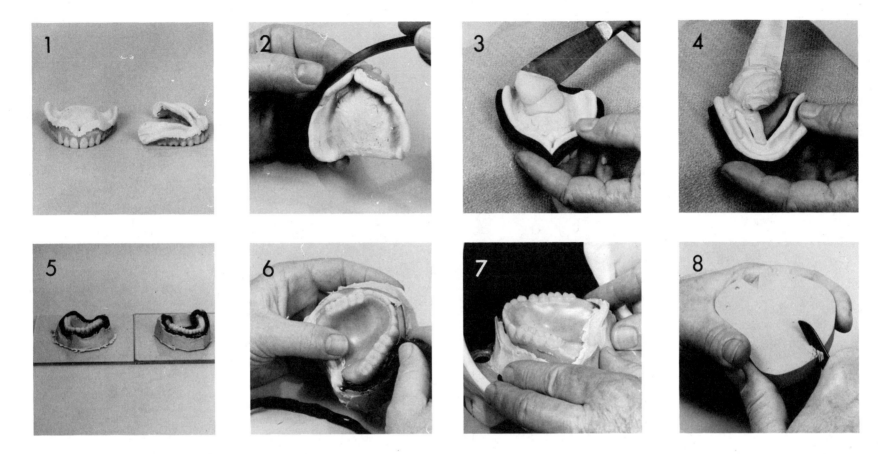

of flexibility in producing an excellent result. The advantages of this technique are that it is neater, small undercuts are no problem because the denture will slip off the cast easily as long as it is not confined, and there is less distortion. The only disadvantage to this technique is the extra time involved which should be compensated for in the fees charged the dentist.

USE OF A HOOPER DUPLICATOR

Figure 1 The dentures containing the reline impressions are sent to the laboratory.

Figures 2 through 5 The impressions are beaded or boxed and poured in the same manner as final impressions. The casts are allowed to set.

Figure 6 The beading wax is removed from the denture and the cast.

Figure 7 The cast is then trimmed on the cast-trimmer. The land area is trimmed in the same manner as was done for master casts for complete dentures.

Figure 8 Index notches are cut in the base of the cast.

Figures 9 and 10 The instrument shown is a Hooper Duplicator. It is a rigid jig which will maintain the relationship of the teeth to the cast.

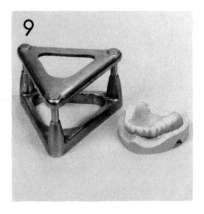 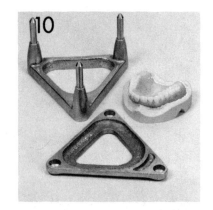 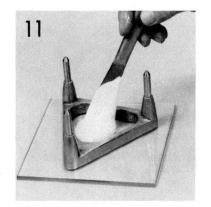 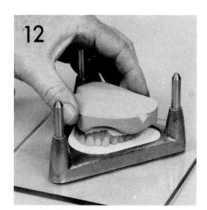

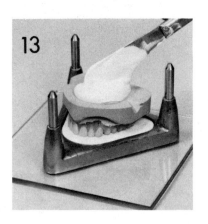 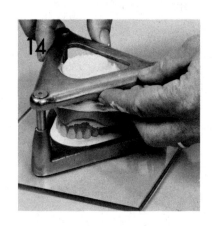 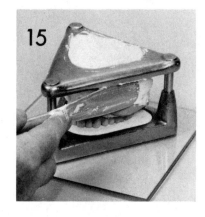 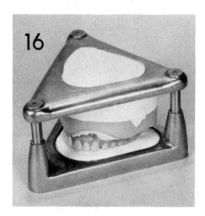

Figure 11   Impression plaster is mixed and is placed in the lower portion of the Hooper Duplicator.

Figure 12   The plaster is smoothed and the teeth are set into the plaster so that an occlusal index is formed. The teeth should penetrate the plaster two to three millimeters.

Figure 13   A second mix of impression plaster is made and is placed on the surface of the cast.

Figure 14   The top of the Hooper Duplicator is placed in position.

Figure 15   The plaster is smoothed on the top of the Hooper Duplicator and around the cast.

Figure 16   The mounting has been completed. The use of the Hooper Duplicator will maintain the relative position of the teeth to the cast surface after the denture is separated from the cast. The occlusal index of the teeth is of a sufficient depth that the teeth may be removed from the denture and a complete new base (rebase) made.

Figure 17   The top portion of the Hooper Duplicator is placed in hot water to soften the impression material so that the denture may be removed from the cast.

Figure 18   The denture is separated from the cast.

Figures 19 and 20   The impression material is removed from the denture.

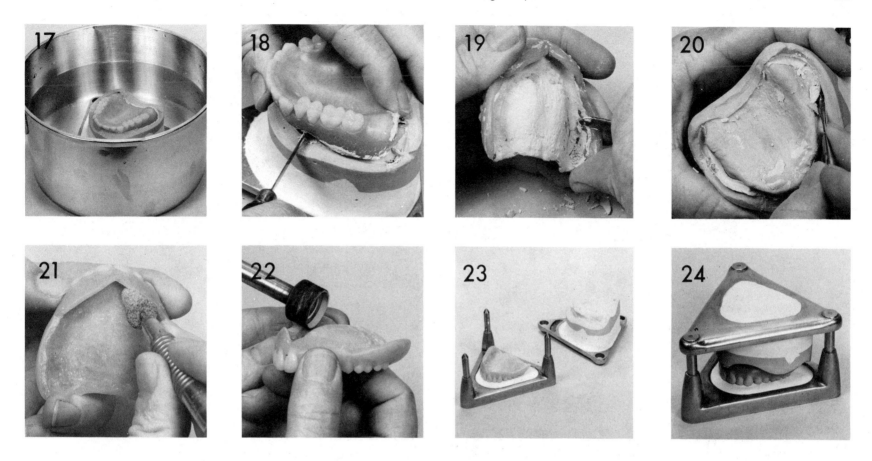

ture and from the cast. A blunt instrument is used to remove the impression material from the cast to avoid scarring the cast.

Figure 21   Any undercuts which remain in the denture base must be removed so that the flask will separate when the dentures are invested.

Figure 22   The border of the denture is beveled in the direction shown here. The purpose of this beveling is to permit the easier application of tinfoil substitute after the denture is invested. (See **Figure 64.**)

Figure 23   The denture is placed in the occlusal index on the Hooper Duplicator.

Figure 24   The Hooper Duplicator is then re-assembled.

Figure 25   This shows the Hooper Duplicator re-assembled with the denture in place. At this point, the denture may be waxed to the cast. No wax should extend onto the polished surface of the denture. The cast is then removed from the Hooper Duplicator and is invested in the usual manner.

VARIATIONS IN THE RELINE/REBASE PROCEDURE

Figures 26 and 27   Less dimensional change will occur in a maxillary reline when the palate is removed. Removing the palate permits the relined or rebased denture to have a palate of uniform thickness. Removal of the palate is one of many variations possible when a Hooper Duplicator or similar jig is used.

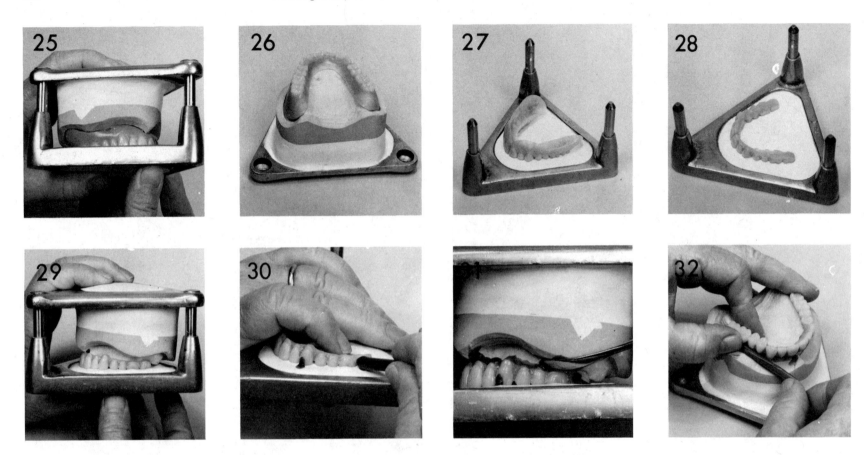

Figure 28   A rebase may be done by removing all of the denture base material from the teeth. When resin teeth are used, the teeth must be left in a horseshoe as is shown in this illustration. If porcelain teeth are used, they may be removed from the denture base by heating them with a waxing torch. This softens the resin around the teeth and permits their removal. The teeth are then placed individually into the index in the bottom of the Hooper Duplicator. However, leaving the teeth in a horseshoe of resin makes re-assembly and waxing easier.

Figure 29   The Hooper Duplicator is assembled to be sure there are no interferences between the teeth and the cast.

Figure 30   The teeth are tacked to the index with sticky wax.

Figure 31   The Hooper Duplicator is assembled and the teeth are sealed to the cast.

Figure 32   After the wax sealing the teeth to the cast has solidified, the Hooper Duplicator is separated. The teeth will adhere to the cast. Additional wax is then placed around the teeth to secure the teeth more firmly to the cast.

Figures 33 through 37   The new base is waxed in the same manner as a complete denture. The Hooper Duplicator is re-assembled to check the occlusal relationships before the cast is removed.

Figure 38   The cast is removed from the plaster mount on the Hooper

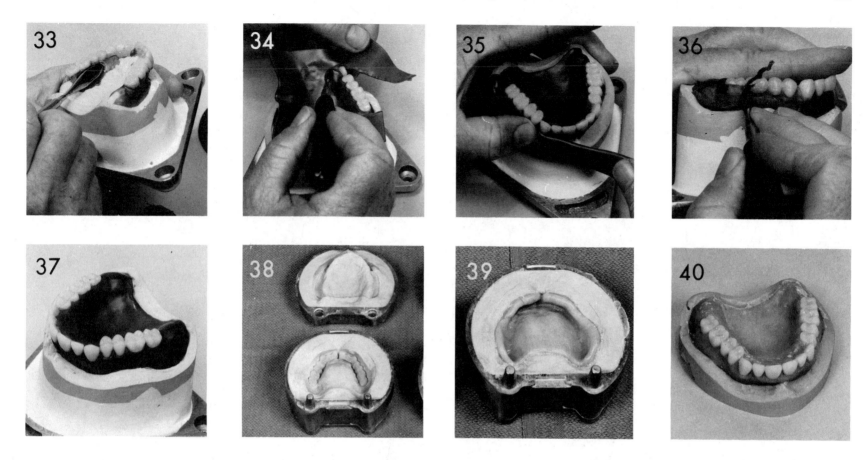

Duplicator and is invested in the usual manner. After the flask is separated and the wax flushed out, the mold is coated with tinfoil substitute in the same manner as it was for the complete denture. The mold is then ready for packing and processing.

Figure 39 The upper half of the flask is shown as it appears before the flask is closed. The same procedures are followed as used for packing complete dentures.

A long cure is used any time new resin is being added to old. In this denture, so little resin was left around the teeth that dimensional change is not a problem. However, as a rule, a flasked reline should never be subjected to temperatures over 165°F. During wax elimination, the flask is placed in 140 to 165°F. water for a prolonged period rather than leaving it in boiling water for a shorter period.

Figure 40 The rebased denture has been cured and recovered from the flask.

Figure 41 The cast is re-attached to the upper member of the Hooper Duplicator.

Figure 42 The upper and lower members of the Hooper Duplicator do not fit together accurately. This is due to the slight processing errors which accompany any processing technique. The processing errors may be removed before the relined or rebased denture is finished.

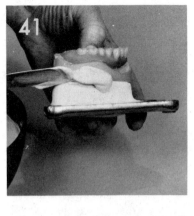
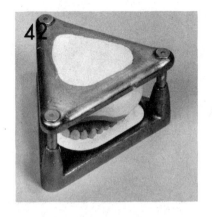
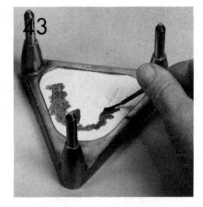
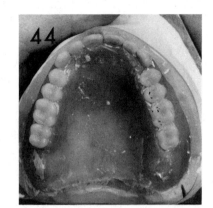

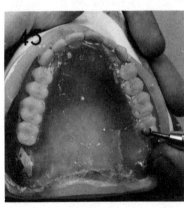
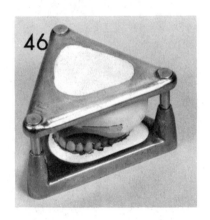
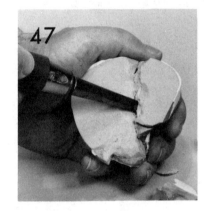
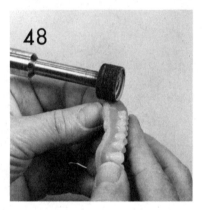

Figure 43   Tracing fluid, which essentially is the same as the marking fluid used by tool and dye makers, is painted onto the occlusal index.

Figure 44   The Hooper Duplicator is then re-assembled and the points on the teeth which make premature contact are marked.

Figure 45   These points are then relieved with suitable stones. This process may have to be repeated several times before the Hooper Duplicator fits together properly.

Figure 46   The processing errors have been removed and the Hooper Duplicator now fits together accurately. Note that the posts of the lower member are flush with the top of the upper member.

Figure 47   The cast is removed from the Hooper Duplicator, and is then removed from the denture.

Figure 48   The denture is trimmed and polished in the same manner as a complete denture.

Figure 49   The completed rebased denture.

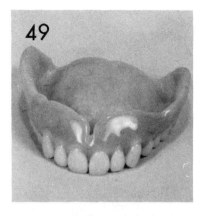
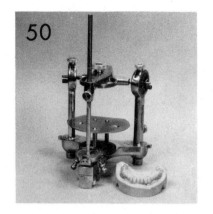
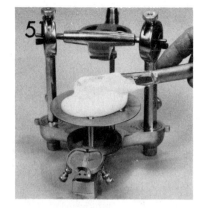
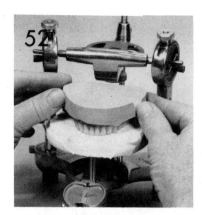
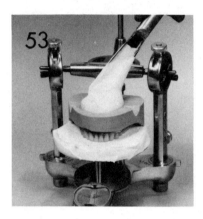
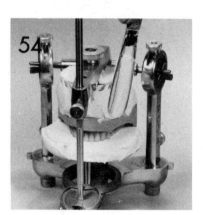
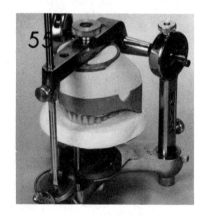
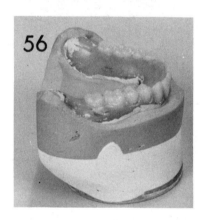

USE OF A HANAU ARTICULATOR IN LIEU OF A HOOPER DUPLICATOR

Figure 50 A Hanau articulator with a remounting jig in place makes a satisfactory instrument for relining dentures.

Figures 51 and 52 Impression plaster is placed on the remounting jig and an occlusal index is made by placing the teeth into the plaster.

Figures 53 and 54 After the plaster forming the occlusal index has set, the upper cast is mounted to the articulator. The articulator must be locked in centric position and the rings secured so that there is no movement except opening and closing. The incisal pin is fastened securely.

Figure 55 The denture is mounted on the Hanau articulator. We now have the same situation that we had when using a Hooper Duplicator. We have a rigid jig which will maintain the relationship of the teeth to the tissue surface.

Figure 56 The cast and its plaster mount are removed from the articulator.

Figure 57 Many mandibular dentures are undercut in the retromylohyoid region. A simple way to insure that this region will not cause fracture of the cast is to place a cut in the denture in the manner shown. This cut extends through the denture to the impression material.

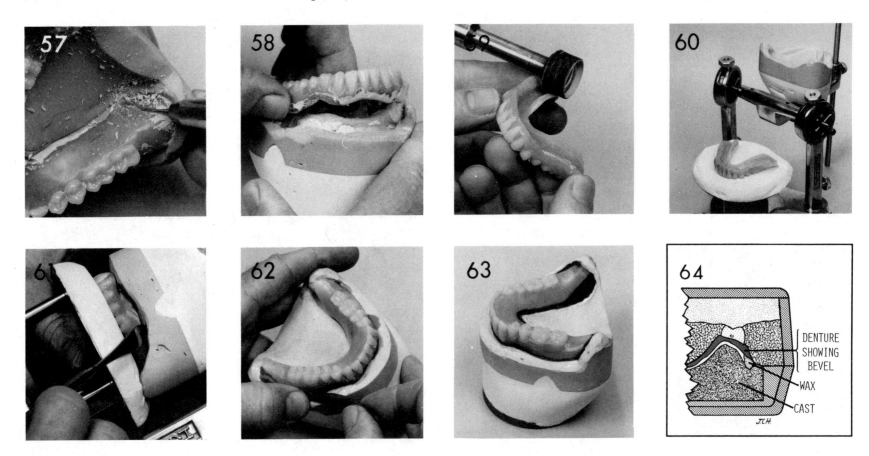

Figure 58 The cast and mounting are placed in hot water and the denture is removed from the cast. The denture and cast are cleaned.

Figure 59 All undercuts are removed from the denture and it is beveled as shown. Beveling permits proper application of tinfoil substitute when the denture is flasked.

Figure 60 The prepared denture is replaced in the occlusal index. At this stage, more of the denture base material may be removed from the denture, or a rebase may be done by removing all the teeth from the denture base and replacing them in the index. In this exercise a simple reline is accomplished.

Figure 61 The articulator is closed and the denture is sealed to the cast.

Figure 62 The cast is removed from the articulator and the borders of the denture are waxed.

Figure 63 The borders of the denture have been waxed and the retromylohyoid region has been replaced. Please note that the wax and the polished surface of the denture meet in a butt joint with no wax extending onto the polished surface.

Figure 64 This drawing emphasizes that the wax around a denture reline should form a butt joint with the polished surface of the denture. A film of wax which extends onto the denture base will form a crevice in the investment when the denture is flasked. It is impossible to paint tinfoil substitute into the crevice, with the result that new resin adheres to the denture and the investment, making separation and finishing difficult.

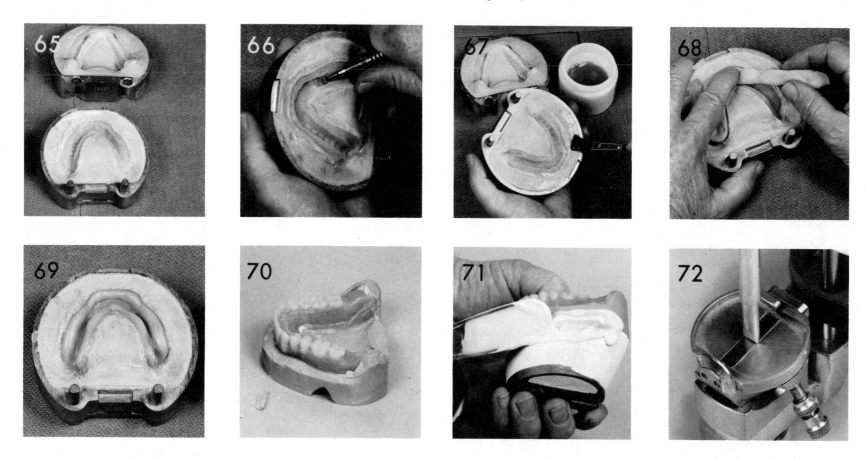

Figure 65   The denture is flasked in the ordinary manner and the wax is eliminated. *Again, it must be emphasized that in order to avoid distortion the denture base must not be heated over 165°F.* The cast portion of the flask may be rinsed in boiling water, but wax elimination should be done at 165°F. or below and the top part of the flask, that containing the denture, should be flushed with clean 140–165°F. water.

Figure 66   Some technicians like to freshen the surface of a reline before packing new acrylic.

Figure 67   Tinfoil substitute is applied to the mold, everywhere except over the denture resin. Do not allow the tinfoil substitute to contact the edge of the denture resin or a white line will be present in the completed reline.

Figure 68   New material, mixed according to the manufacturer's directions, is packed. The same procedures are used as were described in the section on flasking and packing (Section 11). The surface of the denture may be painted with monomer to insure a good bond between old and new resin.

Figure 69   The upper half of the flask is seen as it appears before flask closure. A denture reline must be cured at 165°F. for nine hours. A long, low temperature cure must be used rather than a shorter cure which includes boiling. If a faster cure is needed, it is best to cool the flask and use auto-polymerizing resin. *Under no circumstance should a denture reline be subjected to temperatures over 165°F.*

Figure 70   After curing, the denture and its cast are recovered from the flask.

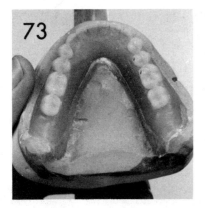
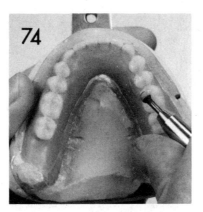
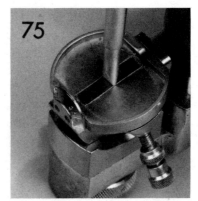
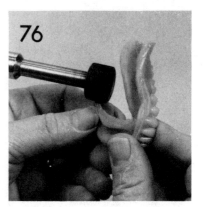

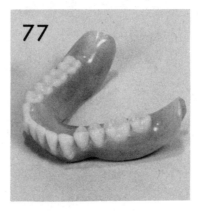
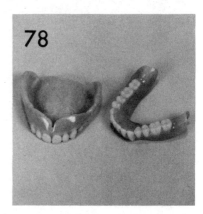

Figure 71   The denture is re-attached to the plaster mount.

Figure 72   The relined denture is checked back to the jig and a slight pin opening is noticed. Marking fluid is used to check for prematurities. (See **Figure 43**.)

Figure 73   This shows a prematurity on the right first molar.

Figure 74   The prematurity is relieved. This procedure may have to be repeated several times until the pin is closed.

Figure 75   The premature contacts have been relieved and the pin now touches the incisal table.

Figure 76   The denture is removed from the cast and is finished in the usual manner.

Figure 77   The reline procedure is now completed.

Figure 78   It is difficult to detect a relined denture if the same brand of resin is used for the reline as was used in the original denture. Even when a different resin is used for a relining, the accuracy will not be altered if proper techniques are followed. Some relines will show a line around a denture where the new resin is attached to the old. This line is usually caused by tinfoil substitute which inadvertently has been painted on the denture base resin before packing the new resin.

Both of the techniques which have been illustrated are essentially the same. In both techniques, a cast is poured into a denture containing an impression. The denture and cast are then mounted on a rigid jig, either a Hooper Duplicator (or similar instrument) or a Hanau articulator.

The rigid jig preserves the tooth-tissue relationship. After the denture is separated from its cast, any portion or all of the denture base may be removed. Thus, after mounting, the technician has many alternatives that may be followed to produce the best possible result. When a denture is flasked directly for relining, these alternate procedures are not possible.

REVIEW QUESTIONS

1. What is the difference between a reline and a rebase?
2. What are the advantages and disadvantages of directly flasking a denture containing a reline impression?
3. Describe the laboratory procedure for refitting a complete denture using a rigid jig.
4. What is the usual recommended curing time and temperature for a denture reline? Why is this important?
5. Why must the border of a denture to be relined be beveled?

SECTION 17

Repairs

Denture repairs probably do more good in less time than most any other dental procedure. The availability of rapid repairs is reassuring to denture-wearing individuals.

Methyl methacrylate denture base material has many advantages. It is easy to work with; the processing methods are simple; it has good color; it may be tinted; it is easy to polish; and it is easy to repair. A broken denture, which is useless to the patient, may be repaired speedily and easily so that it is again a useful prosthetic device.

When methyl methacrylate denture base materials were first introduced, repairs were made with heat-curing resin. Still, the technique was simpler than that used with vulcanite based dentures. Today self-curing repair materials make repairs even simpler. In addition, the use of the self-curing materials prevents the denture from being warped by overheating. The self-curing materials make a better repair and are simpler to use than the older heat-curing methods of repairing dentures.

The key to the repair of all fractured dentures is the accurate re-assembly of the broken parts. When the pieces are re-assembled accurately, the repaired denture will be as good as new. When they are not re-assembled properly, the denture will neither fit nor occlude properly.

Some repair techniques advocate the use of dovetails cut in each side of the fracture line. This is a holdover from the days of vulcanite when mechanical retention was necessary to repair the denture. Dovetails are not necessary because the self-curing material bonds chemically with the original denture base.

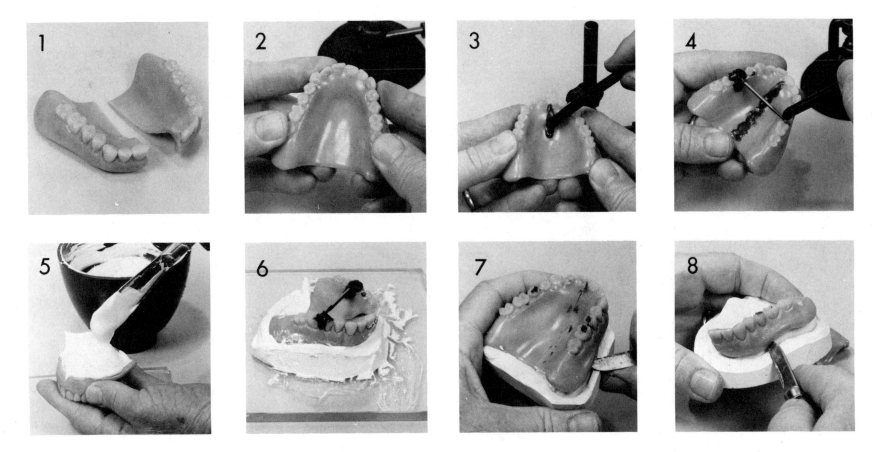

Figure 1 The fractured denture. Mid-line fractures such as this usually are due to poor fit or occlusal problems. If this is true, repairing the denture will alleviate the symptoms, but will not cure the cause. The dentist may have the denture repaired and then reline it to assure a better fit, or remount it to improve the occlusion. Mid-line fractures are often seen on a single maxillary denture against a natural mandibular dentition.

Figure 2 The two halves are assembled.

Figure 3 Sticky wax is applied to the fracture line to maintain the two pieces in correct apposition. Note that a second person is helping in this procedure. It is often necessary to have a helper when joining the pieces.

Cyanoacrylate glue may be used in lieu of sticky wax and reinforcing burs. (See section on cyanoacrylate cements at the end of this Section.)

Figure 4 The denture is reinforced by attaching one or more old burs to the occlusal surfaces of the teeth. A steel bur is better than a wooden stick for this purpose as a wooden stick may warp and cause distortion.

Figures 5 and 6 A cast is poured into the denture using quick-set plaster.

Figures 7 and 8 After the cast is set, it is trimmed and the pieces of the denture gently removed. Caution must be exercised so that the ridge areas of the cast are not broken.

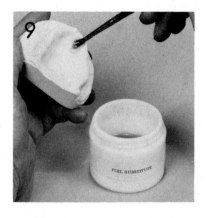

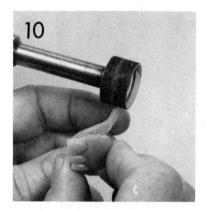

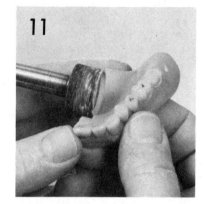

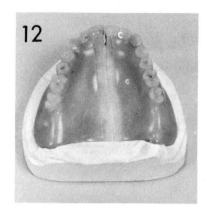

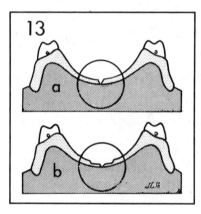

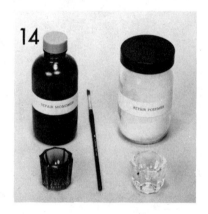

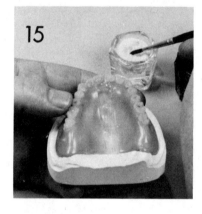

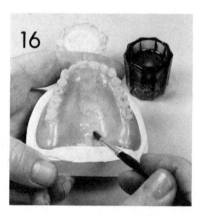

Figure 9   The cast is coated with tinfoil substitute and set aside to dry.

Figure 10   The edges of the fracture are beveled toward the polished surface using an arbor band on a lathe.

Figure 11   The polished surface of the fractured pieces is reduced to form a groove 8 to 10 millimeters wide along the fracture line. Four to 5 millimeters of the groove are on either side of the fracture line.

Figure 12   The pieces of the denture are re-assembled on the cast.

Figure 13   This drawing is a cross-section of a fractured denture prepared for repair: "a" shows the first step in preparation, the creation of a bevel toward the polished surface on each fragment; "b" shows the formation of the groove along the fracture line.

Figure 14   Self-curing repair material is used to repair the denture. Most manufacturers of denture base resins supply repair materials in the same shades as their regular denture base resins. An almost undetectable repair can be made by using the proper material.

Figures 15 and 16   Alternate applications of monomer and polymer are made until the area to be repaired is filled. The area should be slightly overfilled to allow for finishing.

Figure 17   The repair process may be hastened and porosity in the repair material prevented by using a pressure-curing unit. 100°F. water is placed in the curing unit so that it just covers the repaired area.

Figure 18   The curing unit is re-assembled.

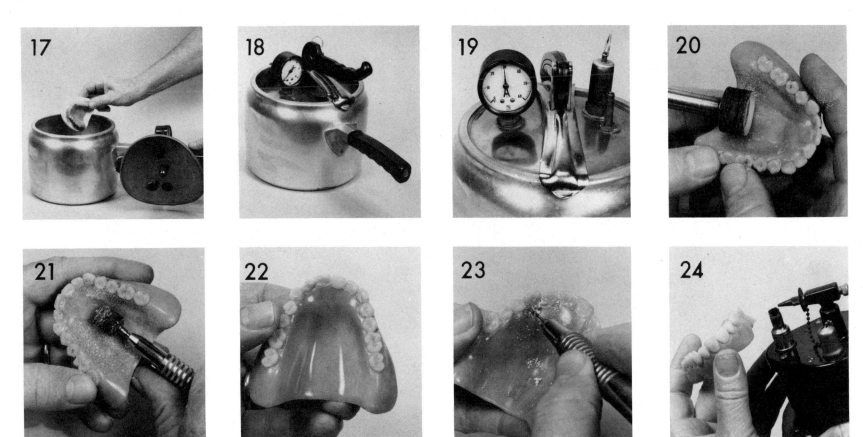

Figure 19   Compressed air is introduced into the curing unit until it contains 30 pounds per square inch pressure. The denture is left in the pressure-curing unit for a minimum of 10 minutes. These curing units are available commercially or may be adapted from inexpensive pressure cookers and parts available in hardware and automobile supply stores.

Figure 20   The denture is removed from the curing unit and removed from the cast. An arbor band is used to remove the excess repair material from the denture.

Figure 21   A small arbor band in a handpiece, or other small instruments are used in hard-to-reach areas. The repaired area is then polished in a conventional manner.

Figure 22   The completed repair.

REPLACING A TOOTH

Replacing a broken tooth is a simple task in a methyl methacrylate based denture. The following technique provides satisfactory results, although there are acceptable variations to this technique.

Figure 23   The area lingual to the fractured tooth is reduced using a fissure bur.

Figure 24   The fractured tooth is then heated with a needle-point flame. Heating the tooth softens the plastic surrounding it.

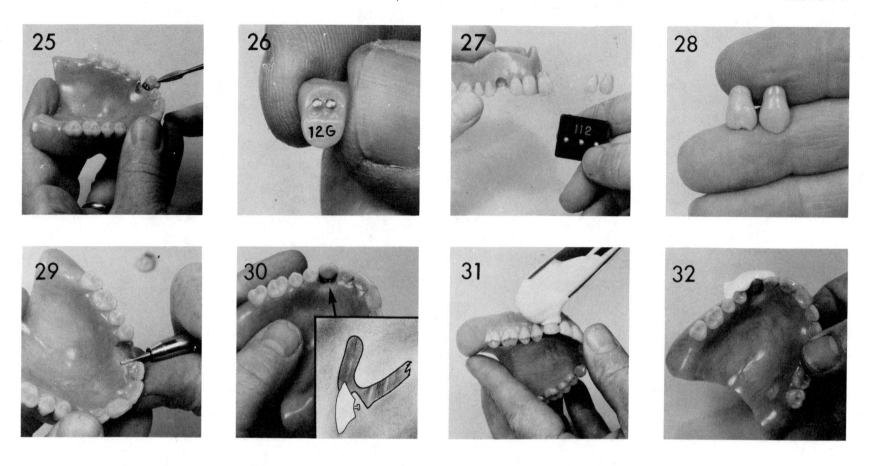

Figure 25   The tooth is pushed out of the denture with an instrument.

Figure 26   The mold of the tooth is determined by inspecting the ridge lap. The mold number is found on the ridge lap of most artificial teeth.

Figure 27   The shade is determined by using a shade guide.

Figure 28   A tooth identical to the one removed from the denture is selected.

Figure 29   The denture is prepared by removing the denture base material lingual to the socket left by the tooth. This reduction must be large enough to accommodate the pins on the tooth without interference. The facial portion of the tooth socket is left intact to aid in repositioning the new tooth.

Figure 30   The new tooth is placed in position.

Figure 31   A matrix of quick setting plaster is made of the facial surface of the new tooth and the adjacent teeth.

Figure 32   The matrix is allowed to set.

Figure 33   The matrix is removed and coated with tinfoil substitute.

Figure 34   The matrix and new tooth are re-assembled on the denture. Some sticky wax may be used to hold the assembly together.

   Note: When a resin (plastic) tooth is being replaced, roughen the surface of the ridge lap to assure a good bond with the repair material.

Figure 35   Self-curing repair material is used to attach the tooth.

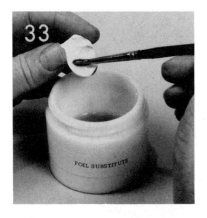
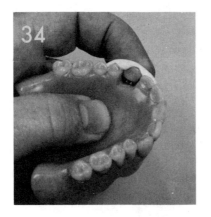
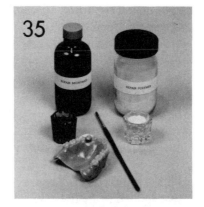
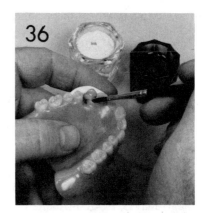

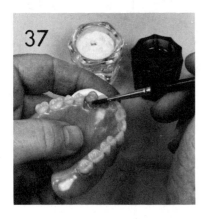
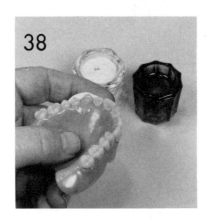
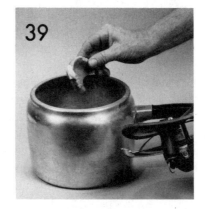
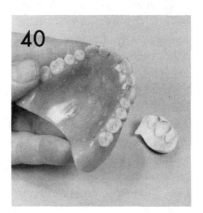

Figures 36, 37 and 38   Alternate applications of monomer and polymer are made until the area lingual to the replaced tooth is slightly over-filled.

Figure 39   The denture is placed in a pressure-curing unit containing 100°F. water. Thirty pounds of pressure are used and the repaired denture is left in the pressure-curing unit for a minimum of 10 minutes.

Figure 40   The denture is removed from the pressure-curing unit and the facial matrix is removed.

Figure 41   The excess repair material is removed with suitable instruments and the denture polished in the conventional manner.

Figures 42 and 43   The completed repair.

CYANOACRYLATE ADHESIVES

Cyanoacrylate adhesives are useful in several removable prosthodontic laboratory procedures but particularly with repairs. These adhesives are readily available in hardware, discount and variety stores as well as dental supply stores. They are sold in small tubes or vials under a variety of names such as Super Glue, Crazy Glue, etc. Some varieties sold in dental supply centers have different setting times although for most uses the usual fast-set type is preferred.

When fresh, these adhesives work very quickly and glue any surface together, even fingers. *Therefore, be careful when these materials are used.* Acetone will dissolve these adhesives so have some on hand in the event you do have an accident. Acetone will take a few minutes to dissolve the adhesive so be patient.

As implied above, these adhesives have a limited shelf-life. Discard the container when the adhesive takes more setting time than usual.

PROCEDURE FOR USE IN RESIN BASE REPAIRS

Cyanoacrylate adhesives make denture repairs simpler and quicker. With simple resin fractures, first determine if the fragments fit together; then practice putting them together.

The cyanoacrylate adhesive may be applied in two ways. The fragments may be held together and the adhesive applied to the fracture line and allowed to penetrate the fracture line by capillary action. This method requires an extra hand. The other method is to apply a small amount to the fracture line and then put the fragments together. With either method be right the first time since the adhesive works almost instantly.

After the fragments have been attached with the cyanoacrylate adhesive, the same procedures are followed as shown in **Figures 7 through 22**. The cyanoacrylate adhesives do not hold up well in the mouth so they are not suitable for permanent repairs.

Note: You may receive some appliances for repair where the patients have repeatedly attempted to repair their own appliances with one of these adhesives; usually this prevents you from accurately aligning the fragments and eliminates the possibility of a good repair.

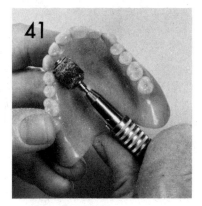
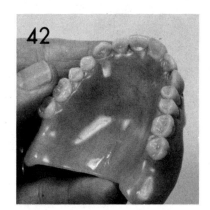
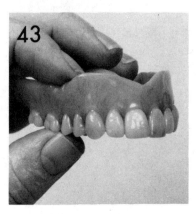

PROCEDURE FOR USE IN SINGLE TOOTH REPAIRS

Cyanoacrylate adhesives may be used in lieu of a plaster matrix, particularly if it is only necessary to reattach an existing tooth. After the denture base has been prepared as shown in **Figures 29 and 30**, a small drop of cyanoacrylate adhesive is applied to the tip of the ridge lap or edge of the tooth and it is placed in the denture. This retains the tooth while the resin is placed in the prepared area lingual to the tooth.

You may find instances where patients attempt to reattach a tooth to a denture base with repeated applications of some adhesive. Often, these accumulations can be removed and the tooth may be reattached properly.

Cyanoacrylate adhesives will help you in many ways. However, do *not* depend on these materials to be permanent; at most they will only last a few days in the mouth. These adhesives are only to be used to hold the pieces together while a proper repair is done.

COMPLICATED REPAIRS

Only lack of ingenuity will prevent you from making complicated repairs—within limits, of course. The following is an example of a repair using cyanoacrylate cements, a plaster cast and matrix, and some common sense.

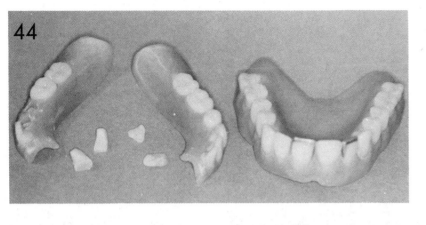

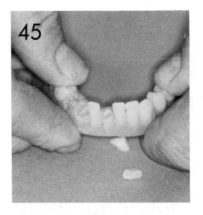

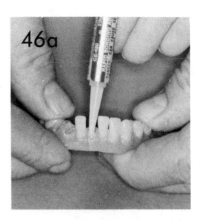

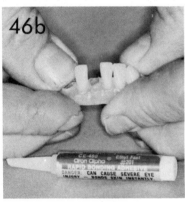

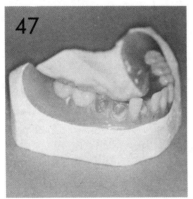

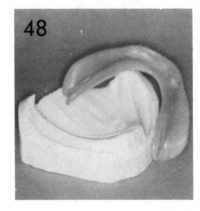

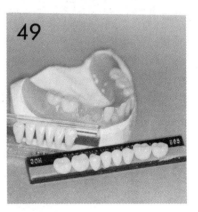

Figure 44 This mandibular denture has been fractured and three teeth have been lost. Note that the maxillary denture is available to the technician.

Figure 45 The fragments are checked to see that they fit together accurately.

Figure 46 a, b The fragments are glued together with cyanoacrylate adhesive. Note that the adhesive is being applied with a "third hand."

Figure 47 Impression plaster is used to make a cast.

Figure 48 The denture is separated from the cast. It is most important that the cast in the area of the fracture be accurate and complete.

Figure 49 New teeth are selected to replace those that were broken.

Figure 50 The area where the teeth are broken is enlarged so new teeth may be placed in the denture base.

Figure 51 The new teeth are waxed into position. It is not important to accurately wax the lingual surface; just seal the teeth in position.

Figure 52 The occlusion is checked with the maxillary denture. For this reason it is most convenient to have the opposing denture in your possession when making a repair.

Figure 53 The teeth are adjusted until they are in correct alignment with the adjacent teeth and the opposing denture.

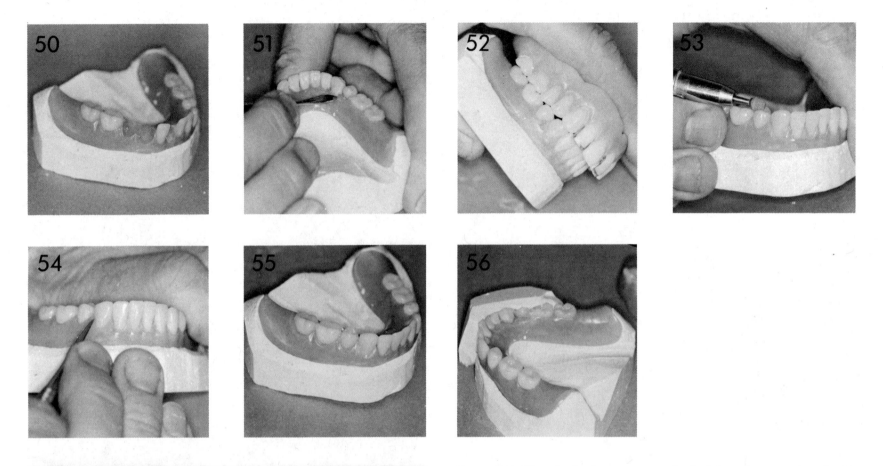

Figure 54   The gingival contours on the facial surface are placed with wax. This needs to be done accurately.

Figure 55   The completed gingival contours.

Figure 56   A plaster matrix is made on the facial surface. This is done by placing either plaster or stone over the facial surfaces of the teeth being replaced and the adjacent teeth. The incisal and occlusal surfaces should also be covered. After the plaster has set, it is removed and the excess removed.

Figure 57   The plaster matrix has been removed and trimmed.

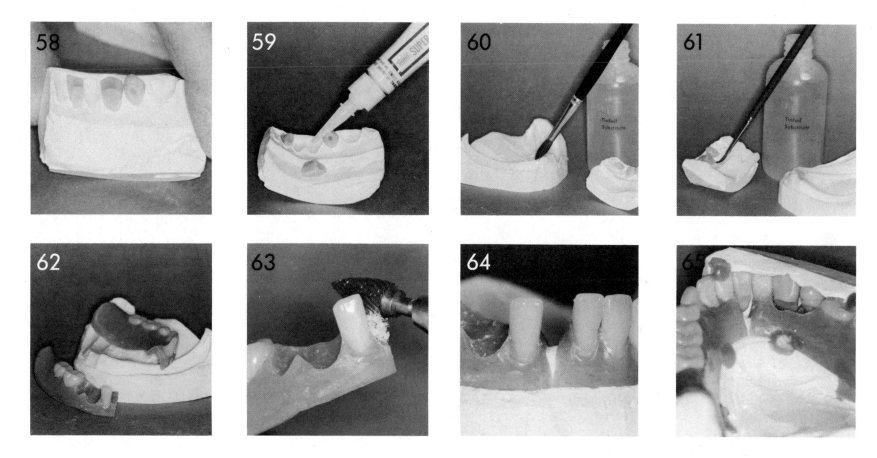

Figure 58   The teeth are cleaned and then placed in the plaster matrix.

Figure 59   If the teeth do not "snap" into the matrix, they may be attached to the matrix with a tiny drop of cyanoacrylate adhesive.

Figure 60   Tinfoil substitute is applied to the cast in the area of the fracture.

Figure 61   The surface of the matrix which will be contacted with new resin is painted with tinfoil substitute.

Figure 62   The matrix assembly is set aside. The denture is removed from the cast and "re-broken."

Figure 63   The surfaces of the fragments which will be contacted by new resin are cleaned and cut back. The object is to "open" the fracture area so new resin can be easily placed later. All traces of wax are removed.

Figure 64   The denture fragments are replaced on the cast. Note how the fracture line has been "opened."

Figure 65   The matrix assembly may be kept in place with, preferably, sticky wax or a small drop of cyanoacrylate adhesive.

Figure 66   Repair resin is placed in and around repair area. A thin mix of resin may be poured into this area or it may be placed with the

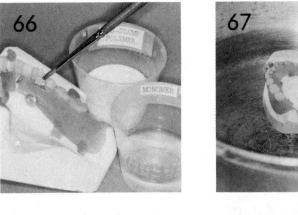
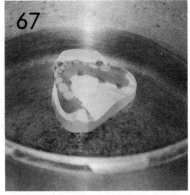
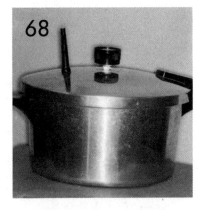
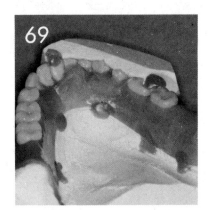

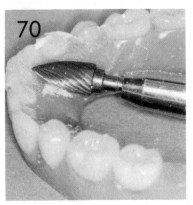
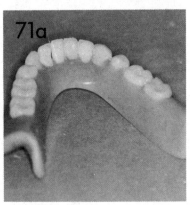
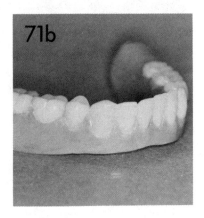

powder-liquid method shown here. A non-slumping viscous type resin is used so the repair area can be built to contour.

Figures 67 and 68   The repair assembly is placed in warm water in the pressure pot. The warm water hastens curing and the pressure prevents porosity in the new resin.

Figure 69   The repaired denture is removed from the pressure pot. The time in the pressure pot is determined by the type of resin and the water temperature.

Figure 70   The repaired denture is contoured on the lingual surface and then polished.

Figure 71 a, b   The repair is completed.

REVIEW QUESTIONS

1. What is the most important step in repairing a broken denture?
2. How can porosity be prevented when using autopolymerizing resins for denture repairs?
3. Describe the laboratory procedure in repairing a mid-line fracture of a maxillary denture.
4. How is a fractured porcelain tooth removed from a denture?
5. How may a cyanoacrylate adhesive be used in denture repair procedures?

SECTION 18

Immediate Dentures

Immediate dentures have saved many people from anguish, embarrassment and loss of income. A patient will rarely reject the opportunity to obtain an immediate replacement for anterior teeth which require extraction.

An immediate denture is "a removable dental prosthesis constructed for placement immediately after removal of natural teeth." (CCDT)

The clinical procedures for making immediate dentures are essentially the same as those involved in making regular (or remote) dentures. Some variations are necessary to work around the remaining natural teeth during impression and jaw relationship procedures.

The advantages of immediate dentures are: (1) a patient does not have an embarrassing edentulous period, (2) the denture acts as a splint to hasten healing, and (3) the contours of the lips and face can be maintained with an immediate denture. Although the patient cannot see how the teeth will appear in the wax stage, the primary disadvantage of an immediate denture is that the denture may need to be refitted sooner than if the teeth were extracted before denture construction.

Immediate dentures are not indicated when the teeth are so broken down or infected that it would be difficult to arrange the teeth in the proper position. Ordinarily, patients with mouths so diseased do not desire immediate dentures, but prefer to wait until their mouths have healed.

IMPRESSIONS FOR IMMEDIATE DENTURES

Many methods are advocated for making impressions for immediate dentures. Some techniques involve the use of two materials, a rigid material for the soft tissue portions and an elastic material for the remaining teeth. Some dentists use custom trays as illustrated here; some use stock trays. Any technique which delivers a complete impression of the tissues involved is acceptable.

LABORATORY PROCEDURES FOR IMMEDIATE DENTURES

The primary difference in immediate dentures in the eyes of the technician is the manner in which the anterior teeth are arranged. It is necessary to remove the stone teeth from the cast and to arrange the artificial teeth in the same position as the natural teeth. This may be done several ways, two of which are illustrated in this section. The first method is illustrated in **Figures 23 through 28**. In this technique the three anterior teeth on one side of the cast are removed and the ridge is trimmed to the anticipated contour of the healed ridge. Then the three artificial teeth are set using the remaining natural teeth as a guide. The opposite side is treated in a similar fashion. Thus, the ridge area is contoured in its final form before the denture is flasked for processing.

The second method requires that the remaining natural teeth be removed alternately. This method is illustrated in **Figures 29 through 36**. The advantage of this method is that it insures each tooth being set

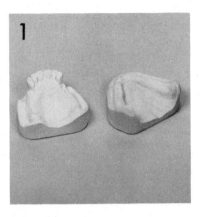
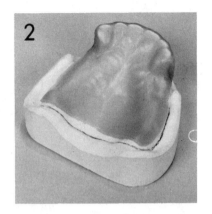
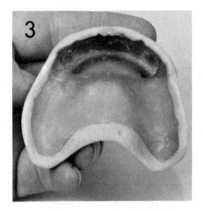
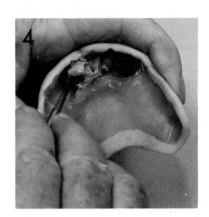

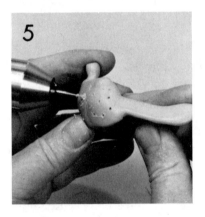
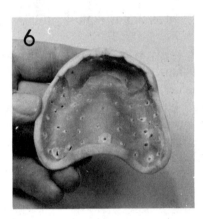

in its proper position. However, the cast must be trimmed further after it has been flasked.

Most dentists use a surgical template when removing teeth at the time of insertion of immediate dentures. This is a clear resin device which enables a dentist to be sure that no spicules of bone remain which might interfere with the insertion of the immediate denture. The surgical template may be made as shown in **Figures 39 through 45**, or with a pressure or vacuum forming machine. (Section 15)

Figure 1   Preliminary impressions are made with alginate impression material and the preliminary casts are poured in the usual manner.

Figure 2   The tray is outlined on the preliminary cast and a thickness of baseplate wax is adapted to the cast so that the wax is 1 to 2 millimeters short of the anticipated tray outline. The wax is removed from the incisal edges of the remaining teeth and is cut so that it is about 4 millimeters short of the posterior border of the anticipated tray outline.

Figure 3   The tray material is prepared and adapted in the same manner as for a complete denture impression tray. The immediate denture impression tray is shown after it has been removed from the cast and the borders trimmed to the predetermined outline.

Figure 4   Some dentists will wish to have all of the wax within the tray removed before it is delivered. Others will want to have only the wax in the area of the remaining teeth removed. When this is done, the tray may be seated accurately in the patient's mouth in order to check the borders. Before the impression is made, the wax spacer will be removed to provide room for the alginate impression material.

Figure 5   Holes are drilled in the tray with a number 6 or 8 round bur. These holes should be spaced approximately $\frac{3}{16}$ inch apart over the entire tray. These holes are not necessary if an adhesive is used to retain the elastic impression material.

Figures 6 and 7   The tray is now ready to be delivered to the dentist. The dentist will check the tray in the mouth and then remove the remaining wax spacer before making the final impression.

Figure 8   This cross section shows a tray with the facial flange improp-

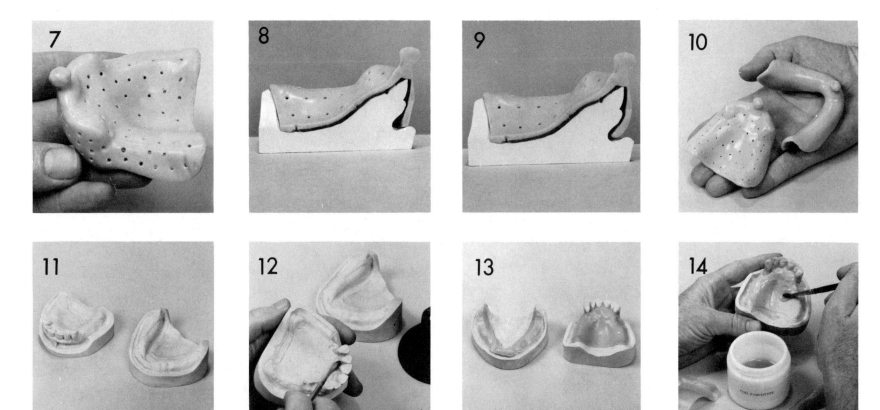

erly contoured. A tray such as this will produce an impression which is overextended in the facial vestibule.

Figure 9 This tray is properly contoured. The anterior border of the tray and the wax spacer are adapted to the facial surface of the teeth and alveolar process. There is enough space in the facial vestibule to permit the impression tray to be seated in the mouth without injuring any soft tissue.

Note that the anterior part of the tray rests against the incisal edges of remaining natural teeth. This and the posterior border (which rests against the palate) form stops which allow the dentist to seat the tray accurately in the mouth.

Figure 10 The completed maxillary and mandibular trays are ready

for delivery to the dentist. A conventional mandibular impression will be made. An elastic impression material is used for the maxillary impression.

Figure 11 The master casts.

Figure 12 The baseplates and occlusion rims are made in essentially the same fashion as they are for a routine denture except that the maxillary baseplate is contoured around the remaining natural teeth. Undercuts on the lingual surfaces of the anterior teeth are blocked out with baseplate wax before occlusion rims are made.

Figure 13 The wax matrices for making the stabilized baseplates are adapted to the casts.

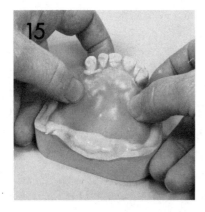
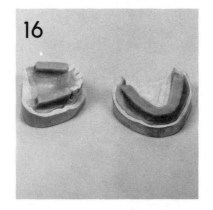
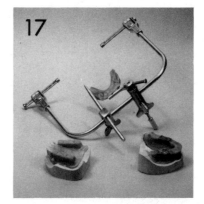
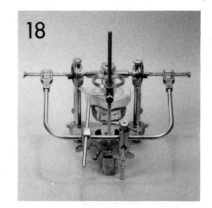

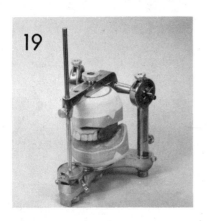
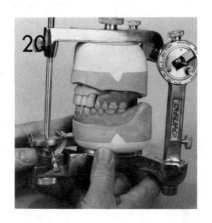
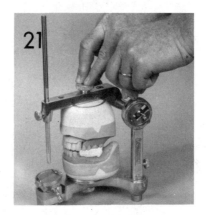
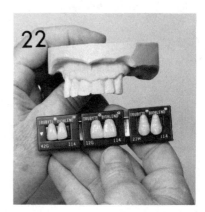

Figure 14   The casts are coated with tinfoil substitute.

Figure 15   A thin mix of self-curing resin, two parts of polymer to one part of monomer, is used to complete the baseplates.

Figure 16   Occlusion rims are built on the stabilized baseplates. The incisal edges of the remaining natural teeth are used to help establish the occlusal plane on the maxillary occlusion rim.

Figure 17   The jaw relationship records and face-bow are returned to the laboratory after these records are made in the dental office. Note that the maxillary occlusion rim fits in a key on top of the bite fork. The bite fork is not inserted into the sides of the maxillary occlusion rim because of the interference of the remaining natural teeth.

Figure 18   The face-bow is placed on the articulator, the maxillary cast and occlusion rim are placed in the bite fork, and the maxillary cast is mounted.

Figure 19   The mounting of the maxillary and mandibular casts is complete.

Figure 20   All of the artificial teeth are arranged with the exception of the teeth which will replace the remaining natural teeth. The set-up is returned to the dentist to check jaw relationships. At this time the dentist checks the vertical dimension, centric relation, esthetics of the mandibular anterior teeth, and makes a protrusive record to adjust the horizontal condylar guides on the articulator.

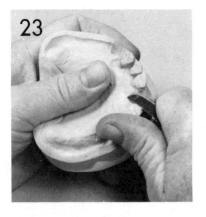
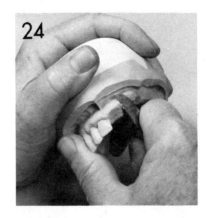
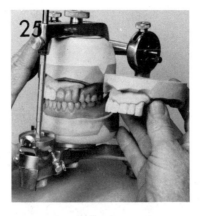
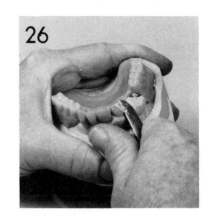
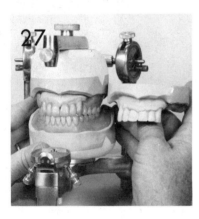
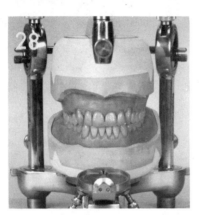
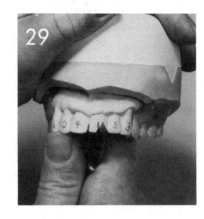
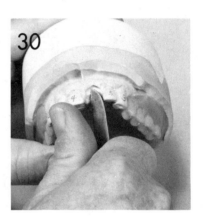

Figure 21   The condylar elements on the articulator are adjusted by use of the protrusive record.

Figure 22   Artificial teeth are selected to match the remaining natural teeth. It may be necessary to recontour the artificial teeth to approximate more closely the shape of the remaining natural teeth. The shade is supplied by the dentist on his prescription.

Figure 23   The cast and its mount are removed from the articulator and the three teeth on the left side are removed.

Figure 24   The ridge area is trimmed to the contour anticipated in the completed denture. The desired form is indicated on the prescription.

Figure 25   The three left maxillary anterior teeth are in position. The preliminary cast and the remaining natural teeth are used as guides. Note that the teeth are set in a more upright position to compensate for the fanning caused by periodontal disease in this patient.

Figure 26   The three right maxillary anterior teeth are removed and the cast trimmed in a similar fashion.

Figure 27   The six maxillary anterior teeth have been set in position and are checked using the preliminary cast as a guide.

Figure 28   The dentures are waxed and are ready to be flasked and processed.

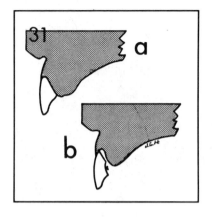
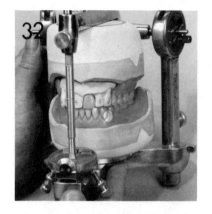
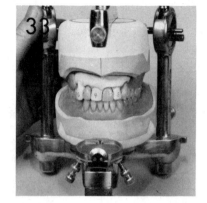
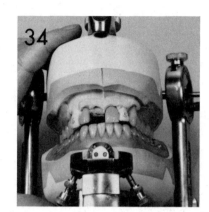
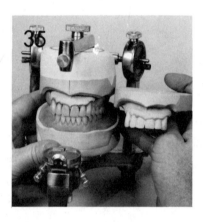
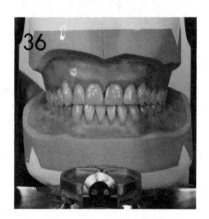
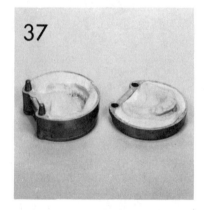
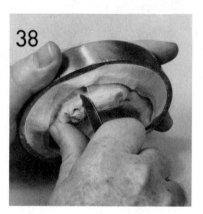

Figure 29   Another method for setting the immediate replacements is to set the teeth alternately. The numbers on the teeth in this illustration show the sequence in which the stone teeth will be removed and the artificial teeth set.

Figure 30   The left maxillary central incisor is removed from the cast and a slight depression carved in the labial region. The gingival area may be reduced if the dentist so indicates on his prescription. No part of the lingual marginal gingiva is removed.

Figure 31   This drawing indicates the proper contour of a tooth socket prepared for setting an artificial tooth in an immediate denture.

Figure 32   The maxillary left central incisor is waxed in position.

Figure 33   The alternate stone teeth have been removed, the sockets prepared and the teeth set in proper position. It can be seen that the remaining natural teeth act as definite guides in the arrangement of the artificial teeth.

Figure 34   The remaining stone teeth are removed one at a time and the artificial teeth placed in position. The easiest way to remove these teeth is to use a fissure bur in a handpiece. The stone teeth can be removed and the socket prepared without disturbing the adjacent teeth.

Figure 35   The six maxillary anterior teeth have been set in position. The arrangement is checked by using the preliminary cast.

Figure 36   The denture is festooned and is ready to be processed.

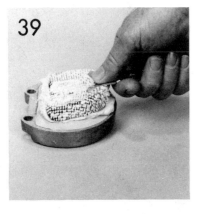

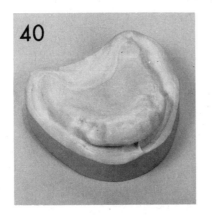

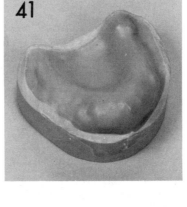

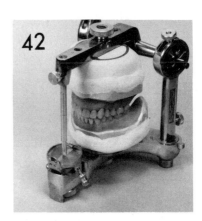

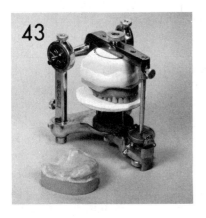

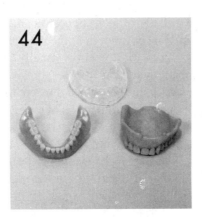

flasked, the wax eliminated, and processed in clear acrylic. The dentures are packed and processed as illustrated in Section 11.

Note: The surgical template may be made in a vacuum forming machine rather than being flasked and processed.

Figure 42 After the dentures are processed they are returned to the articulator and selectively ground to eliminate any processing errors as illustrated in Section 12.

Figure 43 An occlusal index is made before the maxillary denture is removed from the cast for finishing. This figure also shows the clear resin template before it is removed from the cast and polished.

Figure 44 The completed dentures and surgical template are ready for delivery to the dentist.

Figure 37 The flasking procedures are the same as for a conventional denture. This figure shows the maxillary flask after the wax has been eliminated.

Figure 38 The ridge area is trimmed to the desired form, as specified by the dentist on his prescription, or the cast is trimmed by the dentist.

Figure 39 The cast is coated with Vaseline and an impression is made with alginate for a surgical template.

Figure 40 A cast is produced from the alginate impression.

Figure 41 The surgical template is waxed, using one sheet of baseplate wax over the surface with two layers in the border areas. It is

REVIEW QUESTIONS

1. Define immediate denture.
2. List the advantages of an immediate denture.
3. What is the purpose of a surgical template and how is it constructed?
4. When the alternate method for setting teeth for an immediate denture is used, list the sequence in which the stone teeth are removed.
5. Draw a cross-section view of a maxillary cast with a custom tray outline for an immediate denture case.

SECTION 19

Single Complete Dentures

Single dentures are those which are opposed by a natural dentition or a combination of a natural dentition and a removable partial denture. Single dentures produce some unique problems for both the dentist and the dental laboratory technician in that the natural teeth in one arch cannot be changed drastically. Limitations are imposed on function, esthetics, and retention by factors which are basically beyond our control.

One indication of the problems with single dentures is the prevalence of mid-line fractures in single maxillary complete dentures. (For our purposes, a mid-line fracture is one that runs antero-posteriorly between any of the anterior teeth.) These fractures are caused by the relatively strong natural teeth exerting opposing lateral forces on the weaker opposing denture. A combination of a single denture with poor fit often leads to repeated mid-line fractures. It is unusual for such *repeated* fractures to occur except when natural teeth oppose the maxillary denture.

An often over-looked factor in single denture construction is the behavior of teeth which are unopposed by natural teeth or fixed restorations. Such teeth continue to erupt and always disturb the occlusal plane. Two examples illustrate this fact.

First, there is the common illustration of the effects of the loss of a mandibular first molar with the collapse of the adjacent teeth and the extrusion of the opposing maxillary molar. The same phenomena occur when a maxillary molar is lost or when any tooth with occlusal contact is lost. Close examination of diagnostic casts always indicates extrusion of teeth opposing edentulous spaces not restored with fixed appliances or tooth borne removable appliances with metal or porcelain surfaces. (Extrusion is usually seen when resin teeth are used. As the resin wears due to the abrasive action of food, the opposing teeth extrude into the space thus created.)

A second illustration of extrusion is when an individual has six to ten natural lower anterior teeth, a complete maxillary denture, and a mandibular removable partial denture. After a number of years there is a noticeable change with the degree of change determined by the rapidity of resorption in the maxillary anterior region. The noticeable changes are a shortening or disappearance of the artificial maxillary anterior teeth and a lengthening of the natural mandibular anterior teeth. A reverse smile line on the maxillary teeth is often the result with a "fish-mouth" appearance. Contributing to these obvious external changes are changes in the posterior region of the mouth. The mandibular partial denture settles due to resorption and, as the maxillary anterior teeth are pushed up by the strong mandibular anteriors, the posterior portion of the upper denture drops, causing the maxillary tuberosities to grow downward with the tipping denture.

These ravages of time can be helped by cooperation of the dentist and dental laboratory technician. The dentist needs to do all he can to restore the occlusal plane to a reasonable level by "shortening" and recontouring the natural teeth and, where necessary, establishing the correct occlusal plane on a removable partial denture. There may be need to reduce the maxillary tuberosities surgically but this can often be avoided by astute procedures in the dental laboratory. There may also be need for surgical correction in the anterior area of the maxillae.

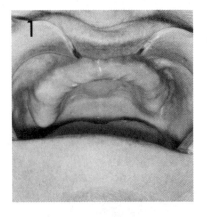
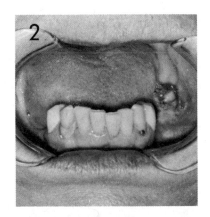
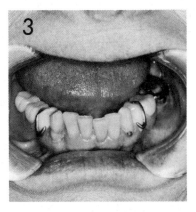
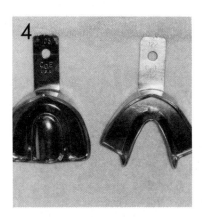

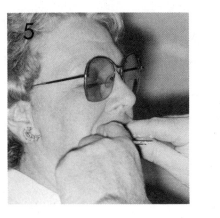
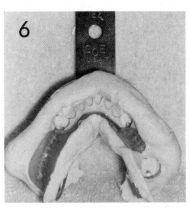

Proper preparation of the mouth will do much to help assure success.

Mandibular single dentures are not common. However, the same principles apply. Many prosthodontists believe mandibular single dentures cause the mandibular ridge to resorb rapidly due to the extra force exerted by the maxillary natural teeth. This is probably true, particularly in those individuals with clamping habits (bruxism) but other factors may influence the retention of maxillary teeth.

The following illustrations show the construction of a maxillary single complete denture. Compare these procedures to those for complete maxillary and mandibular dentures as you progress.

Figure 1   This patient has a good maxillary ridge. Note the difference in the length of the maxillary tuberosities.

Figure 2   The patient's mandibular arch.

Figure 3   The patient's mandibular arch has been restored with a removable partial denture. This is a pre-existing appliance which has been in use for several years. Now, refer to **Figure 1** and correlate the appearance of the maxillary arch with the remaining mandibular natural teeth. You can see that the shorter maxillary tuberosity opposes the existing molar. The larger right tuberosity is most likely due to the action of the maxillary denture being tipped by the mandibular anterior teeth and the lower left molar, causing the right tuberosity to elongate.

When patients have difficulty wearing a single complete maxillary denture, always inspect the mandibular arch. A complete lower dentition is usually essential to provide adequate retention for a maxillary single denture. Otherwise, the denture will tip and lose retention whenever the teeth are brought together. The enlargement of the tuberosity as seen in **Figure 1** will occur even if a partial denture is in place if the partial denture is not maintained and/or the resin teeth on the mandibular partial denture wear and do not provide adequate occlusal support.

Figure 4   Proper trays are selected to make a preliminary impression of the maxillary arch and an opposing cast of the mandibular arch.

Figure 5   The mandibular impression is being made.

Figure 6   The mandibular partial denture stayed in the impression when it was removed from the mouth.

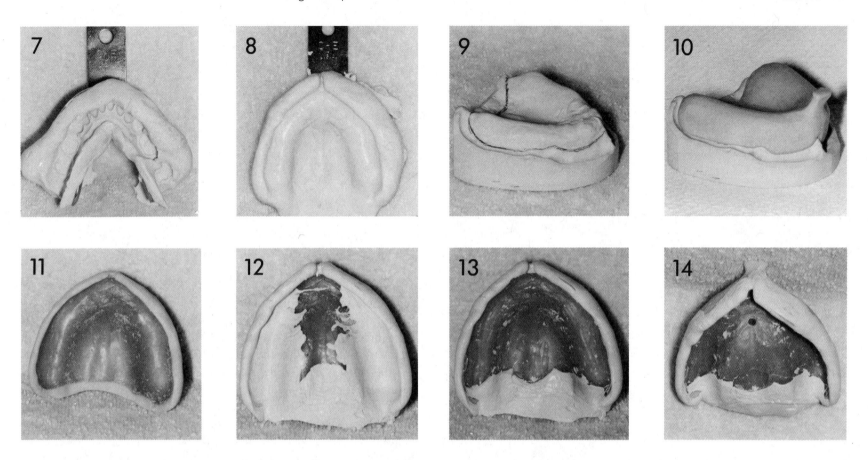

Figure 7   The mandibular removable partial denture has been removed from the impression and returned to the patient. The impression is now ready to be poured.

Figure 8   The maxillary preliminary impression is shown as it appeared when it was removed from the mouth.

Figure 9   The outline for the custom tray has been placed on the cast made from the preliminary impression. (Refer to Section 3)

Figure 10   A custom tray for the maxillary arch has been made. The same procedures are used as described in Section 3.

Figure 11   The wax shim or spacer placed in the maxillary custom tray

may vary in configuration depending upon the desires of a particular dentist. Some dentists prefer to have their trays made without any shim.

Figure 12   Impression techniques vary among dentists and from region to region. This illustration shows the results of border molding, a procedure which defines the border or edge of the impression and the subsequent denture. The material used in this illustration is a heavy bodied zinc oxide-eugenol paste but other materials such as modeling plastic, specially made waxes, or some modified resin materials may be used.

Figure 13   The border-molding material has been removed from the tissue bearing areas of the impression. Note that some material has

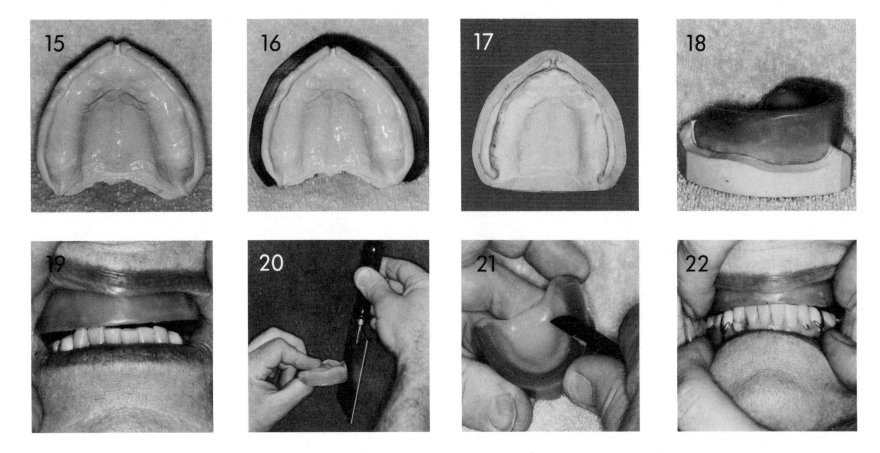

been left in the posterior palatal seal area which will help key the denture in place when the impression is made.

Figure 14 A vent hole is placed in the tray. This serves to relieve pressures which may build up in the palatal area and may distort the impression.

Figure 15 The completed impression. The steps in making this impression are included to demonstrate that often a simple looking impression is proceeded by precise handling of dental materials through several steps.

Figure 16 The impression is prepared for pouring. The same procedures are used in pouring this cast as described in Section 4.

Figure 17 The completed master cast.

Figure 18 A baseplate and occlusion rim have been made on the master cast. Refer to Sections 5 and 6 for the complete technique.

Figure 19 At the third patient visit, the maxillary occlusion rim is placed in the mouth and observed to see what changes need to be made.

Figure 20 The facial surface is adjusted by using a warm hotplate.

Figure 21 The anterior portion of the occlusion rim is reduced.

Figure 22 The occlusion rim has been adjusted so that the anterior teeth touch lightly and the correct vertical dimension has been

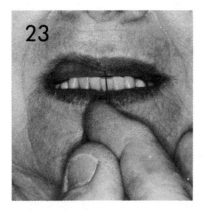
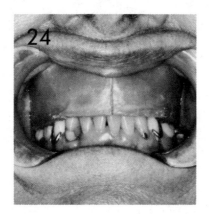
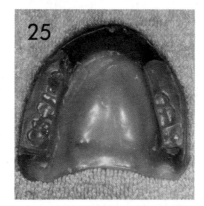
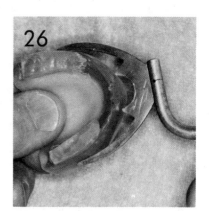

achieved. Note the open space in the posterior region which will be filled subsequently with a soft wax.

Figure 23   The center line is marked on the maxillary occlusion rim with an instrument. Note that the center line coincides with the center of the patient's face and not with the center of the lower anterior teeth. This situation occurs quite often.

Figure 24   An occlusal index or interocclusal record is made by placing warm soft wax on the posterior region of the occlusion rim and having the patient close in centric relation until the mandibular anterior teeth barely touch the wax occlusion rim. After the soft wax cools, it is trimmed so that only the occlusal portions of the mandibular teeth remain in the index. This permits the occlusion rim with the occlusal index to be replaced in the mouth for verification of the correct occlusal relationships.

Figure 25   This illustrates the occlusal indexes left in the posterior region maxillary occlusion rim. If you refer to Section 7, you will see that when complete dentures are made for both arches the occlusal index is made on the mandibular occlusion rim. In this instance, the occlusal index is made on the maxillary occlusion rim because the occlusal plane is determined by the lower natural teeth and existing removable partial denture.

Figure 26   A face-bow transfer is made in much the same manner as for complete dentures. The bite fork is attached to the occlusion rim by heating the bite fork and placing it into the occlusion rim.

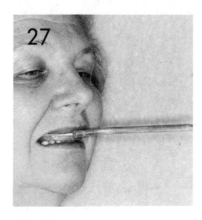
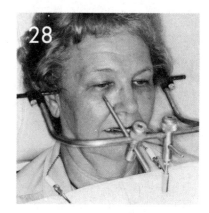

Figure 27   The occlusion rim with attached bite fork is placed in the patient's mouth and the patient instructed to close with only enough force to maintain the maxillary occlusion rim in place.

Figure 28   The face-bow is attached to the bite fork and the orbital pointer placed in the correct location. A complete description of this procedure is found in Section 7.

Figure 29   A shade is determined by using shade tabs of the desired manufacturer's teeth and matching one of them to the existing lower teeth. This procedure varies from the method generally used to select teeth for complete maxillary and mandibular dentures where skin tones are used to select a pleasing color.

Figure 30   The same basic techniques are used in mounting casts as

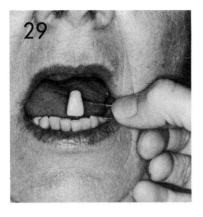
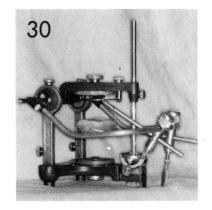
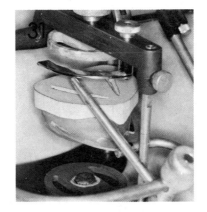
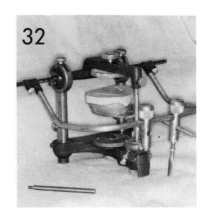

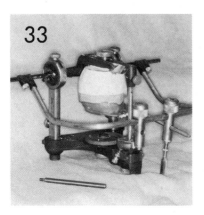
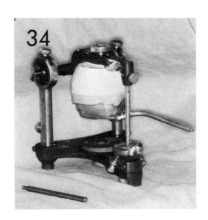
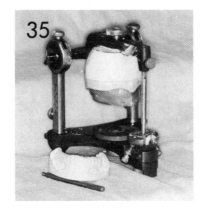
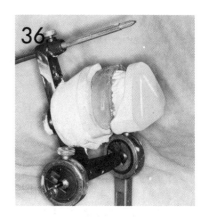

described in Section 7. The face-bow is assembled on the articulator, centering the bite fork on the articulator and adjusting the inferior-superior position until the orbital pointer touches the orbital plane guide.

Figure 31 This shows the correct position of the orbital pointer touching the orbital plane guide of the articulator. Note the indexes which have been cut into the base of the cast.

Figure 32 The orbital pointer is removed from the face-bow at this stage to make mounting the cast easier. The extension pin has also been removed from the articulator.

Figure 33 The maxillary cast is attached to the articulator with plaster.

Figure 34 The face-bow has been removed from the bite fork and set aside.

Figure 35 The bite fork is removed from the maxillary occlusion rim by warming it slightly.

Figure 36 The mandibular cast is attached to the maxillary occlusion rim with sticky wax. This helps assure that the cast will maintain the correct relationship with the maxillary cast during the mounting procedures. Be sure there is no contact between the casts in the "heel" area.

Figure 37 The mounting of the maxillary and mandibular cast is now complete.

Figure 38 This is a close up view of the mounted cast. Plaster has

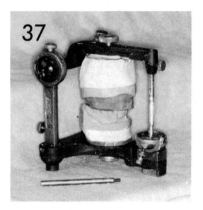
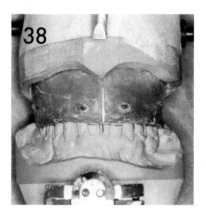
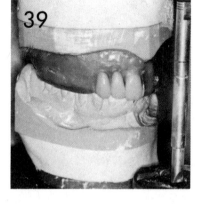
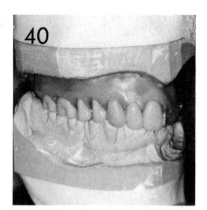

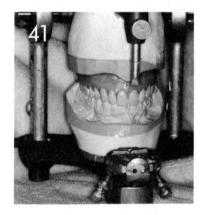
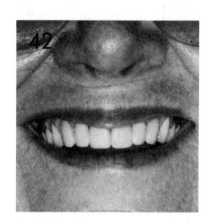

been placed in the center line marked in the mouth making it easier to see. The center line has been transferred to the lower cast along with an indication of the amount of vertical overlap required. This information is furnished by the dentist.

Figure 39 Selection of anterior teeth is the responsibility of the dentist. Some of the factors that are used to select teeth for single dentures are the lower teeth, photographs of the existing natural dentition, the amount of horizontal overlap desired in the completed denture, and the amount of tooth which shows when smiling.

As a guide, the width of the maxillary central incisor should be about 1½ times the width of the mandibular incisor and the size of the six anteriors should be compatible with the mandibular teeth. The relation of the maxillary canine to the mandibular teeth is not correct due to the deviation of the mid-line; these variations must be kept in mind as the teeth are selected and arranged. Proper angulation of the teeth is necessary in order to achieve a natural appearance. Refer to Section 9 for the correct angulations of the maxillary teeth.

Figure 40 The maxillary right teeth have been set in position. Note that the size of the posterior teeth harmonizes with the lower natural teeth and the artificial teeth on the mandibular partial denture. The use of porcelain or resin artificial teeth in single dentures is again the responsibility of the dentist. Some of the factors which enter into this decision are the condition of the remaining lower teeth, the presence of bruxing habits, and the previous experience a patient may have had with a particular type of tooth. Porcelain anterior teeth should not be

used in combination with resin posterior teeth. Resin teeth wear more rapidly than porcelain teeth and when this occurs with a single denture, there is a tripping action with a consequent lack of retention in the denture.

Figure 41 The maxillary teeth have been completely arranged and festooned. They are now ready to be tried in the patient's mouth.

Figure 42 The teeth are tried in the patient's mouth and adjustments made to achieve the best possible appearance. It may be necessary to change the anterior teeth at this point if the appearance (size, color or shape) is not satisfactory. Any changes should be made by the dentist or by the dental laboratory technician in conjunction with the dentist at this time.

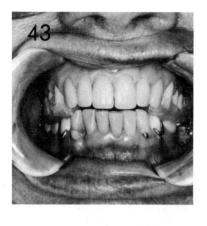 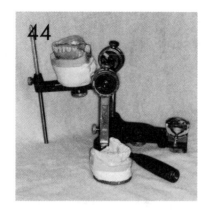 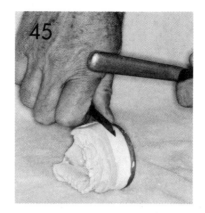 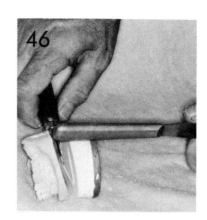

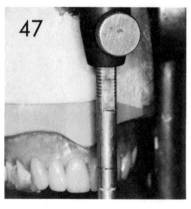 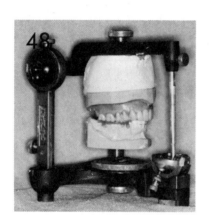 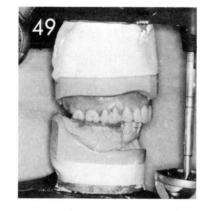 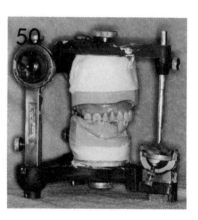

Note the appearance of the denture base in the posterior regions. In order to achieve the best possible appearance, it may be necessary to utilize long posterior teeth and a characterized denture base in this area. This will allow the patient to have a more normal smile.

Figure 43 The try-in appointment is the fourth visit in the sequence of treatment. Another procedure performed at this appointment is a verification of the interocclusal jaw relationship. Some dentists make a new interocclusal record routinely at this time since they feel that a more accurately fitting base, a correct vertical dimension, and the presence of artificial teeth make this record more accurate than the one done at the previous appointment. This illustration shows an interocclusal record being made after the appearance has been verified and approved by the patient.

Figure 44 The waxed denture has been returned to the maxillary cast and the lower cast removed from the articulator.

Figures 45 and 46 The lower cast is separated from the lower mounting. To be safe, this mounting should be soaked for a few minutes before the separation.

Figure 47 A judgment is made relative to the thickness of the wax occlusal index. The pin on the articulator is "dropped" this distance.

Figure 48 The mandibular cast is attached to the maxillary wax denture with sticky wax.

Figure 49 The mandibular cast is reattached to the articulator with plaster.

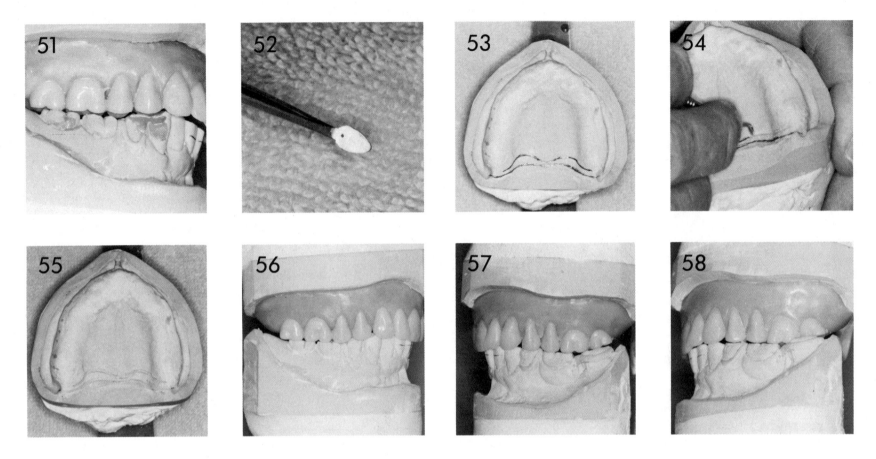

Figure 50 The wax occlusal indexes have been removed from the maxillary waxed denture. The pin is raised and the maxillary teeth are allowed to touch the mandibular teeth. The pin is then lowered until it touches the incisal guide table and is retightened.

Figure 51 This illustrates the amount of discrepancy which existed between the preliminary jaw relation record and that done at the try-in appointment. The posterior teeth will be adjusted to occlude properly with the mandibular teeth before the denture is processed.

Figure 52 The posterior palatal relief is described in Section 10. This instrument is quite satisfactory for placing such relief in the maxillary cast.

Figure 53 The desired posterior palatal relief design is first placed on the cast in pencil. This assures placing the relief in the correct position.

Figure 54 The palatal relief is then scribed in the cast.

Figure 55 The posterior palatal relief is complete.

Figure 56 The teeth have been repositioned into correct occlusion to compensate for the discrepancy observed after the mandibular cast was remounted. The wax base has also been contoured. Note that the dip in the occlusal plane leaves more denture base showing than would occur if the occlusal plane had been straightened.

Figure 57 The left side has also been adjusted. The curvature on the

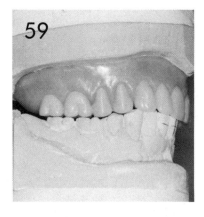
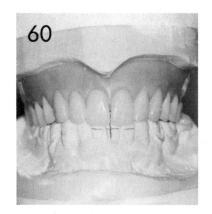
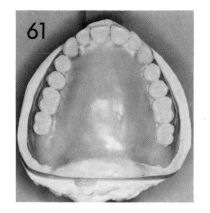
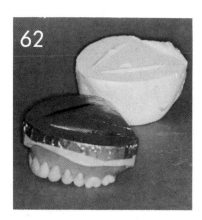

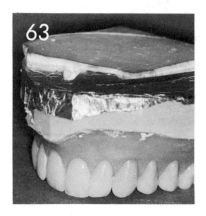
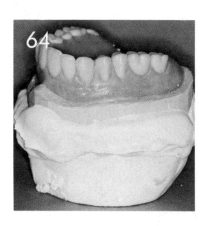

mentioned previously. A better occlusion could have been obtained had the partial denture been available to have the teeth reset.

Figure 60   This shows the teeth in protrusive excursions.

Figure 61   The teeth are waxed and ready to be flasked.

Figure 62   The cast has been separated from its mount and the base of the cast has been covered with tinfoil. The tinfoil is well adapted to the cast. The purpose of the tinfoil is to permit clean separation after processing so that it will go back on the mount easily and accurately. This will save much time later in the procedure. Refer to Section 11, Flasking, Packing, Processing, and Recovery at this time. The procedures used for a single denture are identical to those described in Section 11.

Figure 63   After the cast and denture have been recovered, the plaster is removed. The flasking material separates cleanly from the tinfoiled cast. The tinfoil is removed from the base of the cast.

Figure 64   The cast is reattached to its mount after ascertaining that it fits accurately. Plaster is best used to maintain the cast in position. Waxes do not hold adequately and glue inserted between the cast and the mount may produce inaccuracies.

Figure 65   The occlusion between the newly processed denture and the lower cast is checked. The occlusion is marked with articulating paper

occlusal plane on this side is more pronounced due to the presence of the mandibular second molar. It is evident that if the occlusal plane was more level less denture base would show. The importance of reducing the amount of denture base is evident when you refer to **Figure 42** and note the esthetics of the denture base.

Figure 58   The left lateral excursion and the contact on the posterior teeth is illustrated in this figure. Good lateral excursions were achieved in this single denture by using Anatoline posteriors. These teeth do not require as precise a mesiodistal relationship with opposing teeth as some other types of teeth.

Figure 59   The lateral excursions on the right side are shown. This illustration dramatically shows the discrepancy in the occlusal plane

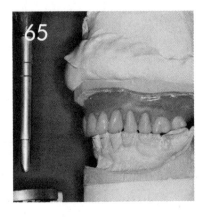
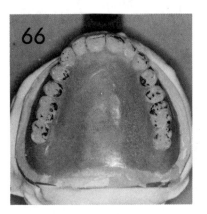
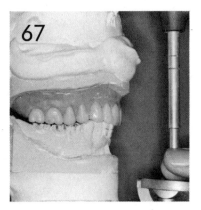
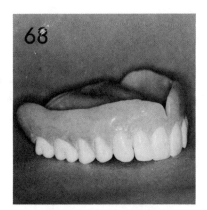

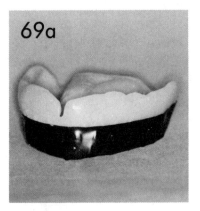
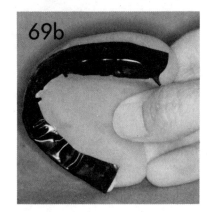

and perfected. Refer to Section 12 for the procedures utilized in perfecting the occlusion and removing processing errors.

One significant difference between the procedures used for a single denture and those described in Section 12 is the elimination of the milling procedure. Milling will simply abrade the mandibular gypsum cast.

The lateral excursions must be carefully developed by observation, use of articulating paper and proper reduction of interfering cusps and fossae.

Figure 66 This shows the distribution of the markings after the occlusion has been refined.

The left lateral excursion has been refined so that there are good working contacts.

The left lateral occlusion has also been refined to develop good balancing contacts.

Figure 67 Protrusive occlusal contacts are not possible to develop with the occlusal scheme present. Note that the occlusion on the posterior teeth is only slightly deficient so that the patient should be able to incise easily.

Figure 68 The denture is removed from the cast as described in Section 13 and finished and polished.

Figure 69 a and b Resin anterior and posterior teeth were utilized on this denture. The greatest difficulty in using these teeth is in the

polishing procedure. One way to avoid defacing these teeth during the polishing procedure is to cover them with tape. Regular black electrical tape was used to cover the teeth during the polishing procedure. Careful use of a brush wheel can help finish the embrasure areas without destroying the anatomy on the facial and lingual surfaces of the teeth.

Figure 70 The teeth are placed in the patient's mouth and facial contours are checked.

Figure 71 The occlusion between the new maxillary denture and the existing mandibular dentition is checked. The excursions are also checked. This illustration shows the teeth in centric occlusal contact. The first contact on closing should be uniform and solid with no skids, shifts or slides. Any interferences in occlusion are removed by marking

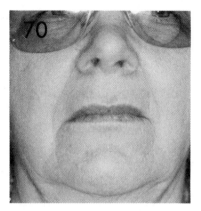
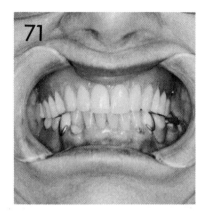
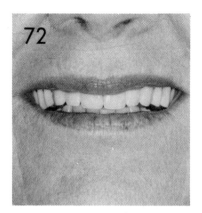

the denture in the mouth or, preferably, doing a clinical remount (Section 14). A new mandibular opposing cast may be needed if any of the teeth are abraded on the original cast.

Figure 72   This shows the patient after the denture has been delivered. The smile shown here is relatively natural and you can see that the denture base is not visible in the posterior parts of the mouth. Part of this is due to the way the patient is smiling and a portion due to the changes made in the teeth and denture base after the try-in.

The successful completion of a single denture is a good illustration of cooperation between the dentist and dental laboratory. The opposing arch must be placed in a relatively good configuration before the initiation of the procedures needed to make a single denture. In the laboratory, special care must be used during all the laboratory techniques in order to avoid abrading the opposing cast; special care must be taken when the teeth are equilibrated in the laboratory to avoid abrading the cast. Also shown are ways to make the resin teeth look better by avoiding over-polishing.

REVIEW QUESTIONS

1. What is the most common cause of mid-line fractures of single complete dentures?
2. Is tooth extrusion more extensive when the opposing tooth is a natural tooth, a porcelain tooth, or a resin tooth?
3. Are maxillary or mandibular single dentures more common?
4. What significant difference exists in perfecting the occlusion of processed dentures between single dentures and complete dentures?
5. If the center line marking on the maxillary occlusion rim does not coincide with the center of the lower anterior teeth has the dentist made an error?

SECTION 20

Introduction to Removable Partial Dentures

Some basic theoretical and practical information is needed before a technician is able to construct a satisfactory removable partial denture. A knowledge of the terminology associated with removable partial dentures is essential.

The term *partial denture* is used to describe many situations and several types of appliances. By definition, a partial denture is "a prosthesis that replaces one or more, but less than all, of the natural teeth and associated structures." (CCDT) The definition makes no mention of material, design, utilization of remaining teeth for retention and stability or whether the appliance is permanently cemented or can be removed by the patient. With the introduction of "acid-etch" tooth replacements, the term "partial denture" becomes even more vague. Therefore, more descriptive terminology is in order for better communication.

A *fixed partial denture* is "a tooth-bone partial denture that is intended to be permanently attached to the teeth or roots that furnish support to the restoration." (CCDT) By common usage this is synonymous with the term *fixed bridge* wherein the teeth to which the restoration attaches are prepared for crowns. However, the term *fixed partial denture* or *fixed bridge* may also apply to other types of permanently attached tooth replacements such as "acid-etched" tooth replacements which require much less tooth reduction.

A *removable partial denture* is "a partial denture that can be readily placed in the mouth and removed by the wearer." (CCDT) Here, also, there is no mention of material, design or how the appliance is retained.

A person who indicates they have a "partial denture" they can remove may mean a simple all-resin appliance with no clasps, a similar appliance with simple wire clasps, a combination resin-cast metal appliance (described in the following sections), or a complicated appliance constructed in conjunction with fixed restorations known as a *precision attachment* removable partial denture. In this manual, the term removable partial denture will apply to appliances with cast metal retentive mechanisms and resin bases.

The term "bridge" is often used by patients. It may mean a "fixed" replacement, a removable partial denture or even a complete denture; (some people just do not like the term "denture"!). Avoid using the term "bridge" unless you modify the word to make it more descriptive.

OBJECTIVES OF REMOVABLE PARTIAL DENTURE TREATMENT

The objectives of removable partial denture treatment are:
1. To preserve and maintain the remaining oral structures.
2. To restore function.
3. To improve or restore appearance (esthetics).

TERMINOLOGY

The following terms are used in the following sections and apply to removable partial denture techniques:

Abutment: A tooth which is used to support or retain a removable partial denture.

Base: That portion of a removable partial denture that contacts the oral mucosa and serves as an attachment and support for the replaced teeth. Usually, the base provides support for the removable partial denture by being in close apposition to the oral mucosa covering the supporting bone (maxillae or mandible).

Direct Retainer: "A clasp, attachment, or assembly applied to an abutment tooth for the purpose of maintaining a removable restoration in its planned position in relation to oral structures." (CCDT) The direct retainers with which we are concerned in this manual are clasps. A clasp usually consists of two arms joined by a body which may connect with an occlusal rest. A clasp is an extracoronal retainer, one that fits over the external surface of the tooth.

Major Connector: "A metal plate or bar (e.g., lingual bar, linguoplate, or palatal bar) used to join the units of one side of a removable partial denture to those located on the opposite side of the dental arch." (CCDT)

Minor Connector: "The connecting link between the major connector or base of a removable partial denture and other units of the restoration, e.g., direct and indirect retainers or rests." (CCDT)

Finish Line: The junction between metal and plastic portions of a removable partial denture. An internal finish line is on the internal or tissue surface and is formed while preparing a cast for duplication. An external finish line is on the polished surface of a denture and is formed in the wax pattern.

Plastic Retention: That portion of a partial denture framework which attaches the resin base to the framework.

CLASSIFICATION OF REMOVABLE PARTIAL DENTURES

Classifications are developed to facilitate communication between individuals. A universally accepted classification permits people to simplify their communications and make them more meaningful. There are many confusing removable partial denture classifications, some based upon the completed appliance, and some based upon the partially edentulous arch. When speaking of removable partial dentures, most dentists and technicians use a short phrase to describe the appliance rather than to use a "Class I" or "Class II" type classification. The primary reason that a universal classification has not evolved for removable partial dentures is that most authorities have promoted their own classifications, all of which are different. This has resulted in confusion.

The simplest and most easily understood classification describes a partial denture in simple terms. In this classification a partial denture is spoken of as (1) tooth borne, (2) tooth-tissue borne, or (3) tissue borne. A *tooth borne* partial denture is one which is supported entirely by the abutment teeth. A *tooth-tissue borne* partial denture is one which is supported by both abutment teeth and the mucosa and underlying bone. This type of appliance is referred to by some authorities as a "true" removable partial denture and has at least one free-end extension. A *tissue borne* partial denture is one which is supported entirely by the mucosa and the underlying bone. An example is a temporary partial denture which has no occlusal rests which is used as a temporary appliance or an immediate replacement (placed at the time of extraction).

SEQUENCE OF TREATMENT

A dental laboratory technician should be familiar with clinical procedures as well as laboratory procedures to understand his important role in removable partial denture construction. The clinical procedures and the subsequent laboratory procedures for each appointment are discussed in Section 1. This section should be reviewed before proceeding. Additional information on clinical procedures is presented in conjunction with the technical phases of removable partial denture construction.

METALS USED FOR REMOVABLE PARTIAL DENTURE FRAMES

The metals used in removable partial denture frames have undergone a significant evolution during the past 50 years. The gold alloys have been displaced almost entirely by the introduction of base metal alloys. Some understanding of how this evolution occurred will make it easier to understand the similarities and differences between the various metals used.

Gold has been used in dentistry since the earliest of times. Reportedly, the Etruscans, an early civilization, used gold and gold wires to attach artificial teeth to natural teeth. As dentistry developed gold continued to be the most common metal used in either cast restorations or as wire and gold plate.

Gold continued to be one of the primary materials used in dentistry as the profession developed in the late 19th and early 20th centuries. Gold foil was used to fill cavities. The foil was gold in its purest form which enabled it to be welded to itself as it was placed in the cavity. There are dentists who still believe that the placement of gold foil restorations is a measure of the highest skills available in dentistry although some dentists believe that the trauma associated with placing of such restorations is injurious to the teeth.

During these times gold continued to be used in the form of wires, plates, and as parts of cast restorations. In some techniques, cast gold and wrought gold were used in combination to make such items as banded cast crowns and Richmond crowns.

What made gold so popular? There are many reasons. Since it was available and had been in use since the earliest times, people knew a great deal about its properties and its manipulation. It melted at a relatively low temperature and it was simple to cast. It could be attached to other gold through soldering, it was easy to polish, and, in the event of breakage, it was easy to repair. In addition, its value was respected by the public.

Another good property of gold is that it is easily alloyed with other metals. These alloys provide a wide range of working properties not possible with pure gold. In dental use, pure gold has little use except in the previously mentioned gold foil restorations. Gold is so soft that it could not be used in pure form anywhere except in the simplest restorations. Therefore, gold alloys became commonly used. Through continued use and experimentations, alloys were developed for specific uses. The United States Bureau of Standards in cooperation with the dental profession established standards in dental materials including dental golds. There are various specifications for dental golds, one being for a hard gold satisfactory for removable partial dentures.

The amount of expansion and contraction which occurs when gold is melted and cast is well known. The effects of alloying metals on gold is also well known. With this knowledge, investments were developed to control the dimensional changes which occur from the production of a wax pattern through the casting and polishing procedure. This knowledge and continuing developments are the reasons why gold continues to be among the most accurate materials available to the profession.

Non-precious alloys for removable partial denture construction were introduced in the 1930's and 1940's. These base metal alloys were composed primarily of chromium and cobalt with some other metallic elements in less quantity. They were more rigid, had a harder surface, and were stronger in small cross sections than gold.

These base metal alloys were promoted to the profession as being superior to gold. The contention was that the stronger material would last longer in the patient's mouth, that it would not tarnish as readily, and would be more acceptable due to its silver color. These metals received wide acceptance by the profession and were in common usage by the 1950's.

When first introduced, these metals were highly promoted; the cost to the dentists was similar to gold with the justification being that the base metals were superior to gold and that the extra time required in fabrication offset the difference in the cost of the metals.

Franchising arrangements were common when these metals were first introduced. Franchises were available on a geographic basis so that each laboratory which had a franchise could be assured of some protection within its area. Of course, there was intense competition between owners of different franchises in any given area.

A laboratory which utilized a base metal in partial denture frames and was franchised needed to have a complete system to handle the particular metal. Special investments, ovens, casting machines, recovery apparatus and finishing machines were required. The extremely high temperatures required to cast these materials and the hardness of the metals rendered equipment normally utilized for casting and finishing gold obsolete. The difference in expansion and contraction from casting to cooling also required investments which were compatible with these different physical properties.

There were some dissimilarities between the various metals. For instance, Ticonium was known as a low heat metal and utilized a gypsum-bonded investment, similar in properties to that used in gold framework fabrication. Even so, investments used for gold could not be used for the low heat base metal alloys. Vitallium was a high heat alloy that required a phosphate-bonded investment. A separate liquid was supplied with the investment rather than using water. The casting machines for both metals were induction type and required electricity rather than an open flame. The temperature range for melting and casting was much narrower and required much more precise equipment than that previously used for gold. (Induction casting machines also became available for use with gold alloys and produced more consistent results than those normally obtained with open flame casting.)

As the base metal alloys became more popular, new franchises and generic forms of these metals became available. Most of the generic metals had similar properties and could be utilized with generic investments which became available as the popularity of these metals increased. With time, most all laboratories that so desired had equipment for making base metal partial denture frames. Those who did not usually had these frames made by a subcontractor.

Eventually, the patents on the most popular base metal alloys expired and this produced a change in the metals as new patents were required for a continuation of the franchise arrangement. The newer alloys and those in present use are composed primarily of nickel. They have some properties which are better than the earlier alloys. They are easier to adjust, easier to polish and less subject to fracture. The earlier base metals had a tendency to break if the appliance was bent or if there was an attempt to adjust a clasp. Clinically, it appears that the newer metals are less scratch resistant and do not have the high luster which formerly was present. Beryllium, a component of some earlier alloys, has been removed from most of the presently used alloys since it is contended by some that this has a deleterious effect upon laboratory personnel. Of course, it is wise to wear a mask when grinding or polishing any of these materials to avoid inhaling the dust produced.

The rise in the price of gold in the late 1970's almost eliminated gold as a metal used in partial denture frames. Today most all partial denture frames are made of base metal alloys and are most satisfactory. It can be easily contended that the profession would not have accepted these alloys had they not been as satisfactory or more so than gold alloys. History seems to indicate that the choice of the base metals for this purpose over the precious metals has been a wise one.

SIMILARITIES IN PRODUCING BASE METAL AND PRECIOUS METAL FRAMES

The basic concept of producing a partial denture frame remains the same regardless of the material used. First, a refractory cast has to be made from the altered master cast. Then, a wax pattern must be constructed on the refractory cast which is subsequently invested. The wax pattern is eliminated through heat and the metal is cast into the mold thus formed. The raw casting is then recovered and finished. These steps are the same regardless of the material used.

These sections on production of the refractory cast, investing, casting and polishing should be viewed as basic knowledge which can be altered to fit whatever materials are at hand. The differences in mixing investment, burnout temperatures, casting techniques and finishing techniques can be noted in margins of the text. In the event that you need to make a gold casting, the information is at hand.

REVIEW QUESTIONS

1. What are the objectives of removable partial denture treatment?
2. Define direct retainer.
3. Define major connector and give examples.
4. Define minor connector and give examples.
5. List the differences in physical properties between gold alloys and non-precious alloys used in partial denture construction.

SECTION 21

Removable Partial Denture Design

The importance of properly designed removable partial dentures cannot be overemphasized. The execution of a removable partial denture design may determine the success or failure of the appliance. Inadequate design assures failure.

The design of a partial denture, including all of its component parts, determines its comfort, its efficiency, and, most important, whether it will be a therapeutic appliance promoting oral health, or will become a destructive influence. All partial dentures must be designed to "preserve and maintain what remains" as well as fill in the missing spaces.

A removable bridge, or tooth borne partial denture, has no significant movement during function if it is properly designed. A "true" partial denture, one with a free-end extension, moves under function because of the resiliency of the underlying soft tissue from which the appliance gains some support. Therefore, all tooth-tissue borne or free-end extension partial dentures are designed with the knowledge that these appliances move during function.

The following principles must be followed when designing partial dentures:

(1) The design of free-end extension partial dentures must compensate for the slight movement which occurs during function so that the remaining oral structures will not be damaged.

(2) The partial denture must be passive, i.e., exert no force, when not in function. Otherwise, the appliance may act as an orthodontic appliance and cause unwanted movement of the teeth.

(3) The partial denture must be comfortable. Without comfort, it will be a failure.

(4) The partial denture must be pleasing esthetically. Excessive display of metal on anterior teeth and premolars may lead a patient to discard the appliance.

(5) With the above principles in mind, the design should be as simple as possible. Simplicity in design helps produce a comfortable partial denture and aids in the maintenance of oral hygiene. Esthetics is generally improved by a simple design.

Before the construction phases of partial dentures are described, it is necessary to have an understanding of the components of a partial denture. The design of these components and their indications and contra-indications will be described before the actual construction phases are undertaken.

SURVEYING

A clasp partial denture is retained by having the tip of the clasp arm engage an undercut on an abutment tooth. An undercut is formed when the base of an object is smaller than the top. Undercuts on abutment teeth are either desirable or undesirable. Desirable undercuts are utilized for retention. All other undercuts are undesirable because rigid portions of a partial denture cannot be placed into an undercut under most circumstances.

Precision casting techniques require that undercuts be located accurately. This is done by using an instrument known as a surveyor. A surveyor is defined as "an instrument used to determine the relative parallelism of two or more surfaces of teeth or other portions of a cast of the dental arch." (CCDT)

As seen in **Figure 1** a surveyor is a simple instrument consisting of a platform with a vertical spindle which is perpendicular to the platform or base. The lower end of the spindle has a chucking device for attaching different instruments. A movable table with a tilting top permits a cast to be mounted and moved in any direction on the base of the surveyor.

Surveyors are manufactured in the United States by several of the larger gold suppliers. The most popular ones are made by the J. M. Ney Company (**Figure 1**) and the J. F. Jelenko Company (**Figure 13**, Section 22). All surveyors are basically the same and accomplish the same jobs. More complex surveyors are available, some through distributors of franchised base metal alloys. Again, these instruments are similar in that they consist of a base with a rod perpendicular to the base and some type of movable table. Some of the complex instruments measure the depth of undercuts by use of dial gauges or electronic instruments.

There are six major uses for a surveyor: (1) surveying the study cast, (2) contouring wax patterns for cast restorations on abutment teeth for removable partial dentures, (3) placement of precision attachments in wax patterns for cast restorations, (4) placement of precision rests, (5) machining cast restorations with the use of a handpiece holder, and (6) surveying the master cast. In this manual we are concerned primarily with numbers (1) and (6).

By definition, a surveyor is used to determine relative parallelism. In doing this the relative height of contour or greatest circumference of each tooth is determined. All of the area below the height of contour is undercut, and this is the area in which a clasp tip must lie in order to provide retention for a removable partial denture. Other undercut areas are undesirable and must be eliminated before a partial denture is made, either by mouth preparation or by blocking out these undercuts on the master cast prior to duplication.

A great deal has been written concerning the "tilting" of a cast while it is being surveyed. Some manuals advocate certain tilts for posterior free-end extensions, other tilts for anterior extensions, and various tilts for removable bridges. Tilting of the cast is probably one of the most confusing factors in surveying and design and accomplishes very little. Tilting determines the path of insertion; that is, the direction in which a

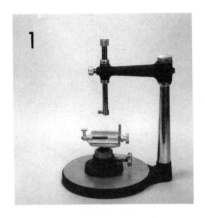

patient places a partial denture in the mouth. Another claim, one that can be disputed, is that tilting will "create" or "produce" an undercut.

After several years of observation and clinical practice, it became evident that a majority of patients placed their partial dentures in their mouth in one manner, regardless of how the cast had been surveyed. This was straight up and down. Odd paths of insertion often caused patients difficulty during insertion and removal. A more important observation was that many clasps, designed to gain retention from undercuts which had been created by tilting the cast, had no retention when they were placed in the mouth. These observations and the confusion surrounding surveying led to a simplified approach which has proved successful, both in the laboratory and in clinical practice.

RULES FOR SURVEYING

1. Undercuts cannot be produced or created by tilting a cast.
2. All casts are originally surveyed with the occlusal plane parallel to the base of the surveyor. (Zero degree tilt)
3. The retentive tips of clasps must engage undercuts which are present when the cast is surveyed in this position.
4. Wherever possible, undesirable undercuts and areas of interference are removed during mouth preparation by the dentist by recontouring teeth or making necessary restorations.
5. The cast may be tilted in the following instances:
   (a) to equalize undercuts,
   (b) to place a clasp tip in a better position for esthetics and

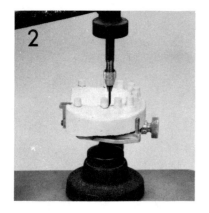

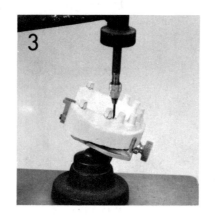

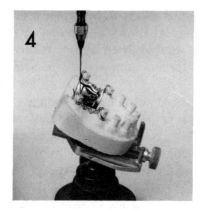

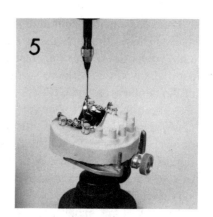

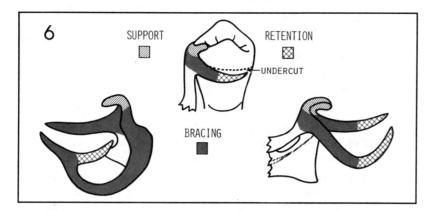

are no undercuts present when this cast is surveyed with the occlusal plane parallel to the base of the surveyor (**Figure 2**). It is seen also that undercuts are present when the cast is tilted (**Figure 3**). A partial denture, made so that the clasp tips engage these undercuts, is retentive as long as the cast is held in this position (**Figure 4**). However, when the cast is again parallel, and most mouths are in this position, the partial denture has no retention (**Figure 5**). It has been said facetiously that tilting a cast is valid if a patient holds his head at the same angle as the cast when it was surveyed.

CLASPS

All properly constructed clasps have three functions: support, bracing, and retention (**Figure 6**). *Support* is achieved through one or more occlusal rests which rest on the occlusal surface of a tooth and are attached with a rigid connector to the appliance. Occlusal rests resist vertical forces and prevent the appliance from moving toward the tissue (settling) and causing injury to the soft tissues adjacent to the teeth. (Rests may be placed on the incisal edge or in *prepared* cinguli areas of anterior teeth.)

Bracing resists lateral forces and is achieved by the rigid portions of clasp arms contacting the lateral surfaces of a tooth.

Retention is derived from the flexible tips of the clasp arms. Retention resists forces tending to displace the appliance occlusally. Clasp retention is possible because the metal used in partial dentures is stiff and resists deformation. The tip of the clasp flexes during insertion so

(c) where six anterior teeth remain which are at such an angle that the survey line is at the incisal edge of the teeth when the cast has a zero degree tilt. In each of these situations, however, it is necessary that the *clasp tip be in an undercut which was present when the cast was surveyed in its parallel or zero degree tilt position.* If the clasp tip is not in such an undercut, it will not be retentive when placed in the patient's mouth.

This system of surveying is simple, easy to understand, and produces uniformly good results. It places the burden for successful partial dentures with the dentist, as it is necessary that he prepare the teeth so that the partial denture will function to its maximum effectiveness.

An illustration of the fallacy of "creating" or "producing" undercuts by tilting a cast is shown in **Figures 2 through 5**. A cast was made in which all of the teeth are represented by cones. It can be seen that there

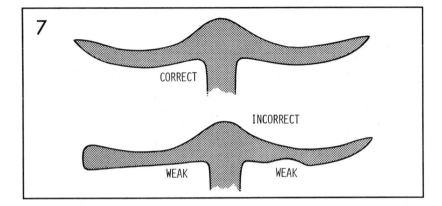

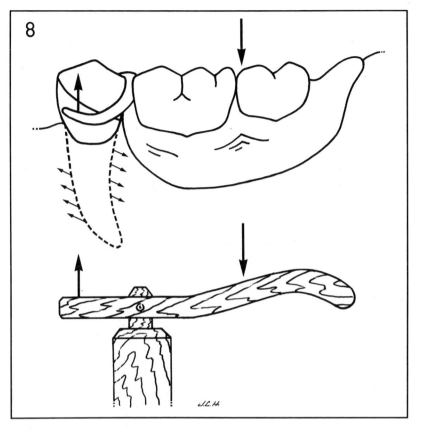

that it engages an undercut on an abutment tooth. Once the clasp is in position, it is passive and exerts no force on the tooth except when the partial denture is removed or when vertical displacing forces are encountered.

The amount of undercut which a clasp engages is determined by (a) the flexibility of the clasp arm, (b) the depth of the undercut, and (c) the amount of undercut utilized. Flexibility depends on (a) the metal used in the clasp, (b) the design of the clasp, (c) the cross-sectional shape, whether it is round or half-round, (d) whether it is wrought or cast, and (e) the length of the clasp arm. Gold has twice the modulus of elasticity and is thus twice as flexible as most non-precious partial denture alloys when the materials are compared in similar clasp situations. A gold clasp can engage twice the undercut to gain the same amount of retention as a similar clasp made of non-precious alloy. Conversely, a non-precious clasp may engage half the undercut used for gold with similar results. These factors must be considered in the design of all clasps.

A clasp arm must taper from its origin to its tip (**Figure 7**). Clasp arms which taper uniformly flex uniformly. Breakage, distortion and inadequate retention may result when thin areas occur in a clasp arm.

There are three basic types of clasps, circumferential, bar, and wrought wire. Circumferential type clasps approach the undercut from an occlusal direction. Bar clasps approach the tooth from the gingival portion of the tooth after crossing soft tissue adjacent to the tooth. Wrought wire clasps are of circumferential design, but differ in the material from which they are made. The chief advantage of round wrought wire clasps is that they flex both vertically and horizontally, whereas cast clasps flex only in a horizontal manner.

There are two basic principles to be followed in designing clasps: (1) the clasp should not traumatize the tooth during insertion and removal, and (2) in free-end extension partial dentures the clasp should not cause the tooth to move when the partial denture moves under function. (There are fewer limitations on clasp design in tooth-borne partial dentures than in free-end extension partial dentures.)

A free-end extension partial denture will act as mild extraction forceps if a rigid, nonyielding clasp is used on an abutment tooth. The action is very much like that of a pump handle (**Figure 8**). For this reason the clasp must be designed so that it can move on the tooth without moving the tooth when the partial is in function. This is done usually by utilizing an undercut adjacent to the edentulous area, a flexible clasp, and may be enhanced by using a mesial rest for better mechanical advantage.

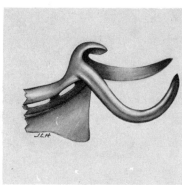

Circumferential (Akers, Class I)

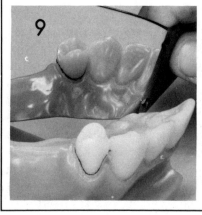

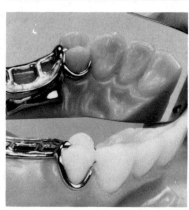

Clasps with two arms may be designed so that both tips are retentive; i.e., engage undercuts. However, it is best to design clasps so that there is one retentive arm and one reciprocal arm. This prevents a clasp from being too retentive and injuring an abutment tooth. The reciprocal arm engages no undercut and opposes any force arising from the retentive clasp. Ideally, both retentive and reciprocal arms should be opposite each other and at the same level on the tooth, and the tooth surfaces contacted by minor connectors and reciprocal arms should be mutually parallel to prevent tooth movement during insertion and removal. This is often impossible or impractical to achieve. Paralleling these surfaces is the responsibility of the dentist and should be done when the mouth is being prepared.

The clasps most commonly used in partial denture construction are listed in atlas form on the following pages. An understanding of these clasps will enable an individual to design partial dentures for most mouths. Components of different clasps may be combined for unusual situations on condition that each clasp provides support, bracing and retention. It must be remembered that any clasp functions more effectively when the mouth has been well prepared by the dentist.

Type: Circumferential
Undercut Utilized: Mesiofacial and/or mesiolingual (.010–.020).
Indications:
1. Removable bridge (tooth borne partial) where there is no movement during function.
2. On free-end extensions where undercut is so small that longer clasp arms will not be retentive.
3. On free-end extensions when minimal undercut is utilized.

Contra-indications:
On free-end extensions except as noted above.

Advantages:
1. Good support and bracing, simple design.
2. Does not distort easily.
3. Easy to adjust.
4. Contacts minimal area of the tooth.
5. Good esthetics.

Disadvantages:
May traumatize abutments when used incorrectly on free-end extensions.

Comment:
Good clasp. May be used on any tooth with proper survey lines. Incorrect use results in slow painless extraction of abutment.

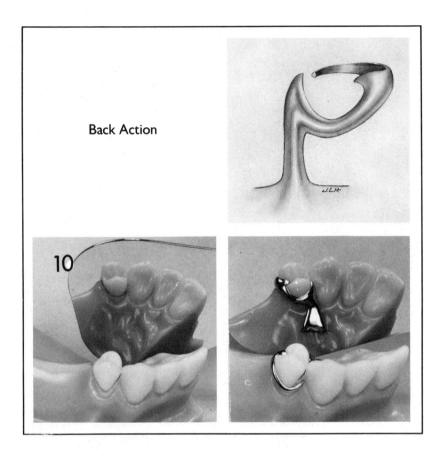

Back Action

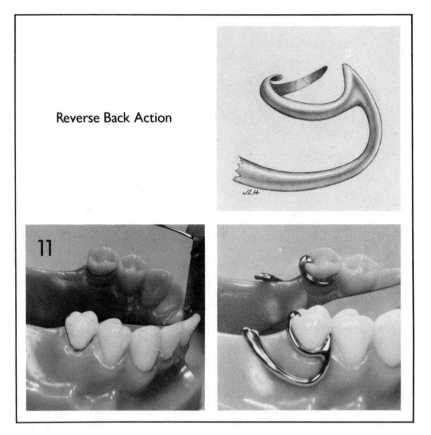

Reverse Back Action

Type: Circumferential
Undercut Utilized:
1. Mesiofacial (.010) and distal (.010).
2. Mesiofacial only (.010–.020).
Indications:
1. Premolar and canine abutments on free-end extensions.
2. On anterior abutments of removable bridges when prognosis of posterior abutment is poor.
3. On short teeth with small mesiofacial and distal undercuts.
Contra-indications:
Not used on molars because of length of clasp arm.
Advantages:
1. Can use small undercut areas.

2. Length of clasp produces resiliency and "stress-breaking" effect on abutments for free-end extension partial dentures.
Disadvantages:
1. Easily distorted because of length. Difficult to adjust.
2. Large tooth area covered.
3. Bracing (resistance to lateral stress) only average.
4. Design produces "food trap" between lingual arm and major connector.
Comment:
"Stress-breaking" action dependent on creation of space between clasp and saddle to permit clasp to flex.

Type: Circumferential
Undercut Utilized:
1. Mesiolingual (.010) and distal (.010).
2. Mesiolingual only (.010–.020).
Indications:
Premolar abutments with lingual inclination on free-end extension partial dentures.
Contra-indications:
1. Maxillary partial dentures for esthetic reasons.
2. When there is a severe soft-tissue undercut inferior to lingual marginal gingiva.

Advantages:
Has "stress-breaking" action similar to "back action clasp."
Disadvantages:
1. Crosses soft tissue.
2. Excessively long clasp, easily distorted, difficult to adjust.
3. Poor esthetics.
4. Contacts large area of tooth.
Comment:
This clasp is a combination of a bar clasp and a back action clasp with none of their advantages and all of their disadvantages. It should be avoided whenever possible.

Half and Half (Split Clasp)

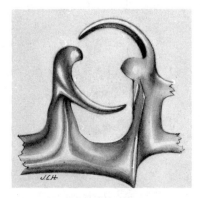

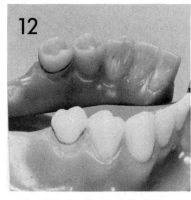
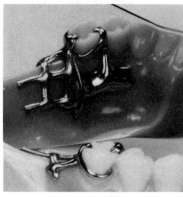

12

Type: Circumferential
Undercut Utilized: Distolingual (.010).
Indications:
1. Premolar and molar abutments for free-end extension partial dentures and removable bridges.
2. Isolated teeth when they cannot be made contiguous with the dental arch by means of a fixed restoration, often for bracing only, with no undercut engaged.

Contra-indications:
None. May be used to avoid trauma to abutment on free-end extension partial dentures.

Advantages:
1. Good support and bracing.
2. Distortion not a problem, easy to adjust.
3. Contacts minimal area of the tooth.
4. Good esthetics.

Disadvantages:
Food trap may be produced between lingual arm and major connector if not executed properly.

Comment:
This clasp is basically a circumferential clasp cut in two. The facial portion is identical to the facial half of a circumferential clasp; the lingual portion originates from a minor connector in the mesiolingual embrasure. This clasp may be used in many odd situations and also lends itself to routine application.

Ring

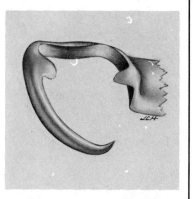

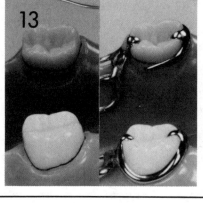
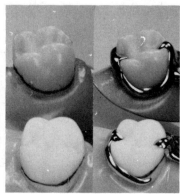

13

Type: Circumferential
Undercut Utilized:
1. Mesiolingual (.020–.030) on mandibular molars.
2. Mesiofacial (.020–.030) on maxillary molars.

Indications:
On molars which are posterior abutments for removable bridges or on tooth borne sides of unilateral free-end extensions.
The molars are usually tipped, maxillary to facial, mandibular to lingual, when this clasp is used. When possible a circumferential clasp is used. However, on maxillary molars, a ring clasp is more esthetic.

Contra-indications:
Not satisfactory when severe distal undercuts are present.

Advantages:
Good support and bracing.

Disadvantages:
1. May distort, difficult to adjust.
2. Contacts large area of tooth.
3. Poor esthetics if lingual undercut utilized on maxillary molar.
4. Accessory arm may cause marginal gingival irritation and act as a food trap.

Comment:
The rigidity of the bracing arm may be increased with a support arm. A support arm is essential when gold is used but is optional with base metal alloys.

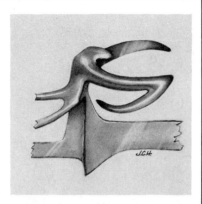

Reverse Action
(Hairpin, C-clasp, Fishhook)

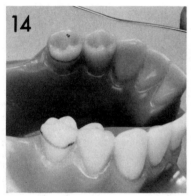

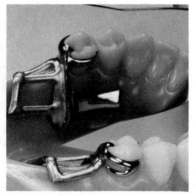

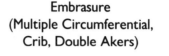

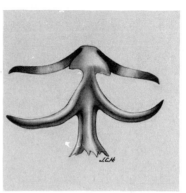

Embrasure
(Multiple Circumferential,
Crib, Double Akers)

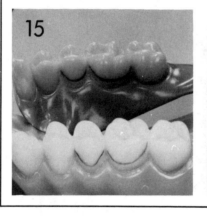

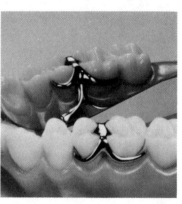

Type: Circumferential
Undercut Utilized: Adjacent to edentulous area (.010–.020).
Indications:
 1. Distofacial undercut on canines and premolars when a sharp tissue undercut prevents use of bar-type clasp.
 2. Undercut near minor connector on molars.
Contra-indications:
 On maxillary teeth where display of metal is objectionable.
Advantages:
 1. Undercut adjacent to edentulous area may be utilized without having minor connector cross soft tissue.

 2. Good bracing and support.
 3. May be used on free-end extension partial dentures or removable bridges.
Disadvantages:
 1. Poor esthetics.
 2. Large area of the tooth surface is covered.
 3. Possible food trap.
Comment:
 May be used instead of a bar clasp on canines and premolars and instead of a ring clasp on molars. Must be made carefully to keep bulk to a minimum.

Type: Circumferential
Undercut Utilized:
 More than one undercut generally is utilized. The number and depth of undercuts are dependent on each situation.
Indications:
 1. To utilize multiple abutments and distribute occlusal support and retention to several teeth.
 2. Where insufficient undercuts are present on a single abutment.
Contra-indications:
 1. Not to be used where clasp would traumatize abutment teeth.
 2. Cannot be used where there is insuf-

ficient space for the minor connector to cross the occlusal surface.
Advantages:
 1. Good support and bracing.
 2. Distributes support, bracing and retention to several teeth.
Disadvantages:
 1. Minor connector usually too thin on occlusal surface resulting in excessive breakage.
 2. Retention may be excessive.
Comment:
 Mouth must be prepared for proper use of this clasp. This clasp is often used where others would be more satisfactory.

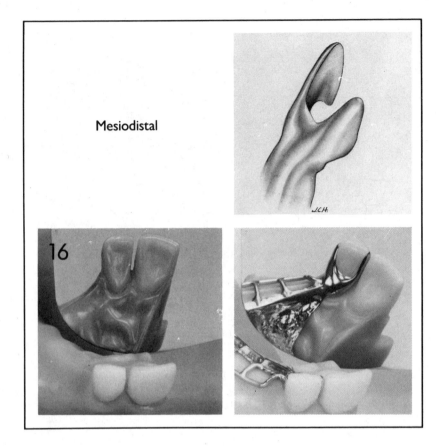

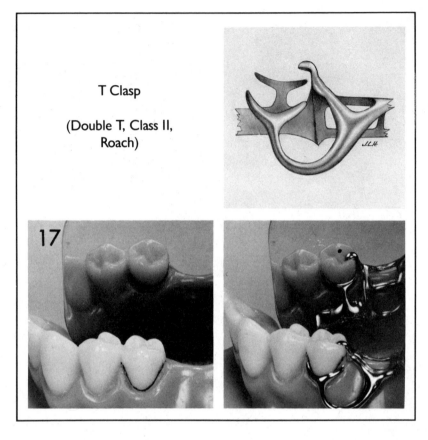

Mesiodistal

T Clasp

(Double T, Class II, Roach)

Type: Circumferential
Undercut Utilized: Retention gained through parallelism and friction.
Indication:
  On maxillary lateral incisors which are abutments for a removable bridge (tooth borne partial) or tooth borne side of a unilateral free-end extension.
Contra-indications:
  1. On free-end extension partial dentures.
  2. On any teeth which have not been properly prepared.

Advantages:
  1. Good esthetics.
  2. Good support and bracing.
Disadvantages:
  Tooth must be prepared by dentist so that proximal surfaces of the tooth are parallel or have slight convergence incisally.
Comment:
  This clasp will traumatize the tooth if used on free-end extension partial dentures. May be used only where distal abutment is present.

Type: Bar
Undercut Utilized:
  1. Distofacial or distolingual on anterior abutments (.010–.020).
  2. Mesiofacial or mesiolingual on posterior abutments (.020).
Indications:
  1. On abutments for free-end extension partial dentures which have distal undercuts.
  2. On posterior abutments when undercut is adjacent to edentulous area.
Contra-indications:
  1. Deep tissue undercuts adjacent to abutment.
  2. Maxillary canines and premolars where minor connectors may be unesthetic.
Advantages:
  1. Utilization of distal undercut prevents abutment from being traumatized in free-end extension partial dentures.
  2. Good esthetics on mandibular canines and premolars.
  3. Small area of tooth contacted.
Disadvantages:
  1. Difficult to adjust.
  2. Bracing not as good as circumferential type.
  3. Poor esthetics on maxillary teeth.
  4. May produce food traps if minor connector crosses tissue undercut.
Comment:
  A mesial or distal occlusal rest may be used; a distal rest is more esthetic. A mesial rest is preferred on free-end extension partial dentures because it produces fewer tilting forces on the tooth.

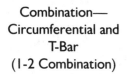

Combination—
Circumferential and
T-Bar
(1-2 Combination)

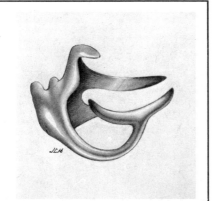

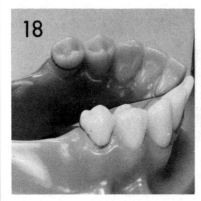

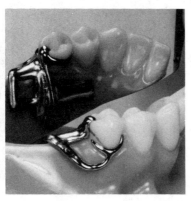

R-Clasp

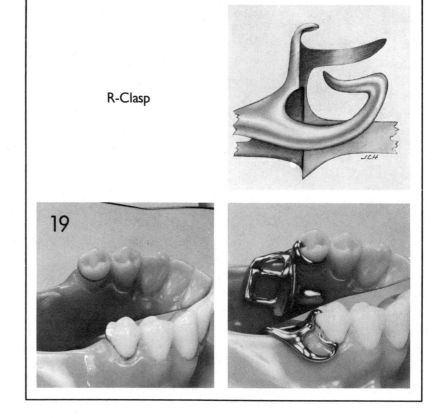

Type: Bar Reciprocated by Circumferential

Undercut Utilized: Adjacent to edentulous area, may be facial or lingual. (.010–.020).

Indications: Same as for T-Bar.

Contra-indications: Same as for T-Bar.

Advantages:
1. Circumferential reciprocal arm makes the design simpler and more comfortable when it is on the lingual surface. There is less chance of a food trap.
2. Better bracing than with two bar type clasp arms.
3. Otherwise, same as for T-Bar.

Disadvantages:
1. Esthetics poor on maxillary canines and premolars.
2. Bar-clasp arm difficult to adjust.
3. Bar-clasp arm may produce food traps if minor connector crosses tissue undercut.

Comment:
This type of design has more applications than a typical bar clasp. Variations may be used on molar abutments to utilize retention adjacent to the edentulous area. Often used on mandibular premolar abutments for free-end extension partial dentures.

Type: Bar or Bar Reciprocated by Circumferential

Undercut Utilized: Same as T-clasp.

Indications: Same as T-clasp.

Contra-indications: Same as T-clasp.

Advantages: Same as T-clasp.

Disadvantages: Same as T-clasp.

Comment:
This clasp is similar to T-clasp except for the shape of the retentive arm. The shape of bar clasp retentive arm is determined by the placement of the undercut and the direction from which the undercut is approached. Note the circumferential reciprocal arm.

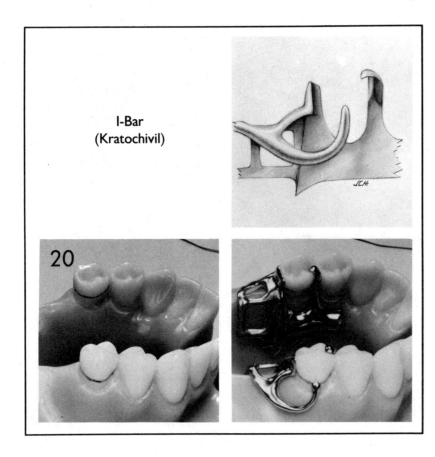

I-Bar
(Kratochivil)

20

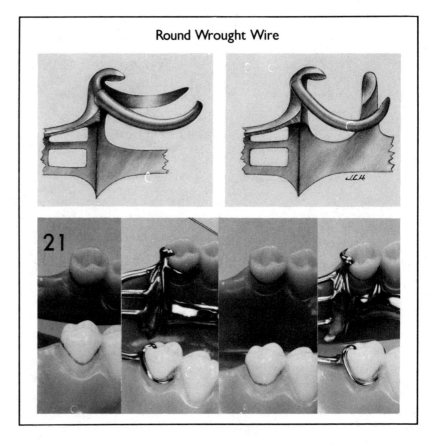

Round Wrought Wire

21

Type: Bar

Undercut Utilized: On center of facial surface at gingival ⅓ (.010).

Indications: On free-end extensions on premolars, usually mandibular.

Contra-indications: On long maxillary free-end extensions.

Advantages:
1. Allows partial to move during function without traumatizing abutment tooth.
2. Good esthetics.
3. Kratochivil system prevents hyperplastic tissue on gingiva distal to the abutment.
4. Minimal tooth area contacted.
5. Least interference with normal tooth contours.

Disadvantages:
1. Relatively poor bracing.
2. Teeth must be prepared by dentist.

Comment: This design consists of several parts:
1. I-bar as described above for retention.
2. Mesial occlusal rest with the minor connector in mesiolingual embrasure to act as reciprocation.
3. Flat metal shoe (with no rest) on distal helps maintain position. Metal over marginal gingiva helps prevent hyperplastic tissue.
4. Abutment tooth must have facial undercut. Distal surface and mesiolingual surface must be prepared to be as parallel as possible.
5. Framework must be tried in mouth without saddles to be sure distal shoe does not bind against tooth.
6. Distal shoe provides definite finish line to which the resin base may be finished.

Type: Circumferential

Undercut Utilized:
   Mesiofacial or mesiolingual (.010–.020).

Indications:
   Canine and premolar abutments for free-end extension partial dentures.

Contra-indications:
   Removable bridges.

Advantages:
1. More flexibility than cast arm. Because it is round, it can flex in any direction (half round cast or wrought arms flex laterally only).
2. Easy to adjust.
3. Good esthetics.

4. Minimal tooth surface contacted—round wire forms line contact.

Disadvantages:
1. Easily distorted by careless handling by patient.
2. Fabrication more time consuming.

Comment:
   In theory, this clasp is advocated for free-end extension partial dentures; when the partial moves in function, the clasp will flex before stress is placed on abutment. The wrought clasp arm may be reciprocated by a cast circumferential arm or a non-retentive I-Bar on mesiolingual surface.

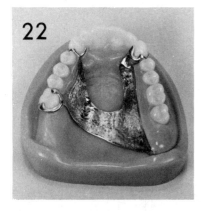
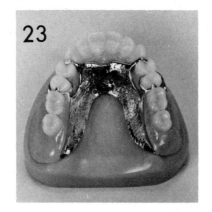
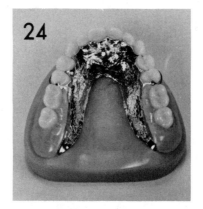
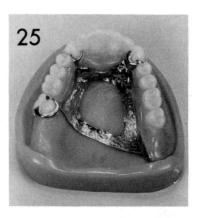

MAJOR CONNECTORS

A major connector is "a metal plate or bar used to join the units of one side of a removable partial denture to those located on the opposite side of the dental arch." (CCDT) Major connectors must be rigid to transmit stresses of mastication from one side of the arch to the other. The forces exerted on a partial denture on one side of the arch are partially transmitted to the teeth on the opposite side by having rigid connectors. This keeps a single abutment tooth from being overloaded.

Major connectors must not impinge on the marginal gingivae. Maxillary major connectors must be at least 6mm. from the marginal gingiva and mandibular major connectors must be at least 2mm. from the marginal gingiva. Maxillary and mandibular lingual plates and mandibular cingulum bars are exceptions to these rules. A major connector must *never* depend on the marginal gingivae for support.

I. Major Connectors for the Maxillary Arch. Maxillary major connectors should be as thin as possible and still be rigid. A wide, thin bar is more comfortable than a narrow, thick bar.

(1) *Single Posterior Palatal Bar* (**Figure 22**). A single posterior palatal bar is indicated for a maxillary tooth borne partial denture (removable bridge), or where there is a unilateral free-end extension. The bar should be wide and nonflexible with the central portion thicker than the edges. This provides strength and yet prevents annoyance caused by the tongue touching a thick bar. The advantage of this type of bar is that it is simple and comfortable for the patient since the tongue seldom touches the posterior portion of the palate. Relief is required when there is a torus palatinus or an enlarged or hard mid-line suture.

The posterior edge must be anterior to the junction of the hard and soft palate (vibrating line).

(2) *Single Anterior Palatal Bar* (**Figure 23**). This connector is indicated when a hard mid-line suture or torus prevents using a posterior palatal bar or a double palatal bar (see below). It usually covers most of the rugae and is designed so that its edges lie in the valleys between the rugae. The corrugations formed by the rugae allow this connector to be made thinner as corrugations add strength. The shape of the anterior palate may cause this connector to have an L beam effect which gives it additional rigidity. The anterior edge should be at least 6mm. from the marginal gingivae.

One disadvantage of this connector is that it may be necessary to make the bar thicker to achieve sufficient rigidity. It covers an area which is the "playground of the tongue" and thickness may cause the patient some annoyance. An anterior palatal bar or "horseshoe" should be avoided when there are other alternatives.

A variation of the anterior palatal bar is the maxillary lingual plate (**Figure 24**). The anterior edge rests on the cinguli of the anterior teeth. The maxillary lingual plate has little value as a splint, but is useful when the vertical dimension of occlusion is being increased and/or when the patient's lower anterior teeth impinge on the lingual gingivae. This connector is useful when anterior teeth are replaced.

(3) *Double Palatal Bar* (**Figure 25**). This connector is the most commonly used major connector in the maxillary arch. It may be used for tooth borne and free-end extension partial dentures and is composed of an anterior and posterior palatal bar. This gives the effect of a circle and is more than twice as strong as either bar would be individually.

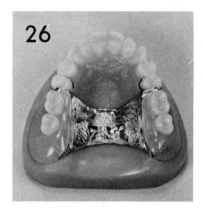
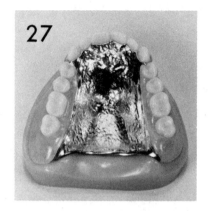
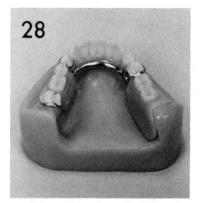
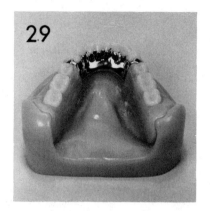

There is a definite L beam effect; i.e., metal in two different planes. The advantage of this type of connector is that each portion; i.e., anterior and posterior, may be made thinner and narrower than single bars and still have sufficient strength and rigidity. The disadvantages are that it covers more tissue and may feel bulkier to the patient than a single anterior or posterior bar.

(4) *Palatal Plate or Strap* (**Figure 26**). A palatal plate is basically a wide posterior palatal bar. Because it is wider, it may also be thinner. The advantages of a palatal plate are that it is less objectionable to the patient and also helps to distribute the stress of mastication over a wider area. A palatal plate may increase retention because of increased interfacial surface tension. The use of a palatal plate may eliminate the need for indirect retention.

(5) *Full Palatal Coverage* (**Figure 27**). Full palatal coverage is used to obtain maximum strength, stability and retention. A full palate is particularly useful when there are only six anterior teeth present and the patient needs a partial denture. Full palatal coverage helps reduce stress on the remaining teeth.

A full palate may be made of either plastic or metal. Metal provides more stimulation to the underlying tissue due to heat transference. Metal is more accurate but rebasing is difficult. Plastic is bulkier but is less expensive.

Note that a metal palate in the illustration includes a lingual plate which terminates on the teeth.

II. **Major Connectors for the Mandibular Arch.** Major connectors are usually on the lingual side of the mandibular arch. Labial bars are necessary only when the teeth have an excessive lingual tilt and to use a lingual bar would necessitate leaving a large space between the bar and the tissue. Labial bars are rarely used.

(1) *Lingual Bar* (**Figure 28**). Lingual bars are the most common mandibular major connector. They; like all major connectors, are rigid to allow cross-arch transference of occlusal loads. Lingual bars are used whenever possible, provided there is no indication for a more elaborate connector.

A lingual bar has a "half-pear" cross-sectional shape. The superior portion of the bar is thin while the inferior portion is thicker. A long lingual bar must of necessity have more bulk but it is advisable to keep the bar as thin as possible and still achieve rigidity. The superior border may contact the mucosa and is always at least 2mm. inferior to the gingival crevice to avoid gingival irritation. The advantages of a lingual bar are that it is simple, does not contact the teeth and hence does not tend to collect food against the teeth. The disadvantage of this type of connector is that it may be flexible if not properly made.

(2) *Lingual Plate (Linguoplate) or Blanket* (**Figure 29**). A lingual plate is an extension of a lingual bar which covers the cingulum of some of the teeth, usually the six anteriors. It may cover the lingual surface of premolars and molars.

A lingual plate is indicated (a) when the remaining teeth need to be stabilized, (b) when a high lingual frenum prevents the use of a simple lingual bar, (c) for indirect retention, and (d) to add rigidity to a long lingual bar. A lingual blanket may prevent the accumulation of heavy deposits of calculus which plague some people.

The advantages of this type of connector are that it helps to stabilize mandibular anterior teeth and does give additional bulk and rigidity to

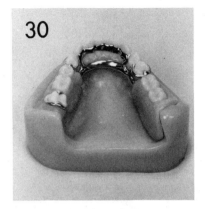

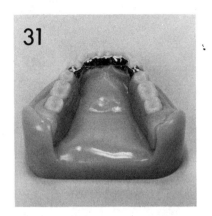

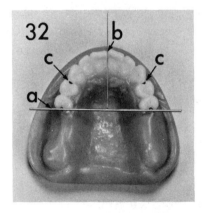

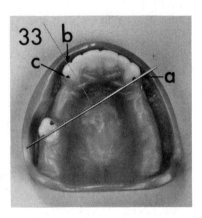

lects food and produces more irritation. A double bar tends to interfere with the tongue and is less rigid than a lingual plate.

(4) *Cingulum Bar* (**Figure 31**). Sometimes a high lingual frenum prevents the use of a lingual bar or a lingual plate. In these instances a bar which covers the cinguli must be used. A cingulum bar must be made with a base metal alloy to obtain sufficient rigidity. They may, like lingual plates, produce decay in susceptible individuals. Cingulum bars are not in general use, but are an ideal major connector for some patients.

INDIRECT RETENTION

When an individual wearing a partial denture chews a piece of sticky candy, there is a tendency for the partial denture to be displaced vertically as the patient opens his mouth. If there is not sufficient retention on the abutment teeth, the denture is dislodged. When the partial denture has a free-end extension and the retention on the abutment teeth is adequate, there is a tendency for a free-end extension to rotate away from the tissue. Indirect retention keeps the free-end extension in place in these situations.

Indirect retention enables a free-end partial denture to resist the "pull of sticky foods." Indirect retention applies only to unilateral or bilateral free-end extension partial dentures and is not a consideration in designing tooth borne partial dentures.

The *fulcrum line* is the line about which a free-end extension partial denture tends to rotate and is determined by joining the most distal occlusal rests in a straight line (a, **Figures 32–34**).

An *indirect retainer* is a mechanical portion of the partial denture which prevents rotation of a partial denture away from the tissue. The ideal location of the direct retainer is determined by bisecting the fulcrum line and placing the indirect retainer as far as possible from the fulcrum line opposite the free-end extension (b, **Figures 32–34**). The logical location of the indirect retainer is often a little different from the ideal location (c, **Figures 32–34**).

An indirect retainer should be a rest perpendicular to the long axis of the tooth or teeth upon which it rests. An indirect retainer which does not have a positive seat perpendicular to the long axis may tend to displace the tooth against which it rests. When a lingual plate acts as an

the major connector. When contoured and fabricated with finesse it will not cause interference with the patient's tongue. The disadvantages are that it may tend to produce decay in susceptible individuals although this is not a common problem. Tissue hypertrophy may occur if there is relief under the plate at the gingival margin. If there is a settling of the distal part of the appliance, the lingual plate will no longer contact the teeth.

(3) *Double Bar (Kennedy Bar)* (**Figure 30**). A double bar is similar to a lingual plate except that the portion covering the marginal gingiva is removed. This results in an inferior lingual bar with a superior bar or strap lying on the cinguli of the teeth.

The advantages of this type of connector are similar to those of the lingual plate. Some people feel that the space allows natural stimulation of the marginal gingiva. Our experience indicates that this space col-

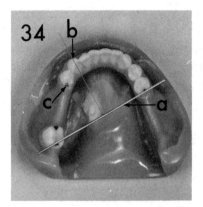
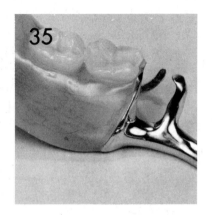
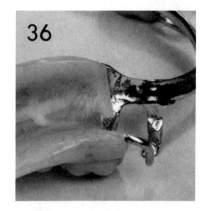

indirect retainer, an occlusal rest should be placed on the mesioocclusal surface of the first premolars. The necessity of indirect retention when only six anterior teeth remain is determined by the dentist and depends on his beliefs and the conditions found in the patient.

An occlusal rest on a clasp may act as an indirect retainer, particularly on a unilateral free-end extension which has a tooth-bound edentulous space on the opposite side. The occlusal rest of the clasp on the anterior abutment on the tooth-bound edentulous space acts as the indirect retainer (**Figures 22, 25, 28 and 30**).

Indirect retention may not be necessary if a broad major connector is used on a maxillary partial denture (**Figure 26**). Other than this exception, it is best to include indirect retention as an integral part of partial denture design.

FINISH LINES

A finish line should be provided on all partial denture frameworks wherever denture base resin and the metal framework join. A finish line allows the resin to terminate in a butt joint (**Figures 35 and 36**). Saliva and debris will accumulate between the denture base resin and the metal when the resin ends in a thin edge.

The technique for providing internal finish lines and external finish lines is discussed in the sections dealing with preparation for duplication and making the wax pattern for a partial denture framework. The utilization of finish lines and their placement are not the sole criteria of success or failure. However, the proper placement and design of finish lines add to patient comfort, oral hygiene, and make a better appearing appliance.

REVIEW QUESTIONS

1. State the two basic principles to be followed when designing clasps.
2. Discuss the three functions of a properly constructed clasp.
3. What are the indications for use of a back-action clasp?
4. What are the indications and advantages of a round wrought wire clasp?
5. Draw in outline form five designs for major connectors for the maxillary arch and state indications for each type.

SECTION 22

Planning, Mouth Preparation, and Final Design

Planning a partial denture is essential so that the mouth may be prepared properly before construction of the appliance is initiated. Successful partial dentures are rarely made without planning and preparation.

Most of the procedures described in this section are the responsibility of the dentist. In many dental practices these procedures are done in the dental office by the dentist or under his direct supervision. This is the best method for determining the design of a partial denture as it places the responsibility directly with the dentist.

In some dental practices the dental laboratory technician pours the preliminary impressions and may make the preliminary survey and design. This is then approved or modified by the dentist, after which he does the necessary mouth preparation and makes the final impressions. This arrangement requires that the dental laboratory technician have a complete understanding of partial denture design, but leaves the responsibility for the design with the dentist. The dentist, knowing the patient's oral condition, must accept this responsibility. In the present day practice of dentistry, a laboratory technician can rarely be blamed for the failure of a partial denture.

Figure A   The first step in any dental procedure is an examination, including X-rays and charting of existing conditions.

Figures B and C   Preliminary impressions are part of the examination procedure when a removable partial denture is indicated. (Many dentists make diagnostic casts for all of their patients.)

Figure D   A simple jaw relation record is necessary to mount the casts. This record is usually made in centric relation so that discrepancies in occlusion may be noted when the casts are mounted.

Figure I   The preliminary impressions are ready to be poured. A simple but adequate jaw relation record should always accompany preliminary impressions.

Figure 2   Before pouring, all saliva should be washed out of the impression. Excess water is removed by shaking the impression, but do not dry. When pouring, place stone in one of the distal corners and allow it to run around the teeth, checking constantly to be sure that air is not trapped. The excess water will be pushed ahead of the stone as it travels around the impression. Allow the excess water to run out of the impression before adding the bulk of stone.

Figure 3   The impression is filled with stone.

Figures 4 and 5   A mound of stone is placed on a glass slab and the impression is inverted into it. The stone is shaped around the impres-

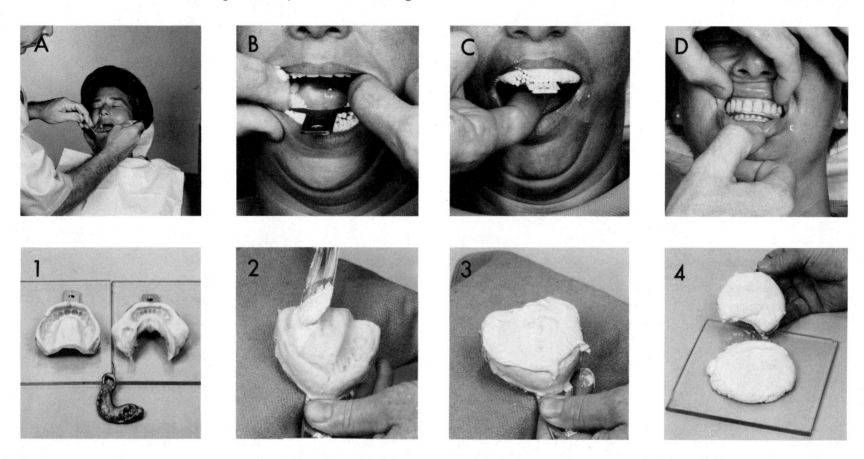

sion in the same manner as was done for preliminary impressions for complete dentures.

Figures 6 through 9 The same procedures are followed for the mandibular impression. Do not press the impression into the stone which has been placed on the glass slab. This prevents excess stone from flowing in the tongue space.

Figure 10 After the stone has set, the impressions are removed from their casts.

Figure 11 The casts are trimmed and are now ready, by means of the interocclusal jaw relation record, to be mounted.

Figure 12 If upon examination there were no occlusal discrepancies, the casts may be mounted on a simple hinge articulator. The selection of an articulator on which to mount diagnostic casts is determined by the desires of the dentist who usually bases this decision on the complexity of the restorative problem. A face-bow transfer will be supplied by the dentist if a more complex articulator is to be used.

At this stage, the dentist should indicate if any teeth associated with the removable partial denture need cast restorations or crowns. The design and contours of such restorations can be developed to enhance the appearance and function of the removable appliance.

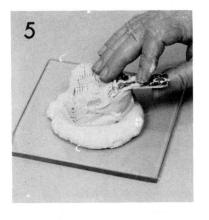
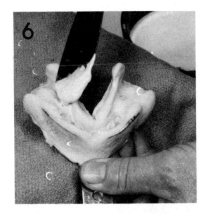
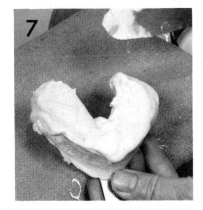
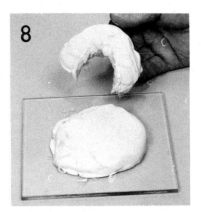
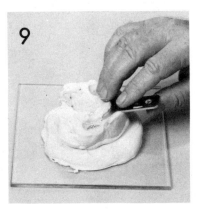
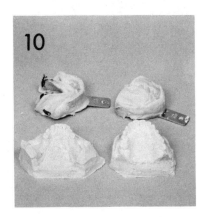
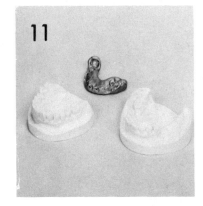
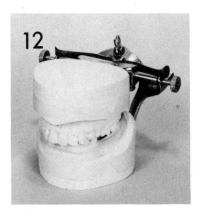

NON-TECHNICAL ASPECTS OF PLANNING FOR REMOVABLE PARTIAL DENTURES

Planning a removable partial denture is a relatively complex procedure. The dentist must assess a number of factors present in each individual patient. The number and location of the remaining natural teeth is one factor; the teeth in the opposing arch must be considered as well as those in the arch needing the removable partial denture. Extrusion of teeth opposite an edentulous space always occurs in time and can complicate dental restorations from simple fillings to complex removable partial dentures.

The caries experience of the patient is also a consideration. Extreme caries susceptibility may influence a dentist to alter his approach to an otherwise simple restorative problem.

Periodontal disease is of importance in planning for removable partial dentures and is usually the most common complicating factor. Often these factors dictate extensive preparation including treatment of periodontal disease and restorations in conjunction with such treatment. Often the abutment teeth for removable partial dentures may be splinted together for additional strength through the use of cast crowns.

The procedures described in the balance of this section assume that the dentist has accomplished all his prior treatment objectives and is now ready to make a removable appliance.

Figure 13 This is a Jelenko surveyor, one of the more widely used surveyors.

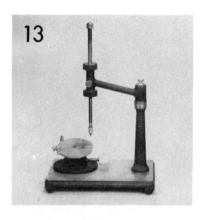
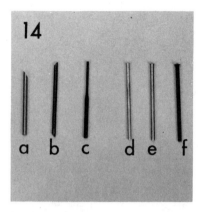
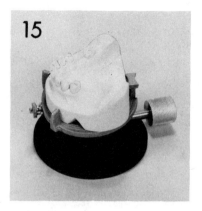
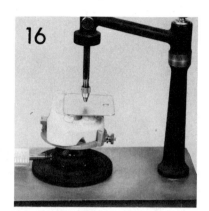

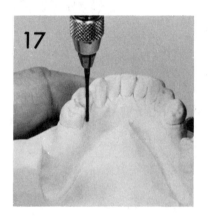
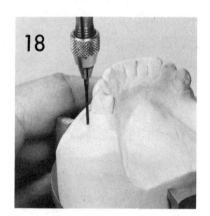
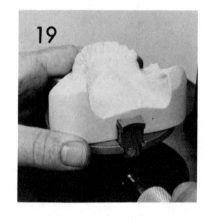
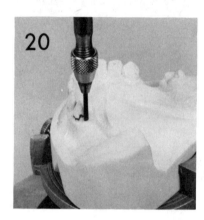

Figure 14   These are the tools which are used in a surveyor:

a is a dental bur which has been beveled and is used as a wax carver.

b is a carbon marker.

c is an analyzing rod which is used to determine undercut areas prior to scribing the height of contour with the carbon marker.

d, e and f are Ney undercut gauges: d is a .010 gauge, e is a .020 gauge, and f is a .030 gauge.

Figure 15   The preliminary cast is placed on the tilt-top surveying table.

Figure 16   The cast is positioned so that the occlusal plane is perpendicular to the vertical rod on the surveyor and is parallel to the surveyor base.

Figure 17   The analyzing rod is placed in the chuck on the surveyor and is used to check the contours of all teeth which may be involved in the partial denture.

Figure 18   Soft tissue undercuts which may influence the design of the partial denture are also checked.

Figure 19   The cast may be tipped slightly to improve undercut areas. It must be remembered that any undercut utilized for retention must be

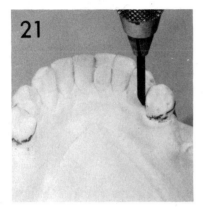

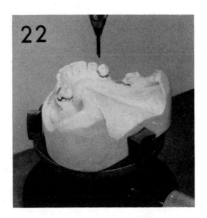

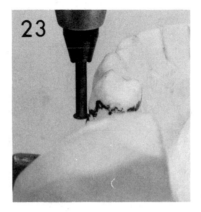

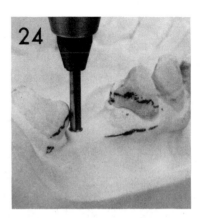

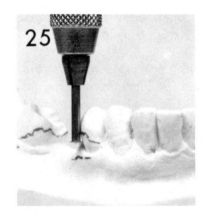

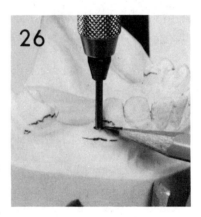

present when the occlusal plane is perpendicular to the vertical rod of the surveyor. Tilting is not often necessary.

Figure 20   The carbon rod is placed in the surveyor and the height of contour is scribed on all teeth involved in the partial denture design.

Figure 21   Beveling the carbon marker allows it to be placed farther into the embrasures.

Figure 22   The survey lines, marking the height of contour of abutment teeth, are completed. Soft tissue undercuts are also marked.

Figure 23   An undercut gauge is used to measure the undercuts on the abutment teeth. In this illustration it is evident that there is very little undercut on the facial surface of the left second premolar.

Figure 24   The .010 undercut gauge is in position against the molar abutment. This shows that the undercut present is greater than .010 inches.

Figure 25   This illustration shows a .020 undercut gauge in position on the right first premolar. This is the correct position of an undercut gauge when measuring an undercut. The shaft of the gauge is touching the tooth at the height of contour, and the flange of the gauge is touching the tooth. This indicates an undercut of .020 inches at this point.

Figure 26   A mark is made with a sharp pencil where the undercut gauge touches the tooth. This indicates the point at which the tip of the clasp will terminate. By terminating at this point the clasp will engage an undercut measuring .020 inches. The position of the other retentive clasp tips is determined in a similar manner. (See Section 21 for the proper amount of undercut.)

Figure 27   The design of the partial denture is drawn on the cast with a colored pencil. A colored pencil prevents the survey line and the design from becoming confused. The dentist making this partial denture decided to use an I-bar on the facial surface of the left second premolar for retention. This type of clasp requires very little undercut. On the lingual surface of the tooth there will be a reciprocal I-bar with a

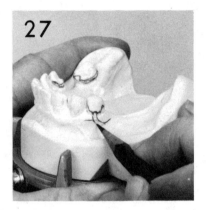

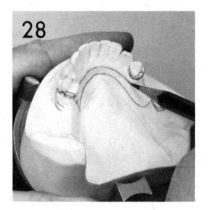

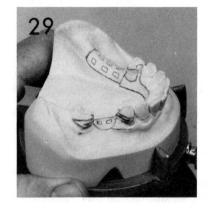

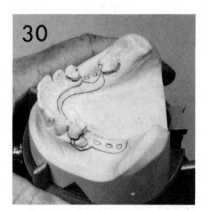

mesioocclusal rest. A distal shoe will complete this clasp. This clasp design is advocated by Kratochivil (**Figure 20**, Section 21).

Figure 28 The lingual bar is drawn in its proper position. The superior edge of the lingual bar must be a minimum of 2 mm. from the marginal gingiva.

Figure 29 The first premolar and second molar are tilted in such a manner that there is a distinct distofacial undercut on the first premolar and a mesiofacial undercut on the second molar. This produces several problems in design which cannot be solved with simpler clasps. It was decided to use a reverse action clasp (**Figure 14**, Section 21) on the facial of each of these teeth. They will be reciprocated on the lingual surface with conventional circumferential arms. Note the position of the lingual I-bar on the left second premolar. It is in an embrasure and will cause a minimum of interference with the tongue.

Figure 30 The circumferential reciprocal arms on the right abutment teeth and the distal shoe on the left second premolar are shown. The distinct facial tissue undercut inferior to the right second premolar can be seen in this photo. This tissue undercut will be blocked out in later stages to insure that the minor connector will not be in a soft tissue undercut. (Leaving the minor connector in such an undercut will abrade the tissue upon each insertion and removal.)

Figure 31 Areas of interference which need to be removed by the

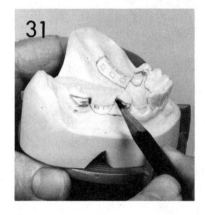

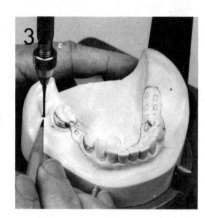

dentist are marked on the cast in a contrasting color. We have used blue pencil to mark the interferences and red pencil to mark the design.

Figure 32 The vertical rod on the surveyor is locked into position and marks are made in three widely separated spots on the cast. These *tripod marks* may be used to reorient the cast on the surveyor if it becomes necessary.

Figure 33 The tripod marks are circled for identification.

Figures 34 and 35 The cast is returned to the articulator to check further the occlusal relationships. The left maxillary molars have extruded because the patient did not have any opposing teeth for some

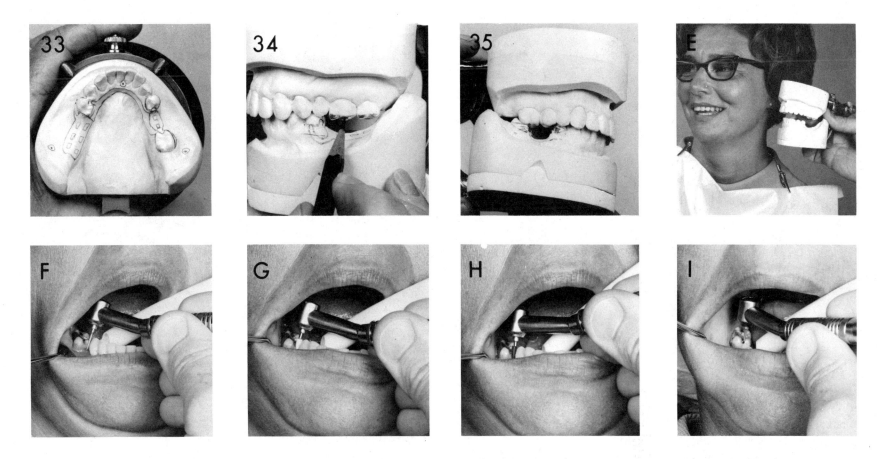

years. It was decided to reduce the occlusal surface of these teeth to provide a better occlusal plane and to increase the intermaxillary space. The teeth on the right side of the cast present a good occlusal plane.

At this stage a tentative design has been determined and the teeth which need alteration have been marked. The contours of any needed restorations would also be decided upon at this time. This patient did not require any restorations.

Figure E The preliminary casts are used as a reference during mouth preparation.

Figures F, G and H The mouth preparation required by this patient was done in one appointment. The mandibular teeth which needed

recontouring were first prepared with a diamond instrument. This leaves a relatively rough area on the tooth which is then smoothed with a fine stone. The area is finally smoothed with rubber abrasive points and polished.

Figure I Occlusal rest preparations are made on the abutment teeth. This is done after the teeth have been contoured to insure that the occlusal rest preparation will not be reduced by the recontouring. Occlusal rest preparations should be ⅓ to ½ the faciolingual distance between cusp tips. The depth should be sufficient to provide strength in the partial denture and shallow enough to prevent penetration of the enamel. Greater depth is possible when occlusal rests are placed in metal restorations.

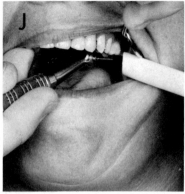
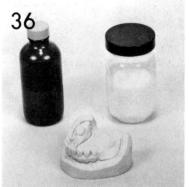
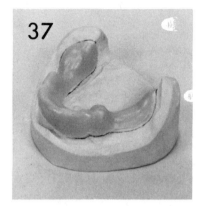
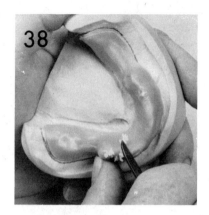

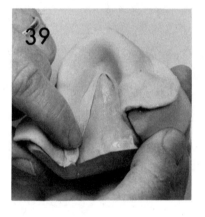
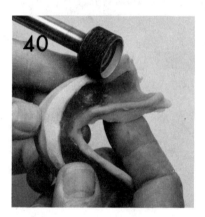

Figure J   The maxillary left molars are reduced occlusally as indicated on the diagnostic casts.

FINAL IMPRESSIONS

Final impressions may be made of agar-agar hydrocolloid in water-cooled trays, of alginate in stock trays modified with wax, or in custom trays. When stock trays are used, the same technique shown in **Figures B and C** is followed. The choice of an impression technique rests with the dentist. The result should be an accurate cast.

Custom trays are made following the same technique used for immediate dentures (Section 18). Alginate in a custom tray produces an impression which is overextended, but not to the degree found in impressions made in stock trays. A stock tray ordinarily is used if a corrected impression (Section 26) is to be made of the free-end extension area.

Figure 36   The outline of the tray is placed on the preliminary cast. Resin tray material is used for making the tray.

Figure 37   A wax spacer is adapted to the cast. This spacer is one thickness of baseplate wax. Any gross undercuts are relieved before the spacer is adapted.

Figure 38   Holes are cut in the spacer on the occlusal or incisal edges

of teeth which are **not** abutments. This produces stops in the tray which help to seat the tray accurately when making the impression.

Figure 39   The resin tray material is adapted to the prepared cast and allowed to set.

Figure 40   The tray is removed from the cast and trimmed to the outline.

Figure 41   The tray is smoothed and the wax spacer is removed. Holes are placed in the tray with a No. 6 or No. 8 round bur approximately ⅛ to 3/16 inch apart. The holes will retain the alginate in the tray. Another method to retain alginate is to use an alginate adhesive.

This type impression tray can be easily modified for use with other

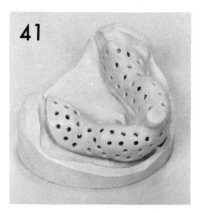
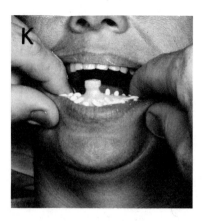
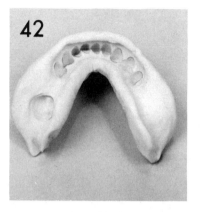
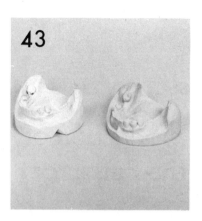

impression materials. After the wax spacer is removed, the interior surface is smoothed. Then the interior surface is coated with an appropriate adhesive for whatever elastic impression material is to be used.

Figure K A custom tray is being used to make a final impression with alginate.

Figure 42 The completed impression.

The master casts are poured in the same manner as the preliminary casts (**Figures 1–10**). This is a satisfactory procedure if a thick mix of stone is used. Some dentists prefer not to invert their impressions; instead they fill the tongue space of mandibular impressions with a wet paper towel to prevent stone from entering the tongue space. (**Figure 22, Section 4**) Another technique is to pour the impression, not invert it, and let the stone reach its initial set. Then the base is poured.

Figure 43 The completed master cast is shown next to the preliminary cast.

REVIEW QUESTIONS

1. What is the analyzing rod on a surveyor used for?
2. Why are tripod marks placed on a partial denture cast?
3. Discuss the preparation of a partial denture preliminary cast prior to making a custom tray.
4. Is the dentist or the laboratory technician responsible for the final design of a partial denture?

SECTION 23

Production of the Refractory Cast

The framework of a removable partial denture is constructed of cast metal and is the backbone of the appliance. The refractory cast is made from the master cast and forms the basis on which the metal framework is made.

The previous steps, examination, X-rays, preliminary casts and mouth preparation, are planning steps. These steps are similar to the preparation which goes into house plans prepared by an architect. The master casts are like the foundation, in that the appliance will be built on them. Producing a refractory cast is the first step in making the cast metal framework.

The master cast must be resurveyed because the mouth preparation done prior to making the final impression has altered the shape of the teeth. The design must also be transferred to the master cast. Before the cast is duplicated, the undesirable undercuts and/or interferences are eliminated with wax. The master cast is also altered so that the resin denture base material can be attached to the metal framework. After this, the master cast is duplicated in a refractory material or high heat investment upon which the wax pattern for the cast framework will be constructed.

Duplication essentially consists of making an impression of the prepared master cast and pouring the impression in a refractory material. This must be done under controlled conditions so that the refractory material expands when heated to compensate for the shrinkage which occurs when the metal cools.

Figure 1 The master cast is placed on the surveyor, is checked with an analyzing rod to be sure it is in the correct position, and the survey lines are placed using a carbon marker.

Figure 2 Tripod marks are placed on the master cast so that it may be replaced on the surveyor if this becomes necessary. The cast is not removed from the surveyor table until the cast is ready for duplication.

Figure 3 The position of the clasp tips is determined with suitable undercut gauges.

Figure 4 The design is placed on the master cast with a red pencil so that the design will not be confused with the survey lines.

Figure 5 The design on the master cast is complete. The final design may be different from the preliminary design if the dentist so directs.

Figure 6 The materials required for preparing a cast for duplication are a Bunsen burner, a Hanau torch, a piece of gauge wax, a small piece of baseplate wax, a bur which has been beveled and will be used as a wax carver, suitable wax carving instruments, and some oil base modeling clay.

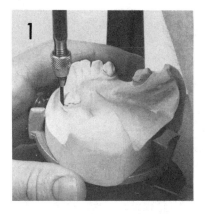
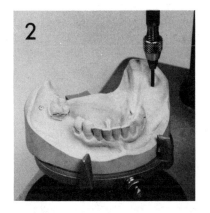
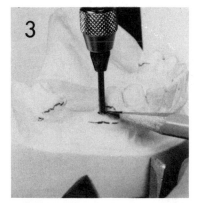
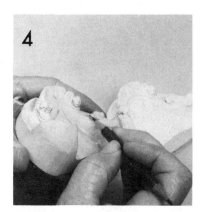
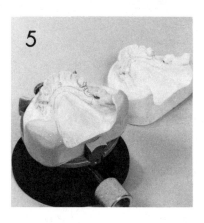
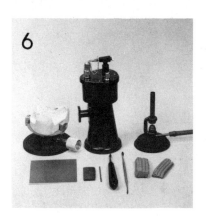
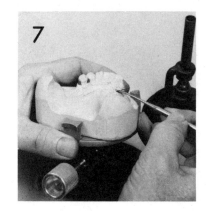
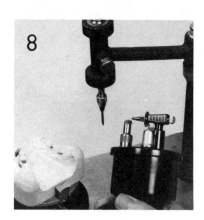

Figure 7 A small amount of baseplate wax is placed in the undesirable undercuts. This includes undercuts on the teeth and soft tissue undercuts which must be eliminated.

Figure 8 The beveled bur shank is placed in the surveyor and heated with a Hanau torch.

Figure 9 The excess wax in the undercuts is removed by moving the teeth against the warm bur shank. The surveyor table will move easily if a few grains of acrylic polymer are sprinkled on the base of the surveyor.

Figure 10 A wiping motion is used to smooth the wax.

Figure 11 A tissue undercut which may be crossed by a minor connector is treated in the same manner as tooth undercuts.

Figure 12 All undesirable undercuts have been eliminated.

Figure 13 Any wax which has flowed above the survey line is removed. Care must be taken not to scratch the surface of the cast.

Figure 14 A small amount of wax is added to the surface of the tooth where the tip of the clasp will lie. A sharp ledge is cut into this wax. This will produce a mark on the refractory cast which will indicate the position of the tip of the clasp.

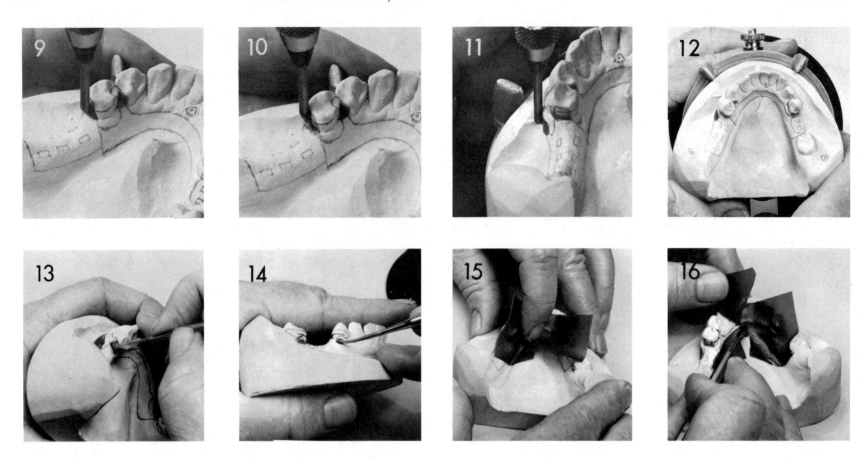

Figure 15 The inferior two-thirds of the lingual bar must be relieved on mandibular free-end extension partial dentures. (It generally is good practice to relieve all lingual bars this way, be they for free-end extensions or tooth borne partial dentures.) This is done by adapting 30 gauge wax in the area of the lingual bar. It must be thoroughly adapted to the cast with no air trapped beneath it.

There may be situations where additional relief is needed. An example is a lingual torus, a bony protruberance lingual to the canines and premolars, which requires substantial relief to avoid irritation in the future.

Figure 16 The wax which extends above the inferior two-thirds of the bar is removed. The design on the master cast may be seen through the wax and acts as a guide for removal of the excess gauge wax.

Figure 17 The superior surface of the lingual bar relief must be feathered into the cast. This prevents a ledge from being formed on the tissue side of the lingual bar.

Figure 18 The superior edge of the lingual bar relief is feathered using a warm, not hot, spatula.

Figure 19 The relief for the area where the free-end extension will lie is made by using a double thickness of 28 or 30 gauge wax. This double thickness of wax is adapted to the edentulous ridge adjacent to the distal abutment tooth. (Note how the anterior edge of this wax overlaps the lingual bar relief.) This relief wax eventually will result in a space between the metal framework and the cast and permits the attachment of the denture base resin to the framework.

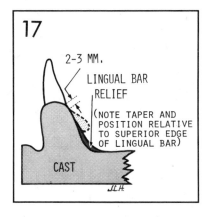
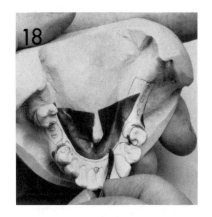
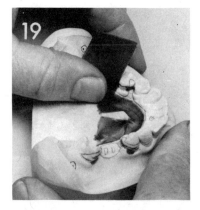
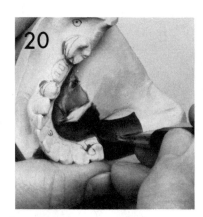
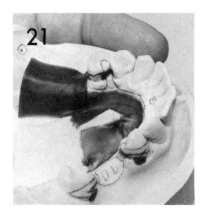
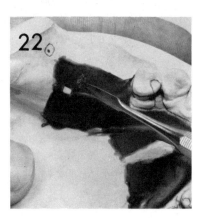
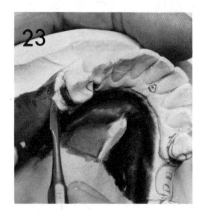
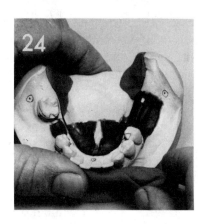

Figure 20 The relief for the plastic retention over the edentulous ridge is trimmed so the anterior edge forms a definite ledge immediately inferior to the distal abutment tooth. This ledge will form the internal finish line on the completed partial denture and should slant slightly posterior from the distogingival margin of the abutment tooth. It should never lean forward; otherwise, the plastic denture base material will lie directly below the abutment tooth.

Figure 21 This illustrates the proper placement of the internal finish line. Note that it is a sharp line or step formed by the relief over the edentulous ridge and the lingual bar relief.

Figure 22 A small square of wax cut out of the relief over the edentulous ridge will prevent the framework being displaced during the

packing procedures. (This step is not necessary but will give some degree of assurance that the framework will not be displaced during packing.)

Figure 23 A small area of wax is removed immediately adjacent to the abutment tooth. This permits metal to lie on the tissue adjacent to the abutment which many dentists feel is healthier than having denture base resin in this area. An additional advantage is that this metal provides a definite place for finishing and prevents excessive space from being created next to an abutment tooth. Such a space can lead to a growth of inflammatory tissue in this area.

Figure 24 A double thickness of 28 or 30 gauge wax is placed over the edentulous ridge between the abutment teeth on the right side of the

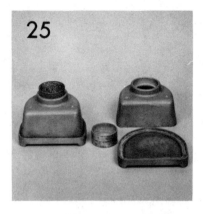
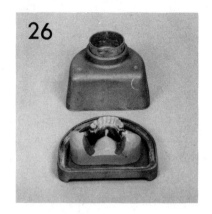
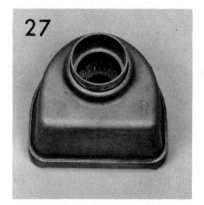
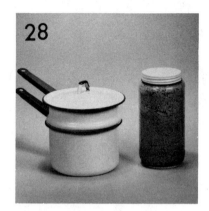

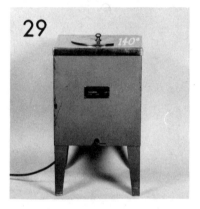
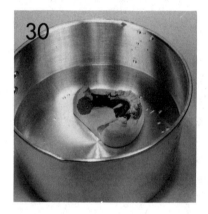

cast. This is trimmed to follow the line on the lingual side of the ridge which is shown clearly in **Figure 23**. This is a sharp ledge as it will become the internal finish line for this small area of denture resin. Note also that a small area of wax has been removed immediately adjacent to each of the abutment teeth.

Oil base modeling clay is used to block out the gross undercuts in the retromylohyoid region and inferior to the anterior teeth. This modeling clay should be trimmed so that it is at least a half a tooth away from the abutment teeth. DO NOT COVER ABUTMENT TEETH WITH MODELING CLAY.

Figure 25   These Ticonium duplicating flasks are one of many satisfactory types of duplicating flasks. (A denture flask may be adapted for duplicating.) One duplicating flask is shown assembled on the left with the three pieces which compose it on the right. The three pieces are the base, the upper portion of the flask, and a reservoir ring.

Figure 26   The cast is checked to be sure that it will fit within the duplicating flask. These flasks are made in various sizes.

Figure 27   The flask is assembled to check that there is sufficient space around the cast for the duplicating material.

Figure 28   Agar-agar hydrocolloid is the most common duplicating material. It is a very accurate elastic impression material which is used in clinical dental procedures as well as in the laboratory. Several manufacturers supply this material for laboratory use. It is usually mixed with water (as per manufacturer's directions), and melted in a double boiler. It should not be melted over an open flame. Agar-agar hydrocolloid melts at 212°F.

Figure 29   This is a Ticonium hydrocolloid storage unit. After the hydrocolloid has been melted, it is placed in a storage unit which is basically a container surrounded by a thermostatically controlled water bath. The brand of hydrocolloid used in our laboratory stores best at 140°F. The hydrocolloid remains molten at this temperature and may be kept in a liquid state in a storage unit.

Figure 30   Before duplication the cast is soaked thoroughly. This usually takes five minutes. Better results are often obtained by inverting the cast so the air bubbles rising from the dried cast are not trapped under the wax.

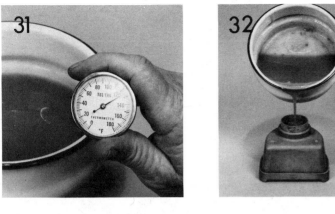
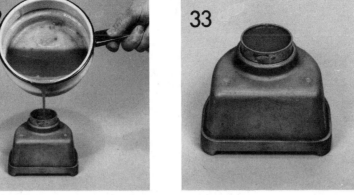
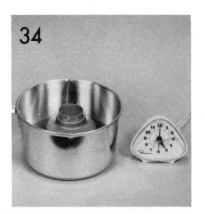

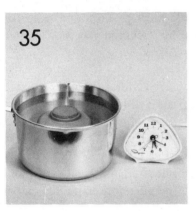
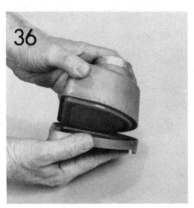
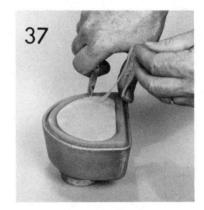
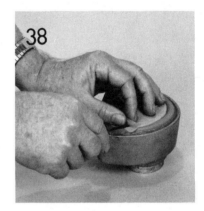

Figure 31 The hydrocolloid is drawn from the storage unit and is stirred until it cools to 125°F. The agar must be cooled to this temperature or it will melt the relief wax which has been placed on the master cast.

Figure 32 Excess water is gently blown off the cast, the cast placed in the duplicating flask and the flask assembled. The hydrocolloid is then poured slowly into the flask. The hydrocolloid rises slowly about the cast and covers its entire surface without trapping any air bubbles.

Figure 33 The flask is filled to the top of the reservoir ring.

Figure 34 The lower one-third of the flask is immersed in cold water for 20 minutes, which cools and solidifies the lower portion of the hydrocolloid while the upper liquid portion acts as a reservoir. This assures close apposition of the hydrocolloid to the cast. Ice may be added to the water to hasten this process. If ice is not used, the water should be changed at intervals. In many localities the temperature of tap water is such that ice becomes necessary during the summer months.

Figure 35 After 20 minutes, the duplicating flask is completely immersed in water. Ice may be used at this stage also. If ice is not used, the pan should be placed under cold running water. The flask is immersed for an *additional 40 minutes to assure that the hydrocolloid is completely solidified.*

Figure 36 The first step in removing the master cast from the duplicating flask is to remove the base.

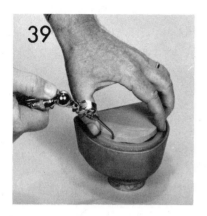
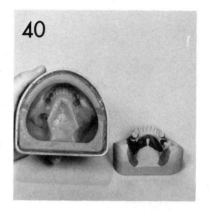
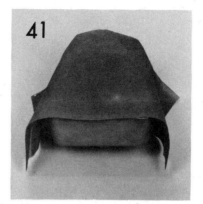
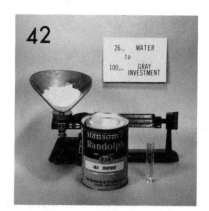

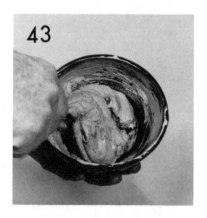
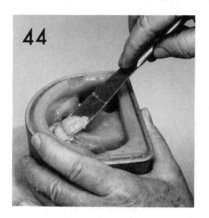

immediately after separation. The mold must be inspected to insure there are no tears or voids. Tears in the hydrocolloid may indicate that the hydrocolloid is old and should be replaced.

Figure 37 Any excess hydrocolloid which has flowed under the cast is removed. Before setting the flask on the bench top, be sure that no hydrocolloid extends above the reservoir ring. If the reservoir ring is removed, cut off the hydrocolloid that extends above the top of the flask.

Figure 41 The hydrocolloid mold is covered with a wet paper towel to prevent evaporation of water. Hydrocolloid will lose water rapidly if it is not covered. It will also take on water if it is immersed.

Up to this point these techniques are similar to those used for low heat base metal alloys. The proper investment for these alloys should be used for production of the refractory cast. High heat base (non-precious) metal alloys may, in addition, require a different duplicating material.

Figure 38 A notch is cut in the hydrocolloid on either side of the cast to act as a finger-hold.

Figure 39 Compressed air is directed around the edge of the cast. This generally lifts the cast from the hydrocolloid. If air is not available, the cast is held by the base and gently removed from the mold.

Figure 42 An investment commonly used for gold partial denture casting is R & R Gray Investment. It is mixed in a ratio of 26cc. of water to 100 grams of investment for investment casts. The proper ratio is very important. One-hundred to one-hundred-fifty grams of investment generally is enough for a refractory cast. The proper proportions of investment and water determine how much the investment cast will expand when it is heated prior to casting. The amount of expansion is calculated to compensate for the shrinkage which occurs when molten gold solidifies.

Figure 40 The hydrocolloid mold and the master cast are shown

Figure 43 Twenty-six grams of investment to 100cc. water makes a thick mix of investment.

Figure 44 The investment is vibrated into the hydrocolloid mold in

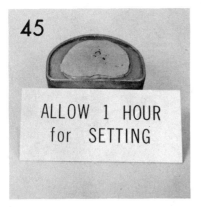
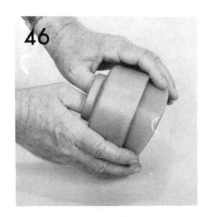
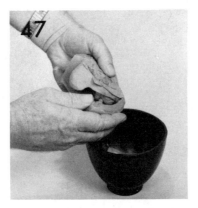
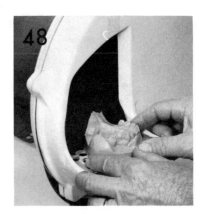

the same manner used for pouring an impression. This mold was poured by placing some investment in the anterior region and letting it flow around both sides simultaneously. The mold is inspected carefully while pouring to be sure air is not trapped. The mold is then filled with investment.

Figure 45 The investment must set for one hour. It is best to cover the top of the duplicating flask with a wet towel while the investment sets.

Figure 46 After the investment is set, the agar is removed from the duplicating flask.

Figure 47 The investment cast is recovered by breaking the agar, which is saved for reuse.

Figure 48 The portion of the cast which is not involved in the pattern is removed on a cast-trimmer. Any slurry from the cast-trimmer must be washed off the cast.

Figure 49 A hole is made through the base of the cast approximately equidistant from all parts of the lingual bar. This hole is approximately ¼ inch in diameter and will hold the main sprue.

Figure 50 The refractory cast must be air dried overnight or placed in a 200°F. drying oven for one and one-half hours. If the cast is left longer in the drying oven, it will disintegrate during later investing procedures.

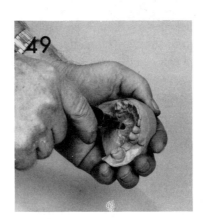
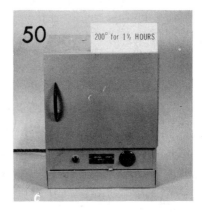

Figure 51 The best results are obtained by dipping the heated cast in beeswax for 15 to 20 seconds. This seals the surface of the cast and will give the tissue side of the casting a smoother surface.

Figure 52 The cast is placed as shown to allow the excess wax to drain. As soon as the cast cools it is ready for fabrication of the wax pattern.

Figure 53 The basic difference between preparing mandibular and maxillary casts for duplication is that a bead line is placed in the master cast around the edge of the maxillary major connector. This bead line is approximately ¾ to 1 millimeter deep and the same width. It should fade out as it approaches the marginal gingiva to prevent tissue displacement in this area. It also fades out over the center of the cast when

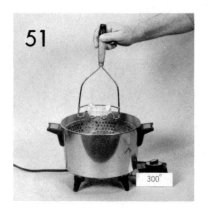
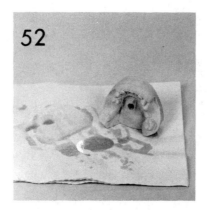
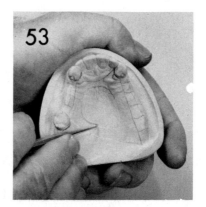
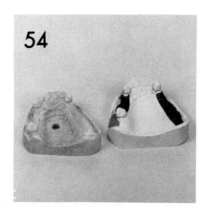

a hard mid-line suture is present. Sometimes a small amount of wax relief may be placed over a hard mid-line suture. This is done at the direction of the dentist. The purpose of the bead line is to keep food from collecting under the maxillary major connector. (A similar bead line under a lingual bar would cause irritation.)

Figure 54 The same basic procedures are followed when preparing maxillary casts for duplication. The undesirable undercuts are relieved in the same manner as for the mandibular cast. Relief is placed over the residual ridges as shown in this illustration to allow for plastic retention. On the lingual side of the ridge the wax is cut to form a sharp ledge which will become the internal finish line.

REVIEW QUESTIONS

1. Describe the preparation of the master cast of a mandibular partial denture before making an impression for pouring a refractory cast.
2. Why is a small area of relief wax removed adjacent to the abutment tooth of a free-end extension ridge?
3. At what temperature is the hydrocolloid material when placed over the master cast for duplication?
4. Describe removing the master cast from the duplicating flask.
5. What is the depth and width of the bead line placed around the edge of the maxillary major connector on the master cast?

SECTION 24

Pattern Construction

The technique of casting into a mold created by making first a wax pattern, surrounding it with a refractory material and then melting the wax, is thousands of years old. Modern technology has refined the technique so that precise castings are easily made.

The "disappearing pattern" technique is used to make the metal framework for a removable partial denture. A substance which vaporizes when heated is used to construct the pattern on the investment cast. The pattern is then surrounded by additional high heat investment which is heated to eliminate the pattern. Metal is then cast into the resulting mold to form the metal framework.

The pattern is made of a combination of pliable plastic patterns and wax. Wax alone was used before the introduction of plastic patterns and some technicians still construct patterns by freehand waxing. However, preformed patterns make fabrication more accurate, faster, and make finishing much simpler. Preformed clasp patterns assure that clasps will have the proper taper and resiliency.

The techniques for pattern construction are the same regardless of the metal to be used. There are some minor variations in the shape of plastic patterns between manufacturers but this makes no difference in the techniques illustrated in this section.

Figure 1   Preformed patterns are available for most partial denture components. They may be adapted to any situation by the addition of wax.

Figure 2   The materials for making a partial denture pattern are: plastic patterns, tacky liquid in an applicator bottle, a Bunsen burner, a Hanau or similar torch, gauge wax, inlay wax, wax shapes for sprues, suitable wax carvers, and the investment cast.

Figure 3   The first step is to outline the framework on the investment cast with a soft pencil to avoid marring the surface of the cast. The master cast is used as a guide. Pay particular attention to the distance of the lingual bar from the marginal gingiva. There is a tendency to get this too close to the abutment teeth.

Figure 4   A lingual bar pattern is removed from the card with a quick motion to prevent stretching the pattern.

Figure 5   Tacky liquid is applied with a small brush or instrument to the tissue surface of the pattern. This liquid forms an adhesive surface on the pattern.

Figure 6   The pattern is placed in position with the external finish line just distal to the abutment tooth. The external finish line on the plastic pattern is placed near or over the internal finish line on the refractory cast. After the finish line has been pressed to place, the lingual bar area is placed using the lines drawn on the cast as a guide. Be sure that the lingual bar is a minimum of 2 millimeters from the marginal gingiva of all the teeth, including the abutment teeth. The plastic retention is then pressed to place with the center bar just lingual to the crest of the ridge.

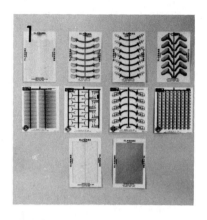
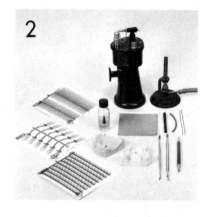
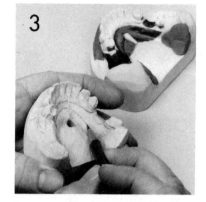
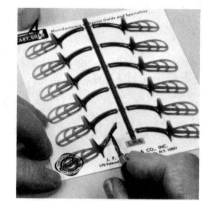

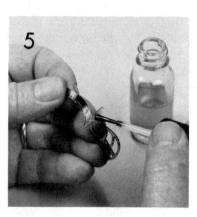
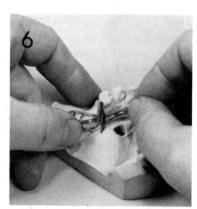
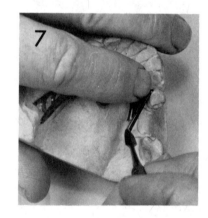
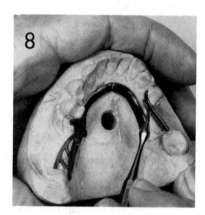

Plastic retention should always extend over the crest of the ridge to prevent mid-line fractures of the denture base. A portion of a lingual bar pattern is placed on the right side of the cast in a similar manner.

Figure 7 The clasp patterns are next placed into position. They are first coated with tacky liquid on the tissue surface and are then adapted to the tooth. The tip of the clasp is always adapted first.

Figure 8 The clasp arm is placed in position.

Figure 9 The excess clasp pattern is removed with a warm spatula.

Figure 10 The clasp patterns have all been placed on the investment cast. The finish line between the abutments on the right side is pro-

duced by freehand waxing. An excess of inlay wax is placed in the area and is carved to proper contour. The finish line is placed with a sharp instrument as is shown in this illustration.

Figure 11 The finish line and plastic retention have been completed on the right side. Note the proximity of the bar clasp to the plastic retention on the left side.

Figure 12 The clasp patterns are joined and the occlusal rests are formed with blue inlay wax. With experience, you will learn the correct temperature at which the wax must be used. If the wax is too hot, it will flow over the surface of the cast. When this occurs, the excess must be removed without marring the cast.

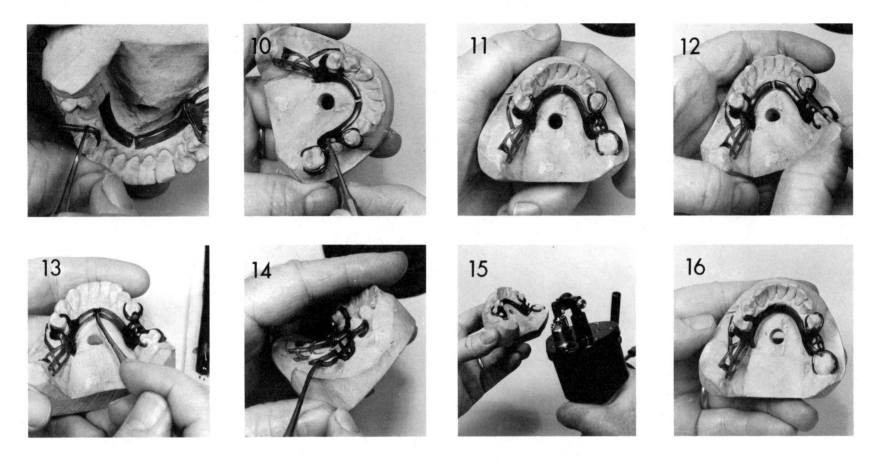

Figure 13　The areas between the lingual bar patterns are joined with blue inlay wax. Note that a stick of inlay wax has been attached to the tongue blade. This method keeps the inlay wax at hand and keeps it clean.

Figure 14　The joints between the clasp arms on the reverse action clasp are joined similarly. Note that the reverse action clasp has been formed by using two separate clasp patterns. It is impossible to make this clasp properly by attempting to bend one clasp pattern on itself.

Figure 15　The completed wax pattern is flamed lightly with a Hanau torch to smooth the wax. This flaming is light and fleeting; otherwise, the surface of the plastic patterns will melt. Excessive flaming also causes the inlay wax to flow over the surface of the cast. After flaming, finish lines made in inlay wax may need to be redefined.

Figure 16　The completed mandibular partial denture pattern. It may be necessary to seal the edges of the lingual bar pattern to the cast. This is particularly true in the area of the internal finish line.

Figure 17　The same procedure is followed for a maxillary partial denture. The first step is to draw the design on the investment cast.

Figure 18　Eighteen gauge round wax is placed in the bead lines. Note the sharp internal finish lines which were produced by proper placement of relief wax prior to duplication.

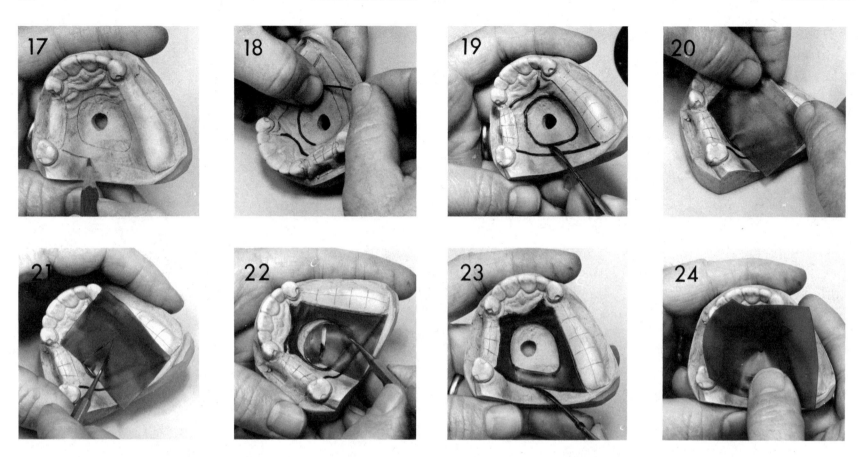

Figure 19 Eighteen gauge round wax is sealed to the cast with a warm spatula. The wax extending above the surface of the cast is removed.

Figure 20 One method of making a palatal bar pattern is to use gauge wax. Do not stretch the wax or there will be thin areas in the bar.

Figure 21 To avoid stretching, a wedge is removed from the wax so that it may be adapted to a concave surface.

Figure 22 The wax is pressed firmly (but gently) to place and the excess is removed.

Figure 23 Another piece of gauge wax is adapted to the right side to complete the palatal bar.

Figure 24 A maxillary major connector should be the thickness of 24 gauge wax or its equivalent. One method to insure that there are no thin spots is to make the maxillary major connector of two thicknesses of 30 gauge wax, which is the equivalent of 24 gauge. By adapting the two layers of 30 gauge wax separately, the danger of thin areas is minimized. This shows the second piece of wax being adapted, after which it is cut back to the outline of the first piece. The edges are then sealed to the cast.

Figure 25 The palatal bar, made of two thicknesses of 30 gauge wax, is complete.

Figure 26 An alternate method of making flat maxillary major connectors is to use a plastic pattern which comes in sheet form. This

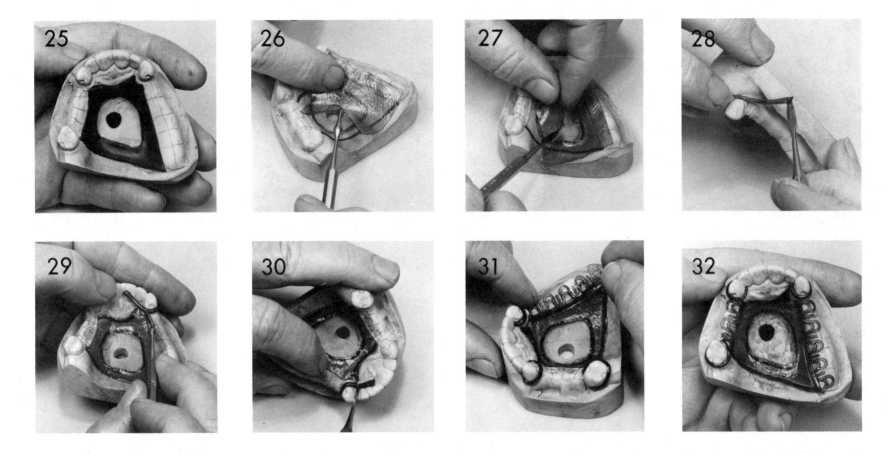

material has a pebbled surface which makes the resulting casting feel natural and is also easier to polish. This material is adapted in much the same manner as the wax, except that the area to be covered *on the cast* is first coated with tacky liquid. This is the only instance when tacky liquid is applied to the cast.

Figure 27   The excess pattern material is removed with a warm spatula. If two pieces need to be joined, a little inlay wax is flowed in the junction.

Figure 28   The clasp patterns are adapted the same way as on the mandibular pattern. The tacky liquid is painted on the flat side of the pattern and the tip is positioned. Note that this clasp is being placed directly against the gingiva. This is often done on maxillary partial dentures for esthetic reasons if the tooth has the proper contour and undercut.

Figure 29   The clasp pattern is then adapted around the tooth as indicated by the design.

Figure 30   The excess clasp pattern is removed with a warm spatula.

Figure 31   All of the clasp patterns have been placed and a finish line pattern is being adapted. This particular pattern has an external finish line and plastic retention loops. The external finish line is placed near or over the internal finish line on the investment cast. The opposing teeth determine the position of the external finish line which should be placed so that a minimum amount of denture base resin is needed on the

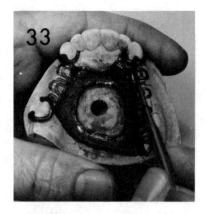

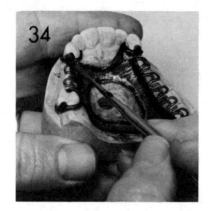

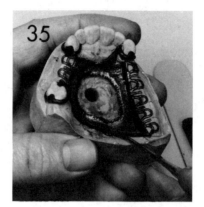

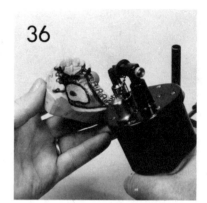

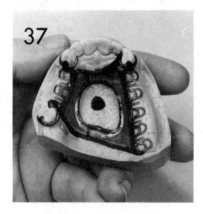

lingual aspect of the teeth. The plastic retention loops should extend over the crest of the ridge.

Figure 32   All of the plastic patterns are in position.

Figures 33 and 34   The occlusal rests are filled with inlay wax and the junctions between the patterns are filled.

Figure 35   The palatal bar pattern is checked to be sure that it is sealed. It is generally best to flow some wax around the edge. The finish line pattern on the patient's left side has been improved by the addition of some inlay wax. The external finish line should run down the minor connector when circumferential clasps are used.

Figure 36   The pattern is lightly flamed to smooth the wax.

Figure 37   The completed maxillary pattern.

REVIEW QUESTIONS

1. What are the advantages of using preformed patterns in preparing partial denture framework patterns?
2. What is the recommended thickness of a maxillary major connector pattern?
3. When adapting a preformed pattern clasp, which part is applied to the cast first?
4. What type of wax is used to fill spaces when preformed patterns are joined?

SECTION 25

Spruing, Investing, Casting, and Polishing

Conversion of a wax pattern into a polished casting is a relatively simple process. Each step must be accomplished precisely to assure good results with minimum effort.

A pathway must be provided through which the molten metal may reach the mold which is formed when the pattern is eliminated. This pathway is formed by sprues. There generally is a main sprue which branches into several auxiliary sprues. The sprues are formed from wax which is eliminated with the pattern. Spruing techniques vary with the type of casting equipment which is to be used.

The pattern and the sprues are invested so that a mold will be formed when the pattern is eliminated. The invested pattern is then placed in a furnace to eliminate the pattern and form the mold. Concurrently, expansion takes place within the mold which compensates for the shrinkage which occurs when the metal solidifies. The metal is then cast into the mold and, after the metal solidifies, the investment is removed, the sprues cut from the casting, and the casting is polished. These procedures complete the steps in making the metal portion of the partial denture framework.

The techniques shown in this manual use gold as the metal from which the partial denture framework is made. The same basic steps are followed with base metal alloys with the exception that different investments and casting equipment are used. The techniques for using base metal alloys are disseminated by the manufacturers of these alloys.

Polishing procedures for the base metal alloys are again basically the same as for gold. A high speed lathe is necessary because of the hardness of the metal. However, the basic principle of removing scratches with finer scratches is followed.

Several variations of investing procedures are shown in this section. A sprue base (crucible former) is used with the maxillary pattern while the mandibular pattern is invested without the sprue base. The maxillary pattern is invested using a "double investment" technique in which a small amount of investment is first painted on the pattern and allowed to reach its initial set. The investing is then completed.

The mandibular pattern is invested with a "single investment" technique which utilizes one large mix of investment. Some is painted on the pattern which is then immersed in the balance of the investment without allowing the "paint-on" portion to set.

These variations may be used in any combination; i.e., the sprue base may be used with a "single investment" technique while the "double investment" technique may be used without a sprue base. Some investing techniques require the removal of the casting ring before the investment is placed in the oven. Variations are acceptable if the basic principles are followed.

Figure 1 Auxiliary sprues are attached to the maxillary pattern. These are made of pink baseplate wax and are arranged as shown in this illustration. The shape and bulk of the pattern determine the size, number and placement of the sprues. They should be attached to the

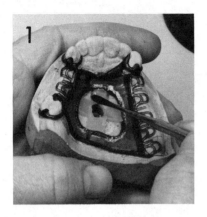
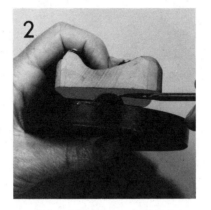
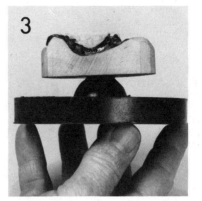
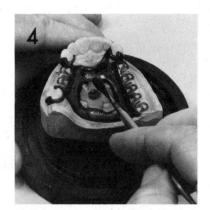

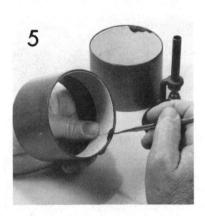
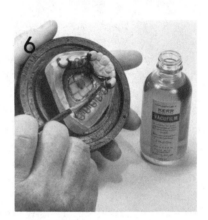
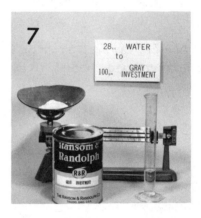
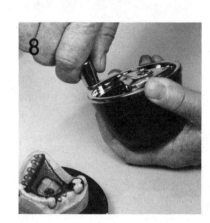

thickest portion of the pattern so that they will solidify last and act as a reservoir. If this principle is not followed, there will be porosity in the framework.

Figure 2   Wax is used to attach the investment cast firmly to the sprue base.

Figure 3   The cast is positioned with the main sprue hole over the center of the sprue base.

Figure 4   The main sprue hole is filled with wax.

Figure 5   The casting ring is lined with a material designed for this purpose. Strips of the material are cut to the proper length, placed in the

ring, sealed with a small amount of wax and the ring is dipped in water to wet the material. The material must be wet so that water will not be drawn from the investment.

The liner permits the investment to expand when it is heated but must be placed so that ⅛ inch of the casting ring is exposed on the top and the bottom of the ring. This keeps the investment from falling out of the ring when it is removed from the oven.

A cast which has not been dipped in beeswax must be soaked in water for 5 minutes before investing. If beeswax, which seals the surface of the cast, is used, soaking is not necessary.

Figure 6   The wax pattern is coated with a surface tension reducing agent. This allows the investment to flow evenly over the pattern without trapping air bubbles.

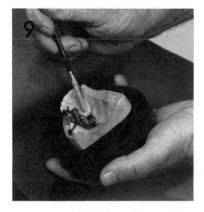

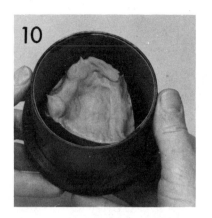

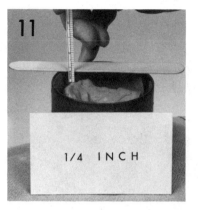

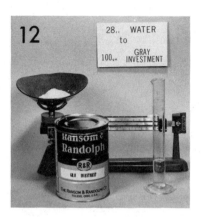

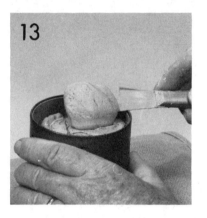

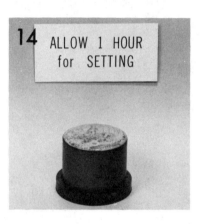

investment is flowed over the wax pattern ahead of the brush to avoid trapping air bubbles. Do not place the refractory cast on the vibrator. This causes particles of investment to settle toward the cast and gives the same effect as a thick mix of investment, resulting in casting fins. The pattern is completely covered and is then set aside until the investment sets.

Figure 10   The casting ring with the wet liner is placed over the sprue base and cast to be sure that it fits within the ring.

Figure 11   The pattern should be one-quarter of an inch from the top of the casting ring. This thickness gives sufficient strength to the investment and allows gases trapped by the molten metal to escape through the investment during the casting procedure.

Figure 12   A 28 to 100 mix of investment is made using 400 grams of investment.

Figure 13   The ring, with the sprue base attached, is placed on a vibrator and is filled with investment.

Figure 14   The investment is allowed to set for one hour.

Figure 15   The auxiliary sprues for the mandibular partial denture are made of 8 gauge round wax. They are attached to the thickest portion of the framework and the junction is rounded to eliminate sharp edges in the mold. This casting, being relatively small, requires only two auxil-

Figure 7   The investment used for the outer portion is the same used for the investment cast. Note that the ratio is 28cc. of water to 100 grams of investment. This produces a thinner mix than was used for the investment cast. Thus, the outer investment expands less than the refractory cast, producing a tight joint between the cast and the outer investment. *Always be certain that the refractory cast is made from a thick mix of investment and the outer investment is a thin mix.*

Figure 8   A small amount of investment (50 grams) is first mixed. A mechanical spatulator produces a smooth, creamy mix which is easily painted on the pattern.

Figure 9   The investment is painted on the pattern with a camel's hair brush. The hand holding the brush is held against a vibrator and the

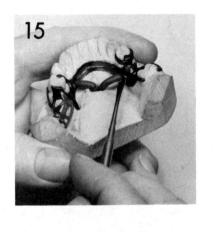

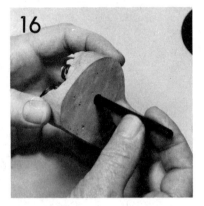

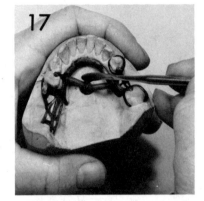

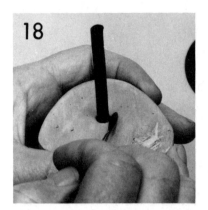

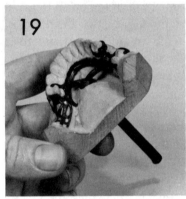

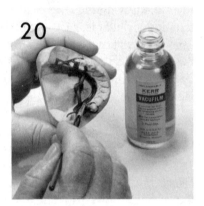

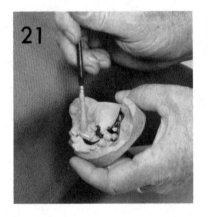

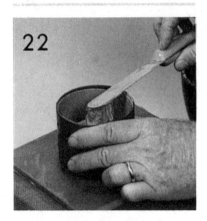

iary sprues which are curved to provide a smooth pathway for the gold entering the mold.

Figure 16 A stick of inlay wax acts as the main sprue. This is placed through the base of the cast.

Figure 17 The main sprue is attached to the auxiliary sprues. The junction is smooth and rounded.

Figure 18 The main sprue is sealed to the base of the investment cast.

Figure 19 The mandibular pattern is ready to be invested (first, see **Figure 24**).

Figure 20 The wax pattern is painted with a surface tension reducing agent.

Figure 21 A single investment technique uses one large mix of investment. The investment is mixed in a 28 to 100 ratio and is painted on the pattern in the same manner as was done for the maxillary pattern.

Figure 22 The casting ring, lined with a wet lining material, is placed on a glass slab covered with a wet paper towel. The balance of the mix is vibrated into the casting ring.

Figure 23 The casting ring and glass slab are held on a vibrator and the mandibular cast, previously painted with investment (**Figure 21**), is

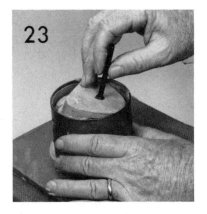

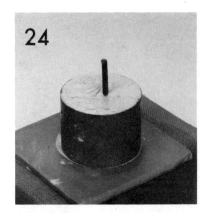

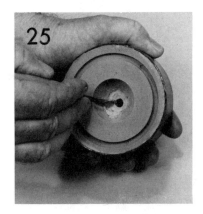

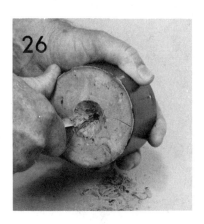

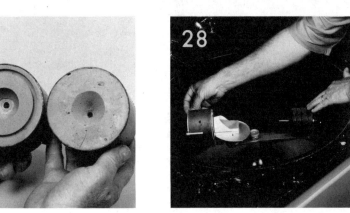

Figure 26 When a sprue former is not used, the depression is carved into the investment with a knife.

Figure 27 This shows a comparison of the two rings, one using a sprue former and one having the depression cut into the base of the investment. The depression is carved so that it is centered in the ring whether or not the main sprue is centered. The depression is 1½ inches wide and 1 inch deep.

CASTING

There are several casting machines on the market which melt metal electrically, and some cast automatically. These machines give consistently superior results, and directions for using them are available from the manufacturers. Equal results are obtained with simpler equipment when it is used properly.

Figure 28 Before the wax pattern is eliminated, the casting machine is balanced by the addition or subtraction of weights. The machine must rotate without vibration.

Figure 29 The invested patterns are placed in an oven with the sprue holes down. The rings are placed so that there is air space beneath them to allow heat to circulate around the ring.

rotated into the investment. The rotation prevents trapping air in the tongue space.

Figure 24 The cast is vibrated into position until the surface of the pattern is ¼ inch from the base of the ring. This is determined before investing by marking the main sprue even with the top of the ring when the wax pattern is ¼ inch from the base of the ring. The investment is allowed to set for one hour.

Figure 25 After the investment has set one hour, the sprue base is removed. This leaves a depression in the investment into which the molten metal will be cast. Any sharp edges are removed to prevent flakes of investment from being incorporated in the casting.

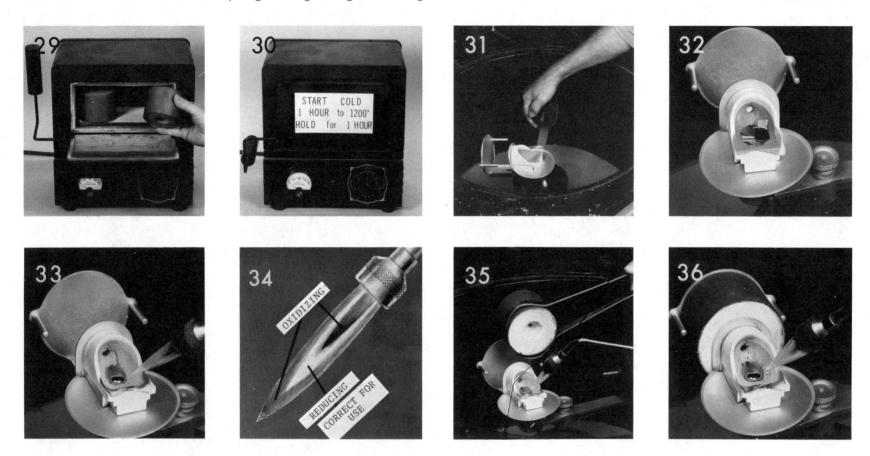

Figure 30   The casting ring is placed in a cold oven. The furnace is turned on and the temperature raised to 1200°F. over a one hour period. The ring is then "heat soaked" for an additional hour to insure that heat penetrates the investment and the pattern is completely eliminated. (Raising the heat above 1250°F. will result in sulfur contamination of the casting if gypsum investments are used.)

Figure 31   The casting machine is prepared. The crucible must be clean. The casting machine is wound and locked in position. Ordinarily two to three turns are sufficient for casting partial dentures. Too many turns may cause casting fins.

Figure 32   The gold is stacked in the crucible so that it will melt uniformly. Twice the amount of gold required for the framework is used to insure that the mold will be filled. This also insures that the sprue will be large enough to act as a reservoir while the casting cools. The average mandibular partial denture casting weighs 7 to 8 dwt. so a minimum of 14 dwt. of gold is needed. As a rule, 14 to 16 dwt. are used for average mandibular castings and 20 dwt. are used for average maxillary castings.

Figure 33   The gold is melted using a gas-air torch.

Figure 34   The reducing area of the flame is used to melt the gold.

Figure 35   The casting ring is removed from the oven and placed in the

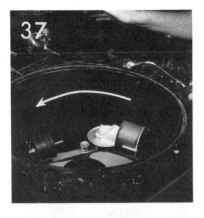
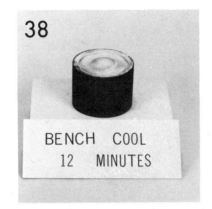
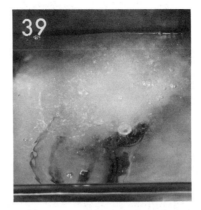
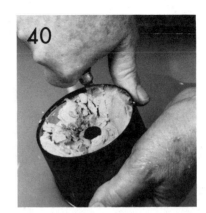

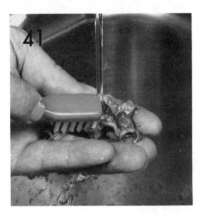
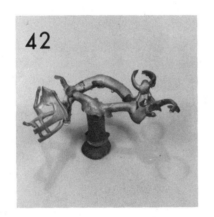
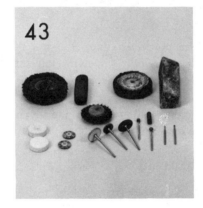
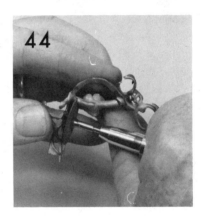

casting machine. It is important not to overheat the gold nor to leave the casting ring in the machine more than two minutes before casting. Overheating destroys some of the components of the gold alloy.

Figure 36   The molten gold has a bright surface prior to casting.

Figure 37   The casting machine is released and the torch removed simultaneously.

Figure 38   The casting ring is allowed to bench cool for 12 minutes from the time of casting. This is one method of tempering a gold framework. Other methods are discussed in the Laboratory and Clinical Dental Materials Manual.

Figure 39   The hot casting ring is then plunged in a sink of cold water. Sufficient water must be present to dissipate the heat in the ring.

Figure 40   After the ring is cool, the investment is trimmed from the edges of the ring. The investment containing the casting is then pushed out of the ring and the investment broken away from the casting.

Figure 41   The casting is scrubbed to remove all traces of investment.

Figure 42   The completed casting with the sprues attached.

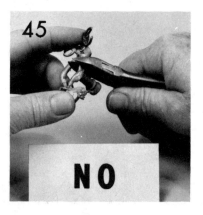
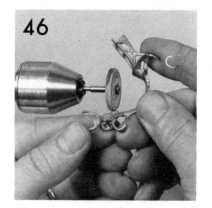
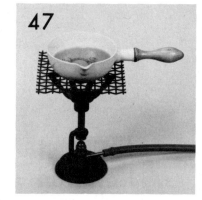
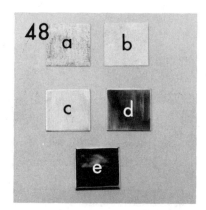

FINISHING

Figure 43   The equipment necessary for polishing consists of stones, separating discs, finishing burs, rubber abrasive wheels, small felt wheels, and polishing wheels for pumice, tripoli and rouge.

Figure 44   A separating disc is used to remove the sprues. They are cut as close as possible to the framework without nicking it.

Figure 45   Pliers should NEVER be used to remove partial denture sprues. This will distort the framework.

Figure 46   After the sprues are removed, the stumps are reduced with a coarse stone. This may be done with a handpiece.

Figure 47   The casting is pickled after the sprue stumps are removed. The framework is placed in the pickling solution and the solution is heated. (Never heat and plunge a framework or the temper will be lost.) Pickling removes surface oxides from the metal and is best done with a commercial pickling solution. Strong acid may be used but it may produce harmful vapors.

Figure 48   The basic principle of polishing is to remove scratches with finer scratches until the final stages when an amorphous layer is formed on the surface by the action of the finer polishing agents. The polishing steps are completed sequentially over the entire polished surface. This prevents repetition of polishing steps.

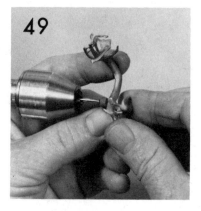
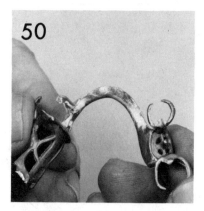

This illustration shows the stages of polishing metal. "a" is a surface after it has been stoned. "b" is a gold surface after a rubber abrasive wheel has been used. "c" is the surface after pumice has been used. "d" shows the surface after tripoli has been used, and "e" shows the luster achieved by using rouge on a chamois buff.

Figure 49   The surface is smoothed using a fine stone. Any flash or irregularity is removed during this step.

Figure 50   The framework has been contoured using the fine stone. Note that the plastic retention areas do not require finishing.

Figure 51   The framework is smoothed using a rubber abrasive wheel.

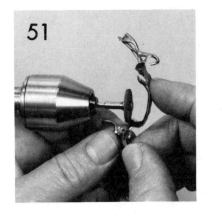
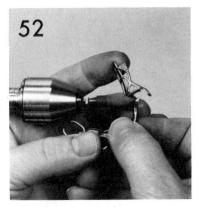
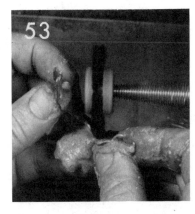
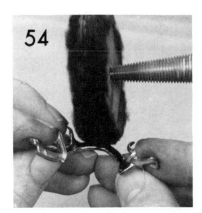

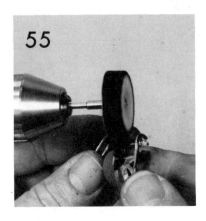
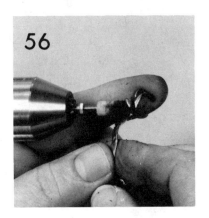
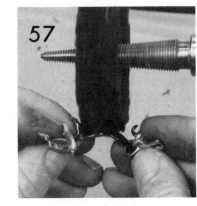
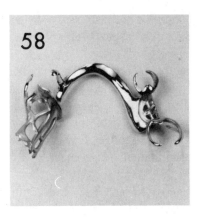

Figure 52 A rubber abrasive point is used to reach less accessible areas.

Figure 53 A brush wheel and wet pumice further refines the framework. The plastic retention is cleaned with wet pumice, and is the only finishing required for these areas.

Figure 54 A rag wheel with tripoli is used to impart a higher polish to the framework.

Figure 55 The less accessible areas are polished with a small felt wheel and tripoli.

Figure 56 The areas around the clasp are polished with a small felt

cone and tripoli. After this step the framework is washed thoroughly with detergent and hot water. Note that throughout the finishing steps, larger polishing wheels are used first, followed by smaller wheels and points. This sequence saves time.

Figure 57 Rouge on a chamois buff produces a high gloss on the surface of the metal. Rouge is used for several minutes and with moderate pressure to produce the proper luster which is a major factor in aiding the patient to keep the appliance clean.

Figures 58 and 59 The completed mandibular framework. Note that the surface has a high luster which reflects light evenly. The tissue surface of the lingual bar has been polished, but very little metal has been removed during the process. The tissue surface of the minor

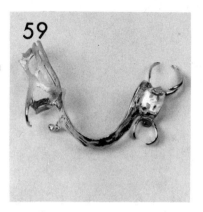

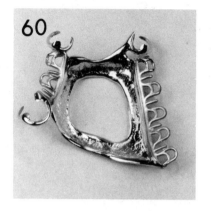

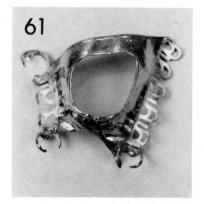

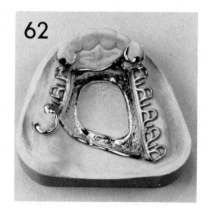

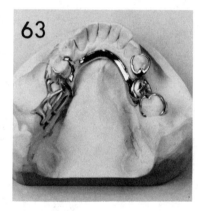

connector has also been polished but the tip of the I-bar which contacts the tooth has not been polished.

Figures 60 and 61   The maxillary framework is shown after polishing. Note the pebbled surface (from the plastic pattern) on the external surface which makes the appliance feel more natural to the patient. The tissue surface of the maxillary partial is finished with wet pumice, tripoli and rouge. It is neither stoned nor rubber wheeled to avoid loss of intimate tissue contact.

Figures 62 and 63   The completed frameworks are returned to the master casts from which the wax for duplicating has been removed. The frameworks are not placed on the master casts until polishing is complete. Note that the superior edge of the lingual bar is in close apposition to the tissue and that both castings fit the master casts well.

FINISHING BASE METAL ALLOYS

The finishing of base metal alloys is essentially the same as that used for gold in that scratches are replaced by ever finer scratches until a high luster is achieved. The basic difference in the procedure is that a high speed lathe needs to be used due to the hardness of the base metal alloys.

Some refinements have been included in the finishing procedures for base metal alloys. In some laboratories, the frames are placed in a large

drum with an abrasive and tumbled to help achieve the initial finish stage. Tumbling is an acceptable procedure if it is not carried out for too long and essential parts of the framework lost.

Another type of finishing is electrolytic stripping. In this procedure the frames are placed in a bath and electricity passed through them to remove metal and make the subsequent finishing steps easier. Stripping is likewise an acceptable procedure if it is used to a minimal extent. Otherwise, the frames may not fit well due to the excessive removal of metal. An understanding of stripping and tumbling procedures will help to assess any deficiencies which may turn up in base metal partial denture frames after they are finished.

Another difference in base metal alloys is that different finishing materials are used. These are required, again, due to the hardness of these metals.

Materials and wheels used for polishing gold should be kept separate from those used for base metal alloys. If wheels utilized for polishing base metals are also used on gold, the gold will be plated with the base metal residue left on the polishing wheel. The gold appliance, be it a fixed partial denture or removable partial denture, will then tarnish in the mouth due to the interaction of the base metal with the precious metal in the presence of oral fluids.

REVIEW QUESTIONS

1. Describe the proper sequence for polishing gold including the sequence of polishing agents and types of wheels, points, etc.
2. What should be the thickness of the investment between the pattern and the end of the casting ring?
3. What is the purpose of painting investment on the pattern prior to full coverage with investment?
4. What is the water:powder ratio for investment used for casting a gold partial denture framework and what is the significance of this ratio?
5. Why are auxiliary sprues attached to the thickest portion of the pattern?

SECTION 26

Corrected Impressions, Jaw Relationship Records, and Mounting Casts

An accurate registration of the soft tissues which help support a removable partial denture is vital to the success of the appliance. A precise recording of the occlusal relationships also is essential.

Sometimes it is necessary to mount the master casts before preparation for duplication. Usually the master casts are not mounted until after the framework is complete. Problems in occlusion are anticipated by the intelligent use of the diagnostic casts before the framework is designed. The master casts must be mounted before duplication if metal occlusal surfaces are to be incorporated into the original casting or if there is a problem of occlusion between natural teeth and parts of the proposed partial denture.

Ordinarily, the partial denture framework is returned to the dentist so that it may be tried in the patient's mouth. At this time, jaw relationship records are made. Many dentists will make a detailed impression of the edentulous ridge area at the same appointment. These impressions are known as corrected impressions, composite impressions, or functional impressions, depending upon the technique and/or terminology used by the dentist.

There are five basic methods by which jaw relationship records may be recorded. The method used will depend upon the conditions present in the patient and the individual desires of the dentist. The five methods are:

(1) *Direct Apposition of the Casts*. If sufficient teeth are present and there are no occlusal discrepancies in the patient, the opposing casts may be fastened to one another using the natural teeth as an occlusal index.

(2) *Simple Wax Registration*. (See **Figure D**, Section 22.)

(3) *Occlusion Rim Separate from the Framework*. This method is illustrated in this section.

(4) *Occlusion Rim Constructed on the Partial Denture Framework*. This method is illustrated in this section.

(5) *Corrected Impression with Jaw Relationship Record Attached*. This method is illustrated in this section.

(6) *Corrected Impression and Functional Chew-In*. This method utilizes a hard wax which a patient chews-in to the proper occlusion. A detailed description of this technique is available in other publications. This method is not in common use.

A great deal of information is contained in the following few pages regarding jaw relationships. It is most important to understand this material and recognize its importance to the finished product, the completed removable partial denture. Failure to recognize interferences between the framework and existing natural teeth and inadequate interocclusal records on the part of the dentist will result in a less than satisfactory result or increased work for the dentist. Likewise, inadequate handling of these records by the technician in the dental laboratory will lead to the same problems. Take time to understand each of the techniques shown in this section.

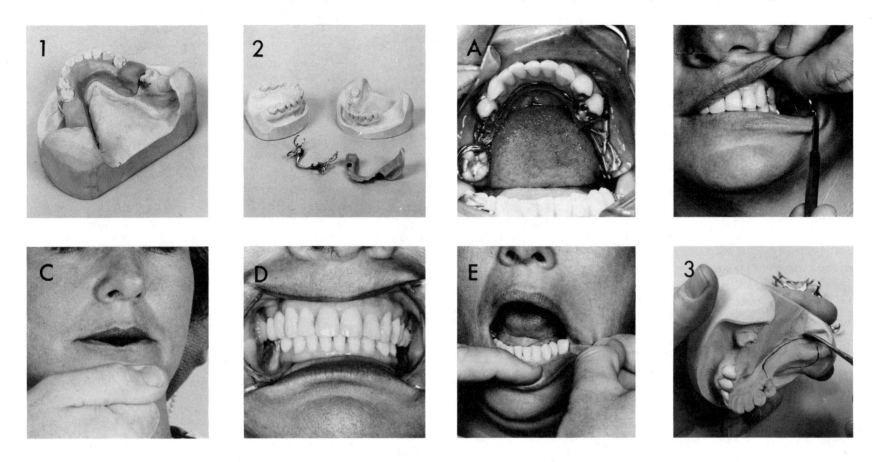

RECORDING JAW RELATIONSHIPS WITH OCCLUSION RIMS SEPARATE FROM THE FRAMEWORK

Figure 1   An occlusion rim separate from the framework may be made to record jaw relationships for a partially edentulous patient. The occlusion rim is made of wax and is lined with self-curing methyl methacrylate resin. (See Section 5.) Notice its close adaptation to the remaining teeth. Depending upon the conditions present in the patient and the preferences of the dentist, it may be necessary to construct wire occlusal rests to stabilize the occlusion rim.

Figure 2   The mandibular and maxillary casts, the partial denture framework, and the occlusion rim are ready to be returned to the dentist.

Figure A   The framework is placed in the patient's mouth and is checked to be sure that it fits and is retained properly. Occlusal rests are checked to see that they are seated and that the bar is in correct apposition to the tissues. Minor connectors which cross soft tissue are checked to see that no soft tissue is displaced.

Figure B   The plastic retention area is checked to insure that it does not interfere with the opposing teeth.

Figure C   The occlusion is checked to insure that no part of the framework interferes.

Figure D   The frame is removed. Then the occlusion rim is checked to be certain it does not interfere with the maxillary teeth upon closing.

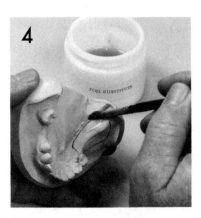
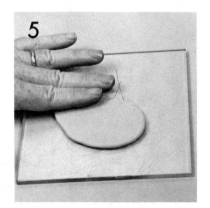
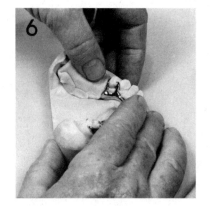
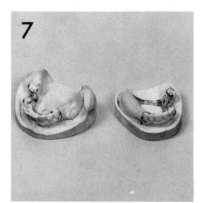

Softened bite wax is then placed on the edentulous areas and the jaw relationship record is made on the occlusion rim.

Figure E   A shade is selected to harmonize with the remaining teeth. A face-bow transfer (**Figures L–N**) is made and is returned to the laboratory with any other pertinent information. The laboratory technician will then mount the casts and complete the partial denture.

CONSTRUCTION OF STABILIZED BASES TO MAKE CORRECTED IMPRESSIONS AND/OR RECORD JAW RELATIONSHIPS

A base may be constructed on the partial denture framework for making jaw relationship records. The base may also be used as a tray for making a corrected impression. The bases are made ordinarily of tray resin or regular self-curing resin. Some dentists use a hard baseplate wax for making the bases but resin bases are more satisfactory.

Figure 3   Undercuts in the ridge area are relieved with baseplate wax.

Figure 4   The area to be covered by the base is covered with tinfoil substitute. Note that a base is not being constructed on the tooth borne side of the cast. A corrected impression is not made in small tooth supported areas of the framework.

Figure 5   Resin tray material is mixed according to the manufacturer's

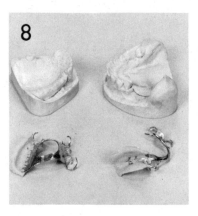
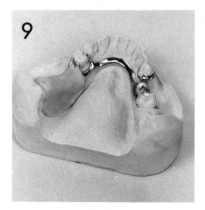

instructions. Only a small amount is needed. The material is flattened on a glass slab which has been coated lightly with Vaseline.

Figure 6   The framework is placed on the master cast and the tray material is pressed through the plastic retention on the framework. It is further adapted around the border area.

Figure 7   The same technique is followed for the maxillary partial denture.

Figure 8   After the tray material has set, the framework and attached trays are removed from the cast. Enough of the tray material has been pressed through the plastic retention to assure that the resin is attached rigidly to the metal framework. The bases are trimmed to the proper

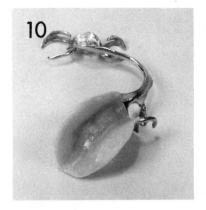

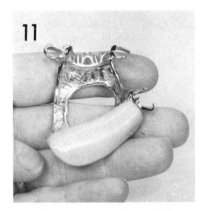

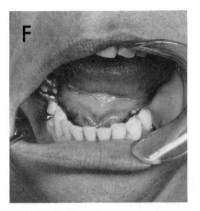

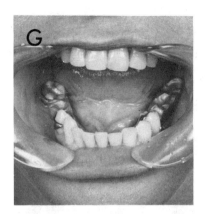

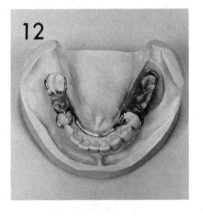

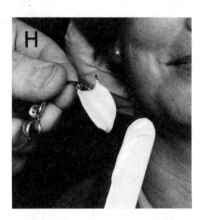

contour and the border areas finished. This type of base on a partial denture framework is best suited for making a corrected impression. Because the tissue surface of the base is not adapted well in the area of the plastic retention, it is not well suited for making jaw relationship records unless a corrected impression is first made.

Figure 9 A resin base made by the sprinkle technique (Section 5) will produce a base which is more closely adapted to the tissue and may be used to make jaw relationship records without making a corrected impression. A sprinkle base may also be used for making the corrected impression. The choice of the press-on or the sprinkle method for making a base is left to the discretion of the dentist. This is a base made by the sprinkle method.

Figure 10 The sprinkle method base is well adapted to the ridge area. Compare this to the base shown in **Figure 8**.

Figure 11 This is a sprinkle method base constructed on a maxillary framework.

RECORDING JAW RELATIONSHIPS ON THE FRAMEWORK WITH A STABILIZED BASE

Figure F The framework with the sprinkle method base is tried in the patient's mouth. Some dentists will try in the framework separately

(**Figure A**) and subsequently make the base. Others will have the base made on the framework before it is tried in the mouth. The occlusion is checked to be sure that there are no occlusal interferences between the framework and/or the base.

Figure G Plaster or softened wax is placed on the base *and* between the abutment teeth on the right side of the arch. The patient is then instructed to close and make the jaw relationship record.

Figure 12 The partial denture framework and base with the attached jaw relationship record is returned to the cast. This, a face-bow transfer (**Figures L–N**), and the shade are returned to the laboratory so the partial may be completed.

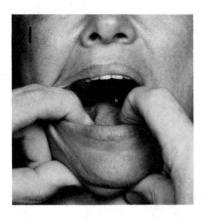

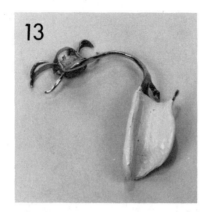

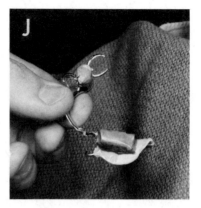

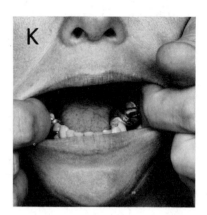

MAKING A CORRECTED IMPRESSION AND RECORDING JAW RELATIONSHIPS

Figure H   Before making a corrected impression the dentist will check the base in the mouth to be sure that it is extended properly but does not displace any soft tissue. Impression material has been placed into the base.

Figure I   The framework is maintained in the mouth by holding all the occlusal rests in position. No force is exerted on the base while the impression material hardens.

A variety of impression materials may be used to make corrected impressions. If it is desired to record the tissues in a resting or nondisplaced state, rubber base impression material or one of the zinc oxide-eugenol impression materials is used. If it is desired to record the ridge area in a functional state, one of the wax impression materials which flow at mouth temperature is used.

Figure 13   The completed corrected impression. Zinc oxide-eugenol impression material was used to make this corrected impression.

Figure J   The framework and corrected impression are returned to the patient's mouth to be sure there are no occlusal interferences. After this, softened wax or plaster is placed on the surface of the base and between the abutment teeth on the opposite side. The framework is returned to the patient's mouth.

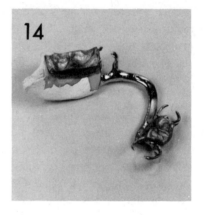

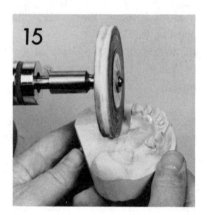

Figure K   The patient is instructed to close and the jaw relationship record is made.

Figure 14   The completed corrected impression with the attached jaw relationship record.

Figure 15   The master cast must be altered so that the corrected impression may be poured in correct relationship to the remaining teeth. The ridge area on the master cast is removed using a coarse stone or a saw. Enough stone must be removed so that no portion of the corrected impression touches the cast when the framework is placed on the cast.

Figure 16   The framework and corrected impression are placed on the

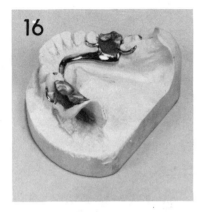

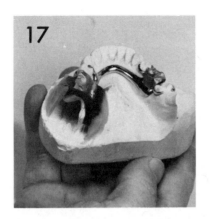

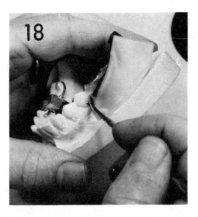

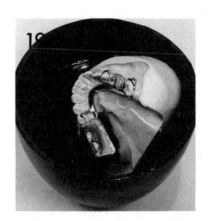

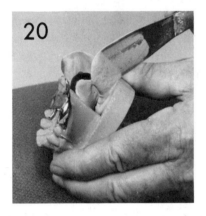

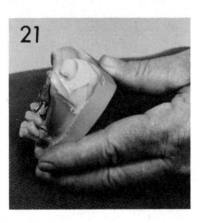

master cast. The cast is scored under the corrected impression to enhance the attachment of the new ridge area to the cast.

Figure 17 A thin rope of utility wax is adapted just above the border of the corrected impression. Baseplate wax is then used to box the corrected impression. The boxing is done in such a manner that the boxing wax does not touch the border of the impression but seals the impression so that stone will not flow outside the confines of the corrected impression area.

Figure 18 The wax is sealed around the anterior aspect of the area to be corrected.

Figure 19 The cast must be soaked before the new ridge area is poured. Failure to do this will prevent stone from reaching the anterior portion of the ridge area and uniting with the cast.

Figure 20 The cast is held on a vibrator and the stone placed in the posterior portion of the opening. The stone is added in small increments to be sure that it reaches the anterior portion of the ridge area without trapping air.

Figure 21 The ridge area has been filled with stone. The cast is then set aside until the stone sets. Note that no stone has been allowed to run on the surface of the jaw relationship record.

Figure 22 After the stone has set, the boxing material is removed. The cast is now ready to be mounted.

The framework and the attached jaw relationship record are not removed from the cast until the cast has been mounted. In other words, the impression material is not removed until after the cast is mounted.

MOUNTING CASTS

Mounting casts for removable partial dentures is similar to the technique for complete dentures. The technique described below utilizes a Hanau articulator with a face-bow, although partial dentures which

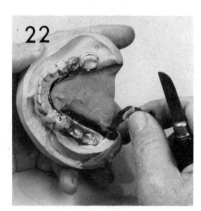
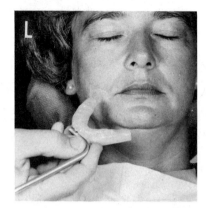
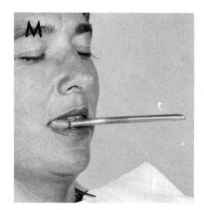
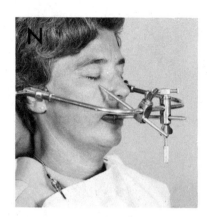

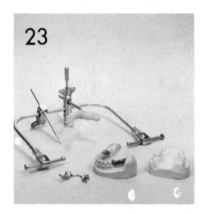
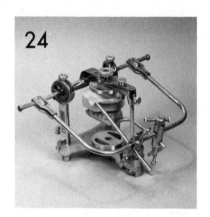

instructed to close. This produces an occlusal index on both surfaces of the wax, one for the maxillary teeth and one for the mandibular. The wax is then chilled. This is *not* a jaw relationship record, but is simply a method to enable the patient to stabilize the bite fork while the face-bow transfer is being made.

Figure M   The bite fork is in place in the patient's mouth. The bite fork is stable because of the indexes produced on the wax which surrounds the bite fork.

Figure N   The face-bow has been positioned on the patient. The entire assembly is removed and returned to the laboratory.

Figure 23   The face-bow, framework, occlusion rim and casts are shown before the casts are mounted.

Figure 24   The face-bow is centered on the articulator and is adjusted so that the orbital pointer touches the orbital plane guide on the articulator. (See Section 7.)

Figure 25   Plaster is applied to the base of the upper cast.

Figure 26   The upper cast is attached to the articulator.

Figure 27   Indexes are placed in the base of the cast so that it may be remounted after processing. The occlusion rim is placed on the cast and

replace a few teeth may be mounted on a simple hinge type articulator. A hinge type articulator is particularly applicable when the occlusion of remaining teeth prevents any lateral movements from being incorporated in the replaced teeth. If a simple articulator is used, it must be rigid so that the jaw relationships recorded in the patient will be maintained.

A face-bow transfer for a partially edentulous patient is made more easily without the framework and/or occlusion rim in the patient's mouth. The technique illustrated for a face-bow transfer is applicable for mounting casts of a natural dentition.

Figure L   Softened baseplate wax is wrapped around the bite fork. The bite fork is then centered in the patient's mouth and the patient is

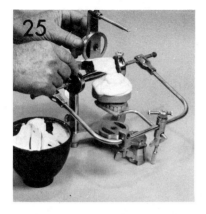
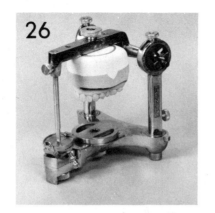
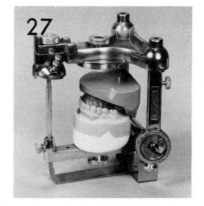
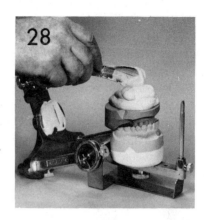

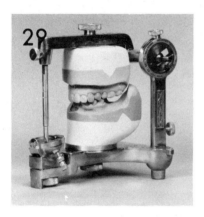
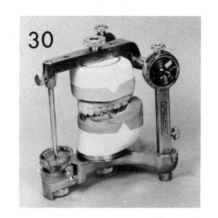
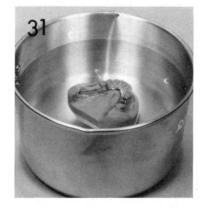
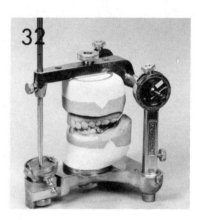

the mandibular cast is placed in its correct relationship to the maxillary cast. A few dabs of sticky wax will help maintain this relationship. Be certain there are no interferences in the posterior region of the casts which could prevent proper apposition of the casts.

Figure 28   Plaster is applied to the base of the mandibular cast.

Figure 29   The mounting of the maxillary and mandibular casts is complete. Note the space between the casts in the posterior region.

Figure 30   This illustration shows a cast with the framework, corrected impression, and jaw relationship records mounted. Note that the

mounting is completed before the impression is separated from the cast.

Figure 31   After the mandibular cast is mounted, it is placed in hot water to soften the impression material to permit the removal of the framework and the resin base. The resin base may be removed from the framework by flaming the resin base with a Hanau torch. This should be done with care to avoid losing the temper in the framework. (Temper is not a problem with base metal frames.)

Figure 32   The maxillary cast and the corrected mandibular cast have been mounted on the articulator and we are now ready to arrange the artificial teeth.

REVIEW QUESTIONS

1. List the five basic methods used to record jaw relationships during partial denture treatment.
2. Describe the procedure for constructing a stabilized baseplate including a partial denture framework.
3. Describe pouring a corrected impression for a partial denture.
4. When are hinge-type articulators acceptable for mounting casts for removable partial dentures?

SECTION 27

Artificial Tooth Arrangement

Commercially manufactured artificial teeth are not made to occlude with natural teeth. A dental laboratory technician will modify the available teeth to meet the situation at hand to produce satisfactory substitutes for the natural teeth.

Posterior teeth selected for partial dentures fill the following requirements: (a) The teeth must have the proper mesiodistal dimension to interdigitate with the opposing natural teeth. (b) The posterior teeth must have the same or a smaller faciolingual dimension as the teeth they replace. Narrowing the occlusal table reduces stress on the remaining natural teeth and/or underlying bone and mucosa. (c) The teeth must not extend behind the anterior border of the retromolar pad or maxillary tuberosity to minimize the lever arm on a free-end extension. However, the artificial teeth must contact all the opposing teeth to help prevent their extrusion. Sometimes a second and/or third molar will be extracted in an arch opposing a removable partial denture to help decrease the length of the occlusal table and thus reduce stress on a free-end extension abutment.

It may be necessary to select teeth other than those lost by the patient to fulfill the requirements stated above. For example, an artificial premolar and a molar may be indicated for a space vacated by two molars. Fewer or smaller teeth are often necessary in a tooth-bound edentulous space because the abutments may have drifted toward one another.

Esthetics is often a factor in the selection of teeth for removable partial dentures. The artificial teeth must be at least as long occluso-gingivally as the abutment teeth to prevent unwanted display of denture base material. This is particularly important on maxillary partial dentures.

The selection of teeth for partial dentures replacing anterior teeth is essentially the same as anterior tooth selection for complete dentures. The shade and mold are selected to match the remaining teeth and/or complement the patient's features. Arrangement of anterior teeth for partial dentures follows the same principles as for arranging anterior teeth for complete dentures.

The occlusal surfaces of artificial teeth in partial dentures usually have to be altered to achieve better interdigitation with the opposing natural teeth. This is essential for proper function and appearance. The occlusal alteration is best done tooth by tooth, or segment by segment as the teeth are being set.

Often space is limited, occlusogingivally and mesiodistally, when setting teeth for partial dentures. In these situations, better results may be obtained by carving the teeth from wax on the cast after an occlusal index has been made by the teeth in the opposing cast. These teeth are reproduced in tooth-colored resin after the cast and appliance are flasked. This technique is illustrated in this and the following section for a single tooth, but the technique is applicable for several teeth and for teeth needed to fill a small space between a clasp and an adjacent artificial tooth.

Figures 1 and 2 The teeth are selected for the mandibular partial denture to fill the existing space. The edentulous space on the right side will be filled with an individually made tooth because of the difficulty

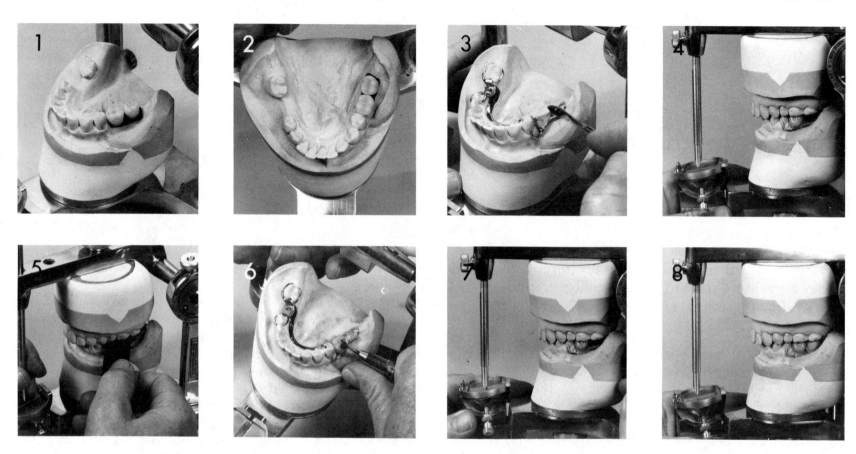

of grinding a tooth to fit this space. A custom-made tooth is easier to make and produces better results.

Figure 3 The partial denture framework is placed on the cast and wax is flowed through the plastic retention of the framework to stabilize the framework while the teeth are being set.

Figure 4 The first molar is set into position. The gingival side of the tooth may need to be reduced but should be "hollow-ground" to preserve the facial surface. The tooth should be set a little high in occlusion so that the occlusal surface may be altered to better interdigitate with the opposing teeth. If it is necessary to contour the tooth around the minor connector, a piece of articulating paper is inserted between the tooth and minor connector and the tooth is wiggled slightly. The

marks on the tooth are then reduced. This procedure is repeated until the tooth is adapted to the minor connector.

Figure 5 The occlusion is checked with articulating paper.

Figure 6 The occlusal surface is altered by reducing the areas marked by the articulating paper.

Figure 7 The occlusion has been refined by occlusal alteration. Note that the incisal pin now touches the incisal guide table.

Figure 8 The second molar is set in similar fashion. The tooth is "high in occlusion" as evidenced by the incisal pin not touching the incisal guide table.

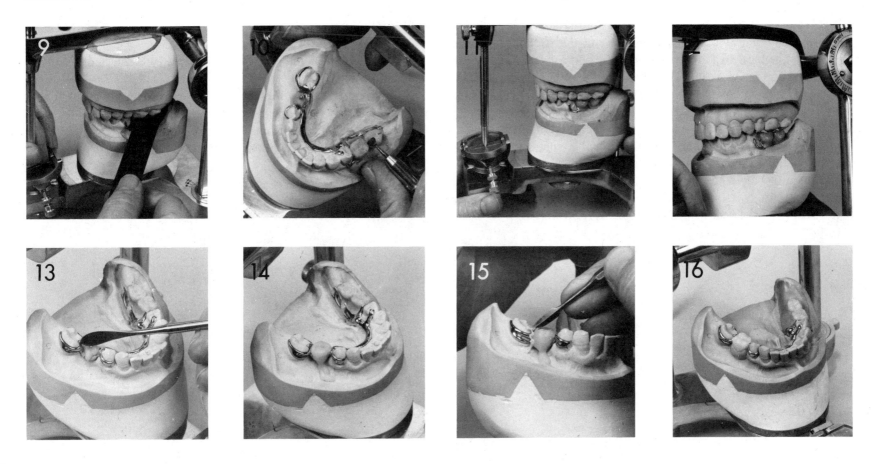

Figure 9 The second molar is checked for occlusion.

Figure 10 The second molar is altered so that it interdigitates with the opposing teeth. *Note that the occlusal alteration is done tooth by tooth.* This is usually easier. However, you may achieve better alignment of the artificial teeth by setting one side and then "grinding in."

Figure 11 The left molars have been set and are shown in centric occlusion.

Figure 12 The amount of tooth contact in lateral and protrusive excursions is determined by the occlusion of the natural teeth, the form of the opposing occlusal surfaces, and the desires of the dentist. The artificial teeth must harmonize with the natural teeth. Occlusal interferences on

the artificial teeth damage the abutments, the soft tissue, and cause pain.

Figure 13 White wax is placed between the abutment teeth on the right side. This wax is built so that it will be high in occlusion.

Figure 14 The opposing maxillary tooth is lubricated and the articulator has been closed to make an occlusal index on the surface of the softened wax.

Figure 15 The tooth is contoured and the occlusal surface refined. The next figure shows a gingival area waxed in pink wax. This is satisfactory or the tooth may be "butted" directly to the cast.

Figure 16 The partial denture is ready to be flasked. The replaced molar on the right side has been carved and the occlusal anatomy perfected. The base area on the left side has been waxed to the correct contour. The gingival carvings and denture base contours are done in the same manner as complete dentures. (See Section 10.) Every attempt should be made to produce the proper contour in the wax base.

Since the framework and wax base are not easily removed from the cast, the base may be thickened slightly (except around the teeth). It is easier to remove a little excess from a small partial denture base than to add resin to the cured base.

All wax must be cleaned from resin denture teeth before flasking. The thinnest film of wax will cause problems (Section 10).

REVIEW QUESTIONS

1. What are the requirements of posterior teeth selected for partial dentures?
2. How is a partial denture framework stabilized on the cast while the teeth are being set?
3. Describe making a custom tooth for a partial denture.
4. When are occlusal alterations done on artificial partial denture teeth?

SECTION 28

Flasking, Processing, and Finishing Removable Partial Dentures

The resin base of a removable partial denture is formed in the same way as bases for complete dentures. The inclusion of the metal framework in the mold requires some alteration in the flasking procedure.

Many of the steps and procedures used for flasking, packing and finishing partial dentures are similar to those used in complete dentures. Most of the variations are simply a matter of applied common sense and will be understood easily if the principles of flasking and finishing complete dentures have been mastered.

The principle of making a mold in which to pack denture resin is the same as discussed in the complete denture section. The pattern is made from wax which is eliminated to form the mold cavity into which the denture resin is packed. The packing procedures are different than for complete dentures in that the denture resin must be packed into both sides of the mold to avoid interference with the plastic retention portion of the framework. This makes it a little more difficult to determine when the mold is properly filled, but a little experience makes this task simple.

Figure 1 The cast and plaster mount are soaked and the cast removed from the mount. The festooned partial dentures and their casts are placed in the flasks to be sure that they fit. The bottom of a cast may not be trimmed or it will be impossible to remount the appliance to eliminate processing errors. The casts must be made thin enough when they are first poured.

Figure 2 Stone is placed in the bottom of the flasks and the partial denture casts are placed firmly in the flasks. The bottom of the cast should touch the bottom of the flask.

Figure 3 The first part of the flasking stone is brought over the entire framework. Only the teeth and the wax holding the teeth are left exposed. There may be no undercuts in the stone or the flasking will break when the flask is opened.

Figure 4 A side view of the lower half of the maxillary flask shows the wax bases are exposed with no undercuts present in the stone covering the framework.

Figure 5 The mandibular partial denture is treated in the same manner.

Figure 6 A plaster separating medium is placed over the entire surface of the first pour. This may be one of the commercial plaster separators,

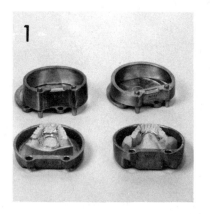
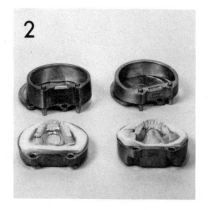
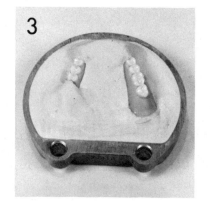
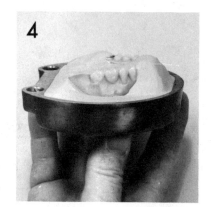

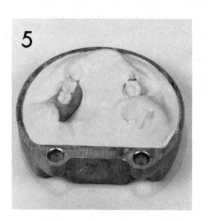
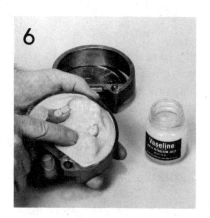
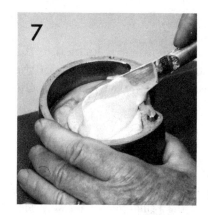
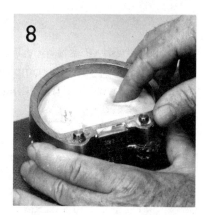

sodium silicate or petrolatum jelly. The separating medium is not placed on the teeth or wax.

Figure 7   The flask is assembled and the second pour of stone is made.

Figure 8   The occlusal surface of the teeth is uncovered. The second pour is then allowed to set.

Figure 9   A plaster separator is placed on the entire surface of the second pour. If petrolatum jelly is used, a thin coat should be applied with *no* excess over the occlusal surface of the teeth.

Figure 10   The third pour, or capping is poured and the lid placed on the flask.

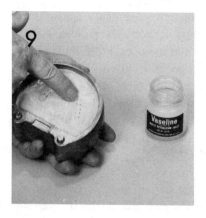
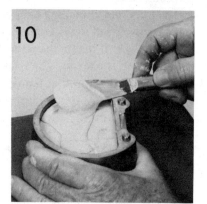

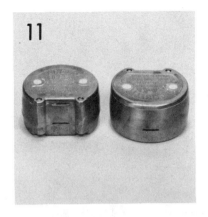
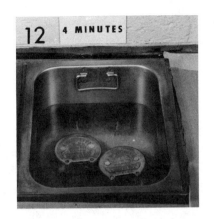
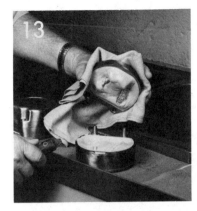
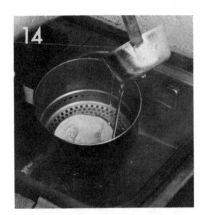

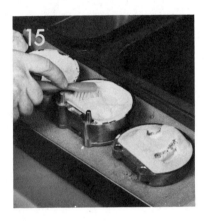
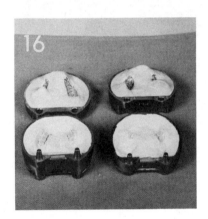
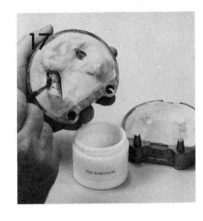
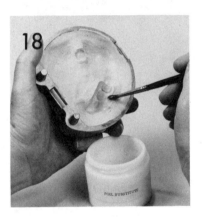

Figure 11   The last pour is allowed to set and the excess removed from the surface of the flask.

Figure 12   The flasks are placed in boiling water for four minutes. The time required for softening the wax will vary depending upon the temperature of the water bath. Four minutes are sufficient in boiling water.

Figure 13   The flasks are removed from the boiling water and are separated.

Figure 14   The wax is flushed from the mold with clean boiling water.

Figure 15   The molds are scrubbed thoroughly with detergent and rinsed in clean, hot water.

Figure 16   The molds are shown immediately after they have been cleaned with detergent and rinsed. They are ready for the application of tinfoil substitute.

Figure 17   The tinfoil substitute is painted on the tissue surface of the cast. It may be necessary to thin the foil substitute with water in order to have it flow under the frame and completely cover the cast. A second coat of the thin foil substitute may be necessary.

Figure 18   The upper portion of the flask is painted with foil substitute, paying particular attention that the material does not run onto the

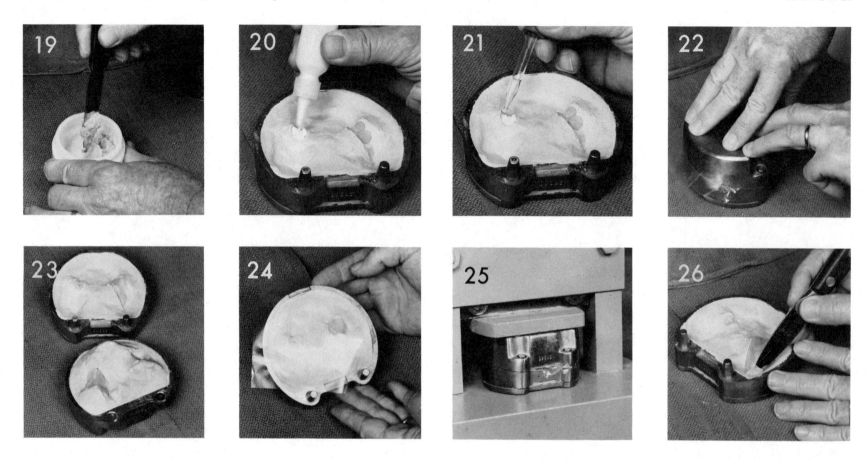

surface of the teeth. This is particularly important when resin teeth are used as shown here.

Figure 19   The denture base resin is mixed according to the manufacturer's instructions.

Figures 20 and 21   While the denture base resin is reaching packing consistency, auto-polymerizing tooth colored resin of the prescribed shade is placed into the cavity formed by the wax denture tooth. The mold cavity is first wet with monomer, then polymer is added and more monomer. These steps are repeated until the tooth cavity is filled.

Figure 22   The two halves of the flask are assembled with cellophane interposed and are pressed together. The tooth colored resin is allowed

to cure. Closing the flask in this manner assures that the new resin tooth will not interfere with the balance of the packing procedures.

Figure 23   Denture base resin is placed in both halves of the flask. It is pressed firmly around the metal framework. This is necessary so that the metal framework will not tear the denture base resin during the trial packing procedures.

Figure 24   Two sheets of plastic are placed between the two halves of the flask and they are assembled.

Figure 25   The flask is placed in a flask press and approximately 800 pounds of pressure are used. A hand press may be used. Only moderate pressure is needed so do not over-tighten a hand press.

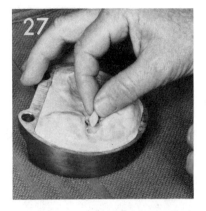

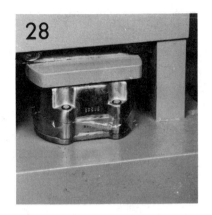

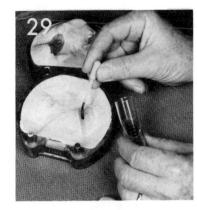

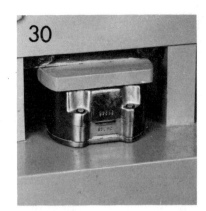

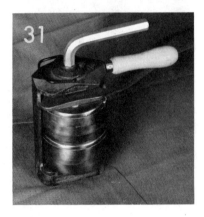

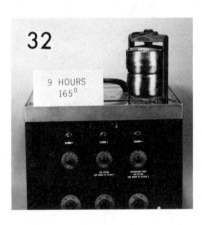

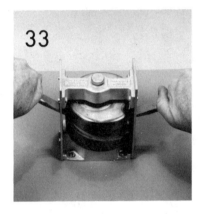

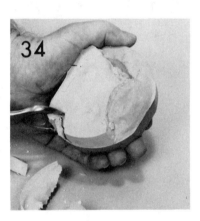

Figure 26 After approximately two minutes, the flask is opened and the excess is trimmed from the edges of the mold. This is done on both the upper and lower halves of the flask.

Figure 27 A small amount of denture base resin is placed so that it will be under the custom-made tooth. If necessary, additional resin is placed on the free-end extension side of the partial denture.

Figure 28 Plastic sheets are interposed between the two halves of the flask and the flask is again test packed. Test packing continues until the flask is filled with denture base resin and good detail is present on all surfaces of the resin.

Figure 29 Some monomer is painted on both halves of the uncured resin before the final closure to assure a good bond.

Figure 30 The flask is closed and is placed in the press with 800 pounds of pressure.

Figure 31 The flasks are placed in a flask clamp and are ready to be processed.

Figure 32 The flasks are placed in a curing unit and are processed for nine hours at 165°F.

Figure 33 The flask is removed from the curing unit, allowed to cool to room temperature and removed in a flask-ejector.

Figure 34 The investment is removed from the partial denture and its cast with a pair of plaster nippers. It is important to preserve the

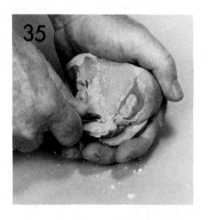

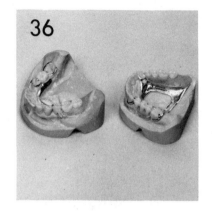

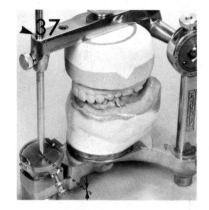

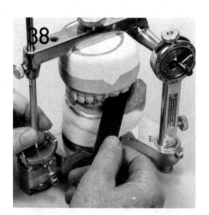

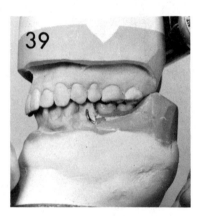

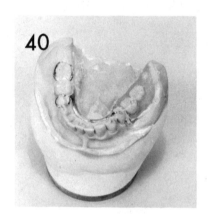

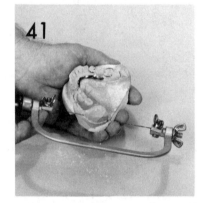

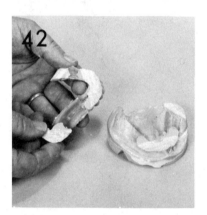

remaining natural teeth when removing the partial denture and its cast from the flask.

Figure 35 The lingual portion of the flasking stone is removed from the mandibular cast with a knife.

Figure 36 The partial dentures and their casts have been recovered from the flask and the casts cleaned preparatory to a laboratory remount.

Figure 37 The mandibular partial is returned to the articulator and secured to the lower mounting with impression plaster. The impression plaster is put around the junction between the cast and the mount. Note

that the pin is not touching the incisal guide table due to the processing error which has increased the vertical dimension.

Figure 38 The occlusion is refined using articulating paper and suitable small stones in a handpiece.

Figure 39 Centric occlusion has been refined and the overall occlusal relationships have been restored. The occlusion is also checked in lateral excursions. In this appliance, the lateral excursions were limited by cuspal interferences in the canine region.

Figure 40 The mandibular partial denture with its cast and mounting is removed from the articulator.

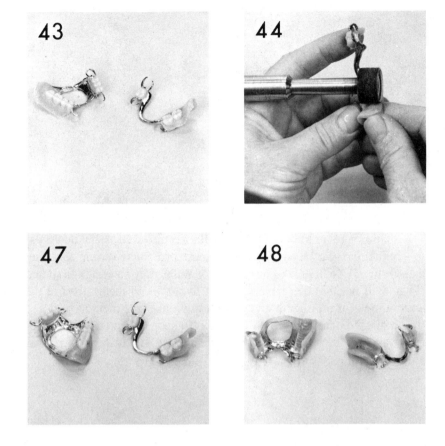

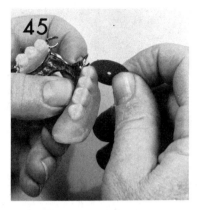

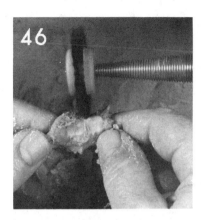

Figure 41   The cast is removed from the mounting and the partial denture is removed from the cast. A satisfactory method for removing the partial denture is to place a saw cut under the free-end extension, another under the anterior teeth, and a third under the posterior portion of the right side. A knife is then placed and gently rotated in the saw cuts to break the cast. This is repeated in each of the saw cuts and is done *with caution*.

Figure 42   Notice the position of the saw cuts in the cast. The remainder of the cast is removed from the partial denture by removing the stone abutment teeth and then removing the stone piece by piece to avoid distortion of the appliance. The same general procedure is followed for the maxillary partial denture.

Figure 43   The mandibular and maxillary partial dentures are shown as they appear before finishing the resin portion.

Figure 44   The flash is removed from the free-end extension and the base is contoured with an arbor band on a lathe or in a handpiece. No trimming should be necessary around the teeth.

Figure 45   A back-action clasp has a stress breaking action only when its entire circumference is free from the denture base resin. The clasp is freed by inserting a lightning disc, held in the fingers, between the clasp and the denture base resin. The safe side of the disc is placed against the clasp with the abrasive side against the denture base resin. The disc is worked back and forth until it slips freely in and out of the space. This produces a space large enough to allow the clasp to flex properly.

Figure 46   The denture base resin is polished in the same manner as a complete denture. The interproximal areas may be polished using a bristle brush and wet pumice. When plastic teeth are used, it is of paramount importance to avoid removing the anatomy of the teeth with pumice or other polishing agents. The junction of the resin and the external finish line must be smooth. It may be necessary to reduce the metal finish line and repolish the junction to produce a smooth surface.

Figures 47 and 48   The completed partial dentures ready for delivery to the dentist. Note the internal and external finish lines which result in

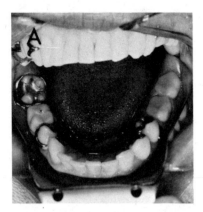
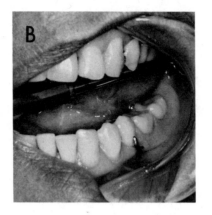
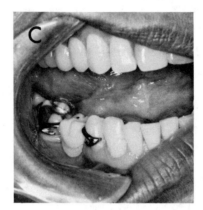
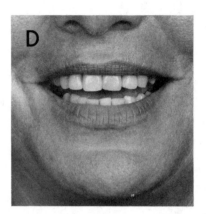

having a butt joint between the denture base resin and the metal framework on both the polished surface and the tissue surface. The resin portion of the denture base is not polished on the tissue surface.

Figure A   The completed partial denture after insertion in the patient's mouth.

Figure B   The left side of the partial denture is shown as it appears in the mouth. Note the small area of tooth surface contacted by the clasp and the adaptation of the denture base to the mucosa. This follows the outline of the corrected impression.

Figure C   The right side of the partial denture as it appears in the patient's mouth. Note the extent of the clasp on this side. This clasp design was indicated because of the position of the abutment teeth. Often a reverse action clasp is unesthetic because of the amount of tooth surface which is covered.

Figure D   This mandibular partial denture does not show when the patient is smiling or speaking. The esthetic qualities of a partial denture are dependent upon close observation and good planning by the dentist to insure that the clasps are not obvious during natural movements. The reverse action clasp on the premolar has been placed low enough so that it is not visible.

Esthetics is more important on maxillary removable partial dentures, in that the maxillary teeth are usually more prominent during speaking and smiling. Usually maxillary partial dentures may be designed so that clasps will not be obvious and so that the replaced teeth blend in the environment of the mouth and are not obvious. One method of doing this in distal extension partial dentures is to keep the anterior portion of the resin base thin, and to start the resin base just distal to the most anterior tooth.

REVIEW QUESTIONS

1. How does the packing procedure differ for partial dentures from full dentures?
2. How many pounds of pressure should be exerted on the flask press during trial packing?
3. Describe the location of the saw cuts in removing the partial denture from the cast after curing.
4. How is a back-action clasp freed from the denture base resin? Why?
5. Is the denture base resin polished on the tissue side when constructing a partial denture?

SECTION 29

Removable
Partial Denture Relines

Relining removable partial dentures maintains the adaptation of the base to the soft tissue support areas. Relining also helps to restore the original occlusal relationships and to maintain the efficiency of the appliance.

In Section 19, Single Dentures, it was observed that there was downward growth of the maxillary tuberosity on the side where there were no natural teeth. This is an example of what occurs when natural teeth are lost regardless of the replacements which are made. The extraction of teeth inevitably leads to changes; these changes may occur rapidly, slowly, be obvious or be subtle, but the changes do occur.

Changes do occur which alter the relationship of a partial denture to the natural teeth regardless of how they are made or who makes them. Naturally, these changes would be much less obvious in a completely tooth borne partial denture with metal occlusal surfaces. Changes are much more obvious in a person with a bilateral distal extension mandibular denture made shortly after the natural teeth were removed.

The changes which occur are due primarily to resorption under free end distal extensions and wear of resin teeth. As the partial denture "settles," the opposing teeth tend to remain in occlusion. When natural teeth are present, they extrude into the space so created. A complete denture will tend to follow the occlusal plane by tipping, with the posterior portion stimulating the growth of hyperplastic tissue in the tuberosity regions and resorption in the anterior region. This sequence was described in Section 19.

Assuming that all occlusal rests remain intact, these changes may produce symptoms in the patient wearing a partial denture. Soreness under a lingual bar on a mandibular partial denture is usually due to the partial denture settling. Relieving the bar may temporarily relieve the symptom but the symptoms recur as the partial denture continues to settle. Similar changes occur in maxillary removable partial dentures but they tend to be less obvious. Resorption may result in having a palatal major connector become sore in the midline.

Refitting a partial denture and restoring the framework to its original relationship to the natural teeth may help to remedy this problem. However, one must compensate for the changes which have occurred (usually through a re-mount procedure) to develop the correct occlusion between the refitted partial denture and the existing opposing occlusion.

In dental circles, discussions often develop regarding the advantages of "closed-mouth" and "open-mouth" impression techniques for relining or refitting partial dentures. Closed-mouth impression techniques, those where the patient keeps their teeth together while the impression material is setting, will make the saddle areas fit better but will do little to change the relation of the partial denture frame to the existing natural teeth. Conversely, open-mouth techniques will help re-orient the framework and return it to a correct relation to the natural teeth but will also develop disturbances in the occlusion. The closed-mouth approach is simpler while the open mouth approach is much more complicated but is more likely to bring long-term satisfaction to the patient provided the occlusion is checked.

Many relines for removable partial dentures are done with materials which cure in the mouth and do not require laboratory support. Many of

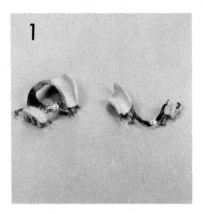 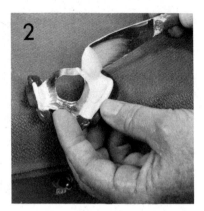 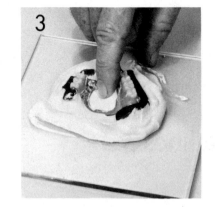 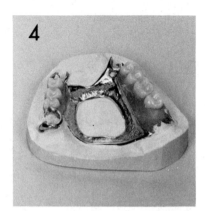

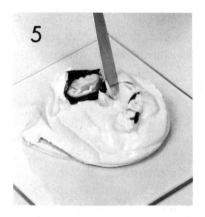 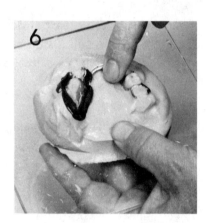

the materials used in this fashion do not last as long as a heat cured laboratory reline so that laboratory support is often essential for a long lasting result. The laboratory phases for producing a heat cured reline in a partial denture are shown in this section.

The technique for relining removable partial dentures in the laboratory differs in several details from complete dentures. A Hooper Duplicator or an articulator may be used in the same manner as when relining complete dentures. However, partial denture relines may be handled more simply by the following technique.

Figure 1   Maxillary and mandibular partial dentures with reline impressions are shown as they appear when delivered to the laboratory. Reline impressions are made in the same manner as corrected impressions and with the same materials. Many dentists will reline a partial denture at the time of delivery rather than make corrected impressions, although this involves an additional visit by the patient.

Figure 2   The impression is surrounded with a bead of utility wax and stone is vibrated into the reline impression. Only the relined portion of the denture is filled with stone.

Figure 3   Additional stone is placed on a glass slab and the partial denture is inverted into it. *Care must be taken that the stone does not surround the clasp or does not overlap the framework in any place, but the framework must contact the stone throughout as much area as possible.* The framework will act as a key for replacing the partial denture on the cast after the impression material has been removed.

Figure 4   The partial denture and the cast are shown as they appear after the beading wax has been removed and the cast has been trimmed. Note that no stone extends over the framework or engages any of the clasps.

Figure 5   The mandibular partial denture is poured in the same manner.

Figure 6   Care is taken that the stone does not cover the lingual bar but *the lower border of the lingual bar must contact the stone.* The clasps are not engaged by the stone.

Figure 7   The completed mandibular cast is shown after the beading wax has been removed. You will note that the single tooth on the right

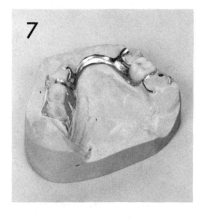
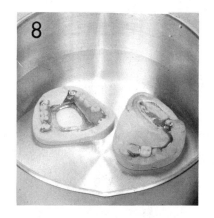
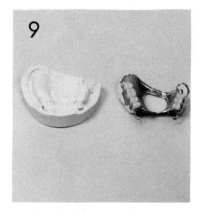
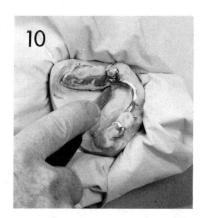

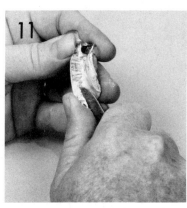
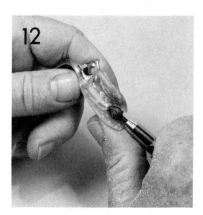
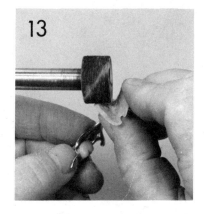
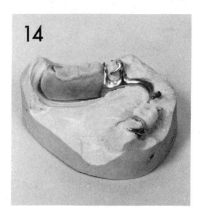

side of this partial denture has not been relined because tooth borne areas generally do not require a reline if this area is well healed before the appliance is made. Relining of this area is left to the discretion of the dentist.

Figure 8 The casts are placed in 160°F. water for 7 to 10 minutes to soften the impression material.

Figure 9 The maxillary partial denture as it appears after it is removed from the cast.

Figure 10 The mandibular partial denture is removed from the cast by teasing it gently with a knife or other suitable instrument.

Figure 11 The impression material is removed with the knife.

Figure 12 The tissue surface is cleaned and all traces of impression material are removed with a coarse acrylic bur.

Figure 13 The borders of the denture are beveled in the same manner as complete dentures being relined (Section 16).

Figure 14 The partial denture is replaced on the cast. The lower border of the lingual bar fits into the groove on the cast and acts as a positive index for the proper repositioning of the partial denture on the cast. Enough of the resin base must be removed so the appliance slips on and off the cast without interference.

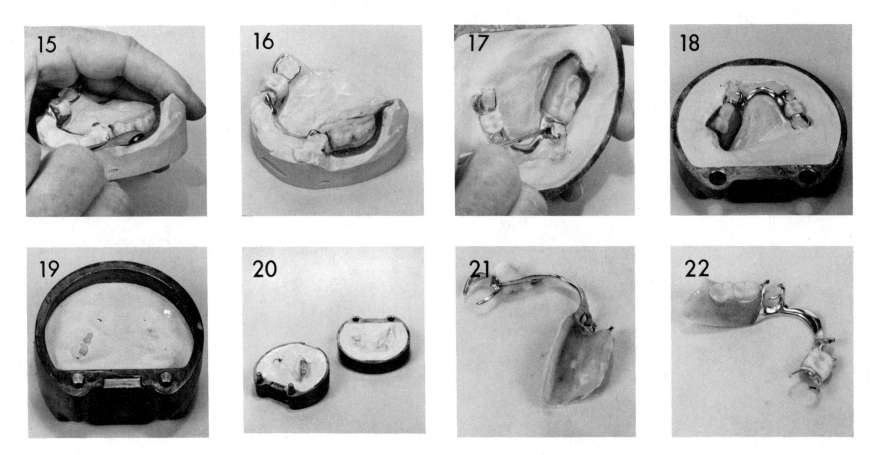

Figure 15 The borders of the free-end extension are filled with wax.

Figure 16 The borders of the mandibular partial denture have been waxed and the appliance is ready to be invested. Note that the wax and denture base meet in a butt joint and no wax extends onto the polished surface of the partial denture. This also is evident in **Figure 17**.

Figure 17 The partial denture is flasked. The framework is exposed so that the upper half of the flasking stone will engage the framework and hold the partial denture in the upper half of the flask. Stone may be teased under but not around the clasps to make deflasking easier. Common sense will dictate the proper method of handling clasps to avoid their distortion.

Figure 18 The lower half of the flasking is shown with the upper half ready to be poured. Note that there are no undercuts in the flasking stone and that the clasps are free of the lower stone, but that stone has been contoured so that the clasps may be disengaged easily after processing.

Figure 19 The second pour of the flasking has been made. Note that the occlusal surface of the teeth is exposed.

A plaster separator is applied to the surface and the flask is filled with stone. The stone is allowed to set.

Figure 20 The flask is placed in boiling water for 4 minutes to soften the wax. The flask is then opened and the wax is flushed from the mold.

The wax may be removed using a wax solvent and then scrubbing the mold thoroughly with detergent and hot water. In a partial denture of this size, distortion of the denture base resin is not a problem. However, good practice dictates that the portion of the flask containing the partial denture should be flushed with water not exceeding 165°F. The mold is then packed in the usual manner and is processed at 165°F. for nine hours.

Figure 21　　The partial denture is removed from the flask. Care is taken not to distort any of the clasps.

Figure 22　　The partial denture is polished as described in the previous section and is delivered to the dentist.

REVIEW QUESTIONS

1. In pouring casts for partial denture relines, how is the metal framework treated?
2. Are tooth-borne or tissue-borne partial dentures in need of more frequent relines?
3. In preparing a mandibular cast for a partial denture reline, why must the lower border of the lingual bar contact the stone?
4. When a partial denture flask is separated, in which half will the framework appear?

SECTION 30

Removable
Partial Denture Repairs

Dental laboratory technicians share techniques with other industries. The same methods of electro-soldering are used successfully by both jewelers and dental laboratory technicians.

Fractures in the resin base portion of a removable partial denture and broken teeth are repaired using the same techniques described for complete dentures. Breaks in a metal partial denture framework are repaired by soldering.

Partial denture repairs may also take many other forms from the simple replacement of a clasp arm to the addition of a tooth and new clasps to a partial denture. All of these procedures require cooperation between the dentist and the dental laboratory technician and understanding on the part of the patient. An attempt is made to make a repaired partial denture as good as the original but often this is impossible.

A relatively common occurrence is the addition of a tooth and/or clasp to a partial denture when a natural tooth is extracted. This may involve the making of a new clasp and attaching it to the partial denture or may simply mean the addition of a wrought wire clasp imbedded in the resin base. Regardless, an impression containing the partial denture must be made by the dentist and delivered to the laboratory before any repair or addition can be made.

Any successful repair requires that the occlusal rest on the partial denture be intact. If the occlusal or incisal rests are not intact, the partial denture will settle and will cause serious gingival problems around the remaining natural teeth. It is the dentist's responsibility to decide whether it is worthwhile to repair a partial denture or to suggest the construction of a new one. It is the laboratory technician's responsibility to follow the instructions for the repair which may be of a temporary nature to hold the patient for a period of time until a new appliance can be made.

When making a new clasp for an existing partial denture, impressions are made, an investment or refractory cast is produced and the new clasp is waxed on this cast. A retentive mechanism is incorporated on the clasp so that it may be imbedded in resin which will be added to the existing partial denture. There are times when such a clasp can be attached in the mouth but it is usually done in the laboratory utilizing the same impression upon which the clasp was designed. Such new clasps should always have occlusal or incisal rests.

In the event that a clasp arm breaks and the occlusal rest is still present, a clasp may be soldered to the existing partial denture. Most gold solders will adhere to base metal frames and produce good results. However, you may wish to contour a wrought wire and imbed the end of this in the resin base rather than make a new cast clasp or to solder. Solder may cause changes in the structure of the metal which render it much more likely to fracture so that the repair may not last as long as an imbedded wrought wire. An intelligent decision on the part of the dentist and the laboratory technician will indicate which procedure is best in any given situation.

There are many ways to repair partial dentures; so many that an entire text could be developed showing just the various methods of repairing partial dentures. The basis of all repairs should be an adequate impression with the partial denture in place and an understanding of

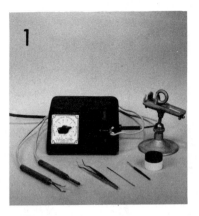 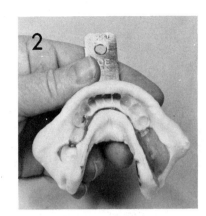

methods to preserve the proper occlusal relationship already present on the removable partial denture.

Fractures may occur in a partial denture framework because of metal fatigue, improper contour of the component parts, or faulty castings. Faulty castings may be due to inclusions of bits of investment in the metal, crystallization of the metal, or improper casting techniques. Many times it is impossible to know that these defects are present when the partial denture is delivered. When a patient is unfortunate enough to bend a lingual bar, the partial denture may need to be sectioned and the halves rejoined. The procedures involved in joining the two halves are the same as for repairing a framework.

Partial denture repairs may be done by soldering with an open flame. When the fracture is near a saddle, it is necessary to remove the teeth and saddle from the framework before the soldering operation. This is a major procedure which is not required when electro-soldering techniques are used.

Electro-soldering techniques are widely used in the jewelry industry. The same principles and techniques used in soldering jewelry are used to repair the metal portions of partial denture frameworks. The technique for soldering is the same whether the framework is made of gold or base metal alloys. Gold solder is used with base metal alloys in the same manner as for gold, with the exception that white solder is used.

There are many electro-soldering machines available. The directions for using the machine should be followed exactly. The directions must be read thoroughly to determine any variations in technique required of the individual machine.

The principles of soldering described in the Laboratory and Clinical Dental Materials Manual (in this series) are followed with electro-soldering machines. The surfaces to be joined must be cleaned and accessible to the contacts of the soldering machine. The work must be arranged so that gravity favors the flow of solder. One of the advantages of electric soldering is that intense heat is located at the site of the fracture rather than throughout the framework. However, if the fracture occurs adjacent to a resin portion of a partial denture, the resin should be protected with wet asbestos.

Figure 1 This electric soldering machine was designed to repair jewelry, but is equally useful for repairing partial denture frameworks. The machine includes a double prong ground, a ¼ inch carbon rod and a foot pedal, which is not shown. The amount of heat applied to the work is varied by adjusting the dial. The stand at the right is used to hold the work to be soldered, and is a convenience, not a necessity. The top tilts so that the cast may be oriented for better accessibility. The other instruments are a fine pair of tweezers for placing the solder, a strip of triple-thick solder, a brush and flux.

Figure 2 The dentist must make an impression of the mouth with the broken appliance in place. It is impossible to replace a partial denture on a cast made of the mouth without the appliance in place because of the displaceable nature of the tissues under the partial denture base. (When a major connector needs to be repaired, the fragments of the partial denture must be stabilized in the patient's mouth and an impression made.) A cast is poured in the usual manner with the partial denture still in the impression.

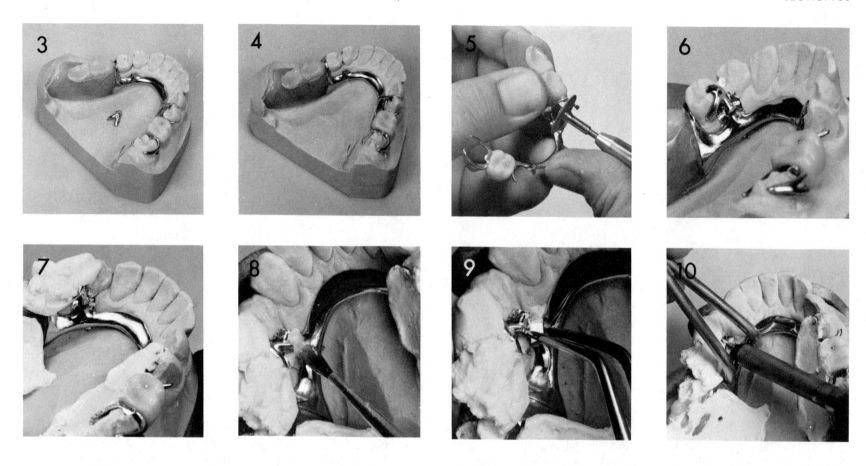

Figure 3   The fractured clasp is shown in the middle of the cast.

Figure 4   The abutment teeth not involved in the repair are trimmed to permit the removal of the partial denture from the cast. The partial denture is removed from the cast in order to permit the proper preparation of the joint and the adaptation of platinum foil under the repair site.

Figure 5   Each side of the fracture is beveled at a 45° angle with suitable stones in a dental handpiece. The bevels create a space into which the solder flows readily and also cleans the surface of the metal.

Figure 6   Prior to the replacement of the partial denture, platinum foil is adapted accurately to the cast under the repair site. It is essential to use platinum foil because of its high melting point. Note that both

fragments have been beveled to provide a space for the solder.

Figure 7   Impression plaster is used to stabilize the partial denture and the fragment on the cast.

Figure 8   Electric soldering flux is painted into the area to be soldered. Borax may not be used in electric soldering because as it melts it forms a non-conductive surface which prevents the heat from reaching the area.

Figure 9   A piece of triple-thick solder adequate to fill the prepared area is placed in the fracture site.

Figure 10   The double pronged ground is placed on either side of the

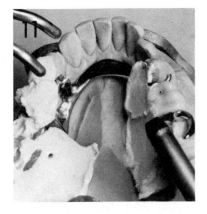
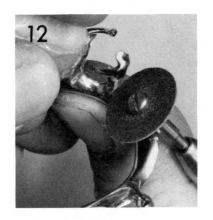
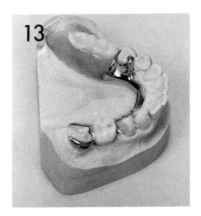
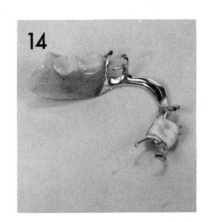

repair site. A ¼ inch diameter carbon rod is placed on the solder and the foot control depressed. The solder will flow almost instantaneously when current is applied. **Note:** The soldering machine is set to deliver enough heat according to the volume of solder and the thickness of the area to be repaired. This machine was set at number 8 on the scale of 1 to 10 to repair this area. The machine would be set at a higher level to repair a bulkier fracture, such as a lingual bar. A certain amount of experimentation and experience is needed before an individual will be competent with the electro-soldering machine.

Figure 11 As soon as the solder melts, the foot pedal is released and the carbon point is withdrawn. It is important to release the foot pedal first or an arc will form which causes pitting in the solder joint. If it is necessary to resolder an area because insufficient solder was used during the first operation, the partial must be removed from the cast and the surface ground to remove oxidation. This is necessary to be sure that the second melt of solder will flow properly.

Figure 12 The partial denture is removed from the cast; the soldered area is ground to contour and polished.

Figure 13 The repaired partial denture is replaced on the cast to check the accuracy of the repair. Note that the clasp and rest are in correct apposition to the tooth.

Figure 14 The repaired partial denture is ready to be returned to the dental office.

REVIEW QUESTIONS

1. What may cause faulty framework castings?
2. What is the main advantage of electro-soldering over open flame soldering in repairing a partial denture framework?
3. What is the purpose of 45° angle bevels on each side of the fracture?
4. Why is borax not used as a flux in electro-soldering?
5. What are the differences in broken tooth repairs for partial dentures and complete dentures?

INDEX